SEEING SUFFERING IN WOMEN'S LITERATURE OF THE ROMANTIC ERA

For Emma

Seeing Suffering in Women's Literature of the Romantic Era

ELIZABETH A. DOLAN
Lehigh University, USA

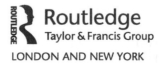

Routledge
Taylor & Francis Group

LONDON AND NEW YORK

First published 2008 by Ashgate Publishing

2 Park Square, Milton Park, Abingdon, Oxon OX14 4RN
711 Third Avenue, New York, NY 10017, USA

Routledge is an imprint of the Taylor & Francis Group, an informa business

First issued in paperback 2016

British Library Cataloguing in Publication Data
Dolan, Elizabeth A.
Seeing suffering in women's literature of the Romantic era
  1. Smith, Charlotte Turner, 1749–1806 – Criticism and interpretation 2. Wollstonecraft, Mary, 1759–1797 – Criticism and interpretation 3. Shelley, Mary Wollstonecraft, 1797–1851 – Criticism and interpretation 4. English literature – Women authors – History and criticism 5. English literature – 18th century – History and criticism 6. English literature – 19th century – History and criticism 7. Suffering in literature 8. Literature and medicine 9. Vision in literature 10. Romanticism – Great Britain
  I. Title
  820.9'353

Library of Congress Cataloging-in-Publication Data
Dolan, Elizabeth A.
  Seeing suffering in women's literature of the Romantic era / by Elizabeth A. Dolan.
    p. cm.
  Includes bibliographical references and index.
  ISBN-13: 978-0-7546-5491-9 (alk. paper)

  1. English literature—Women authors—History and criticism. 2. English literature—18th century—History and criticism. 3. English literature—19th century—History and criticism. 4. Smith, Charlotte Turner, 1749–1806—Criticism and interpretation. 5. Wollstonecraft, Mary, 1759–1797—Criticism and interpretation. 6. Shelley, Mary Wollstonecraft, 1797–1851—Criticism and interpretation. 7. Suffering in literature. 8. Literature and medicine. 9. Vision in literature. 10. Romanticism—Great Britain. I. Title.

  PR448.W65D65 2008
  820.9'353—dc22

                                                          2007042382
  ISBN: 978-0-7546-5491-9 (hbk)
  ISBN: 978-1-138-27535-5 (pbk)

Contents

List of Figures

Acknowledgments

Sociability and sympathetic gazes—major themes in this book—also made the writing possible. Thanks first and always to my parents: to my mom who sets the standard for love and generosity, and to my dad who has always thought his daughters could do anything. I'm grateful also for the encouragement and good humor of my sisters Emily Murray and Patricia Dolan, both of whom I admire and cherish. And my dear Emma, to whom this book is dedicated, I love you.

I'm indebted to Jeanne Moskal, another kind of parent, who helped birth the early stages of this project and who continues to be a most generous advisor and mentor. Her on-going influence will be apparent in my citation of her work on travel literature and on Mary Shelley. I've learned much from Patricia Clare Ingham in all arenas of life, including the profession. Her research on trauma and narrative greatly influences chapter 5 of *Seeing Suffering*. I'm deeply grateful to Jan Fergus for reading the book as it unfolded, offering brilliant advice, and urging me on at every stage. Many thanks also to my insightful colleagues and friends both at Lehigh and elsewhere who read sections of the manuscript: Kate Crassons, Stuart Curran, JoAnn Dolan, Patricia K. Dolan, Suzanne Edwards, Tim Fulford, Scott Paul Gordon, Jill Heydt-Stevenson, Dawn Keetley, Jacqueline Krasas, A. A. Markley, Rosemary Mundhenk, Monica Najar, Kathy Olson, Lynda Payne, Jennifer Phegley, Barbara Traister, Gina Luria Walker, Sarah Wascura, and Stephanie Powell Watts. I count myself lucky to have had the exceptional support of Alexander Doty and Barry Kroll, chairs of my department while this was a work in progress. Somewhere in the substrata of the prose bubble the insights of two groups from whom I've learned a great deal: the members of my graduate school writing group—Marya DeVoto, Kathryn Schmidt, Holloway Sparks, and Kathryn Walbert—and my dissertation committee members—Judith Farquahar, Wil Gesler, Laurie Langbauer, and John McGowan. Thanks to Judith Stanton for loaning me her manuscript of Smith's letters many years ago and for her continued encouragement. I'd like to thank D. L. Macdonald and Judith Pascoe for sharing their proofs of the *Complete Works of Charlotte Smith* in advance of publication. The expert eyes of Kristina Fennelly, Jim O'Brien, and Paul Sisko have made this a better book than it might have been. Finally, I offer special thanks to the Wascura family and to the Jai Yoga community for their steady and open-hearted support, and to Christina Raiser and Colleen Martell for caring for Emma during key moments of the writing process.

Sections of chapter 1 appeared as "British Romantic Melancholia: Charlotte Smith's *Elegiac Sonnets*, Medical Discourse, and the Problem of Sensibility" in *The Journal of European Studies* 33.3/4 (December 2003) 237–54. A less developed version of chapter 3 appeared as "Mary Wollstonecraft's Salutary Picturesque: Curing Melancholia in the Landscape" in *European Romantic Review*, 13.1 (2002) 35–48, under the name "Beth Dolan Kautz." Finally, part of chapter 5 was published as "Spas and Salutary Landscapes: The Geography of Health in Mary Shelley's

Rambles in Germany and Italy" in *Romantic Geographies: Discourses of Travel 1775-1844*, Ed. Amanda Gilroy, Manchester, UK: Manchester University Press, 2000, 165–81, again under "Beth Dolan Kautz." Taylor-Francis/Routledge, Sage Press, and Manchester University Press have kindly granted me permission to use these materials here.

I'd like to acknowledge the financial support I received at various stages of the project from the PEO Foundation, the University of Missouri-Kansas City Faculty Research Fund, the Lehigh University Franz and Class of 1968 Junior Faculty Fellowship Fund, and the Gipson Institute for Eighteenth-Century Studies at Lehigh University. I'm grateful especially to the Gipson Institute for granting me the reproduction fees for the images in *Seeing Suffering*. I offer thanks to the librarians who aided my research at the following institutions: the British Library; the Wellcome Library for the History of Medicine; the Historical Medical Library at the College of Physicians of Philadelphia; the Clendening History of Medicine Library; the Linda Hall Library of Science, Engineering, and Technology; the University of Pennsylvania Rare Book and Manuscript Library; the Louis Round Wilson Library at the University of North Carolina; the Duke University Rare Book, Manuscript and Special Collections Library; and the Lehigh University Special Collections.

List of Abbreviations

CLCS   *The Collected Letters of Charlotte Smith*. Ed. Judith Phillips Stanton. Indianapolis: Indiana University Press, 2003.

CLMW   *The Collected Letters of Mary Wollstonecraft*. Ed. Janet Todd. New York: Columbia University Press, 2000.

JMS   *The Journals of Mary Shelley: 1814–1844*. Eds. Paula R. Feldman and Diana Scott-Kilvert. Baltimore: Johns Hopkins University Press, 1987.

LMWS   *The Letters of Mary Wollstonecraft Shelley*. Ed. Betty T. Bennett. 3 vols. Baltimore: Johns Hopkins University Press, 1988.

MTWW   *Mary and The Wrongs of Woman*. Ed. Gary Kelly. Oxford: Oxford University Press, 1998.

WMS   *The Novels and Selected Works of Mary Shelley*. Gen. ed. Nora Crook. 8 vols. London: Pickering & Chatto, 1996.

PW   *Posthumous Works of the Author of A Vindication of the Rights of Woman*. In four volumes. Ed. William Godwin. London: J. Johnson, 1798.

WCS   *The Works of Charlotte Smith*. Gen. ed. Stuart Curran. 14 vols. London: Pickering & Chatto, 2006–07.

WMW   *The Works of Mary Wollstonecraft*. Eds. Janet Todd and Marilyn Butler. 7 vols. New York: New York University Press, 1989.

Introduction

"*Esse* is *percipi* (To be is to be perceived)."

George Berkeley

"The question is not, Can they *reason*? nor, Can they *talk*? but, Can they suffer?"

Jeremy Bentham

From the glittering eye of Samuel Taylor Coleridge's Ancient Mariner to the watery eyes of Mary Shelley's creature in *Frankenstein*, from Ralph Waldo Emerson's Transparent Eyeball to the narrator's obsession with the old man's twitching eye in Edgar Allan Poe's "The Tell-Tale Heart," the organ of visual perception haunts Romantic literature on both sides of the Atlantic. A philosophical and psychological interest in perception, that long-standing theme in Romantic studies, underlies this intense interest in vision. Different in their significance, the literary examples I cite above nonetheless share a peculiar physicality, an explicit focus not just on vision but also on the eye itself. While vision is certainly one of the most over-determined categories in literature, this unusual emphasis on the physical nature of looking and of being seen, I argue, does particular cultural work in the Romantic era. Just as the late twentieth-century medical focus on the immune system inspired, as Emily Martin posits, the dominant trope of flexibility in popular culture, late eighteenth-century society relied on philosophical and medical conceptions of vision to mediate a number of concerns related to subjectivity, including the relationship between gender and literary authority, the tension between rationality and sensibility, the contrast between solitude and sociability, and the difference between sympathy and judgment. Based on this connection between vision and subjectivity, *Seeing Suffering in Women's Literature of the Romantic Era* ultimately argues that two seemingly divergent late-eighteenth-century cultural preoccupations—the materiality of vision and pressing social justice issues—created new modes of "seeing" (and thus of expressing and alleviating) suffering in the Romantic era.

Philosophical theories of perception, especially those articulated by John Locke, David Hartley, and George Berkeley, deeply influenced many Romantic era writers.[1] In *A Treatise Concerning the Principles of Human Knowledge* (1710), for

---

1 For decades critics have analyzed Romantic-era poets' interest in philosophical theories of perception, focusing particularly on the responses of Coleridge, William Wordsworth, and Percy Bysshe Shelley to the theories of Berkeley, Locke, and Hartley. See Locke's *Essay Concerning Human Understanding* (1690), Berkeley's *An Essay towards a New Theory of Vision* (1709) and *A Treatise Concerning the Principles of Human Knowledge* (1710), and Hartley's *Observations on Man, his Frame, his Duty, and his Expectations* (1749), republished and abridged by Joseph Priestley as Hartley's *Theory of the Human Mind, on the Principle of the Association of Ideas; with Essays Relating to the Subject of It* (1775). For helpful studies of the connection between these philosophical theories of perception and the Romantic poets, see Abrams, de Man, Hartman, Hayden, Kharbutli, Lamb, Malekin, Miall, and Perry.

example, Berkeley puts forward his famous principle "*esse* is *percipi*"—to be is to be perceived (78). Because objects are collections of ideas, Berkeley argues, an object exists only in the mind that perceives it. Berkeley's idealist philosophy in part inspired William Wordsworth and others to explore the creative ramifications of subjective perception. However, recent interdisciplinary scholarship suggests that Romantic-era writers were interested in theories of the body as well as philosophies of perception.[2] In *British Romanticism and the Science of the Mind*, Alan Richardson urges Romanticists to augment our knowledge about Romantic-era philosophies of mind with renewed attention to the late-eighteenth-century interest in corporeality: "[L]iterary Romanticism," he argues, "has most often been associated with idealistic and transcendental conceptions of mind," yet the "many points of contact between scientific and literary representations of the embodied psyche help remind us of an antidualistic, materialist register within Romantic writing" (36). In this spirit of inquiry, *Seeing Suffering* explores Romantic-era ideas about the physiological and embodied properties of vision, thus resituating sight—the sense most closely linked with Romantic transcendence—within a "materialist register."

Indeed, the Romantic-era fascination with subjective perception emerges as much from medical theories about the physiology of vision in individual bodies as from idealist philosophy. Examples of these medical theories that I discuss at greater length below include the theory of color vision put forward by Thomas Young and the exploration of the eye's "morbid anatomy" by John Vetch, James Ware, and James Wardrop. These medical re-conceptions of vision add a physiological dimension to debates about perception. The eye, previously thought of in optics as a stable instrument transmitting images to the brain, was redefined as a physiological entity subject to the caprices of individual anatomy and physical function. Thus, two people might look at the same object and see it differently based on variations between their bodies. Several decades after Berkeley published his idealist treatise, then, this new understanding of ocular physiology's influence on individual vision offered a physical metaphor, or perhaps metonym, for Romantic-era subjective perception.

To consider eighteenth-century philosophical and medical understandings of subjective perception as cognate rather than as merely resonant is to place beside the transcendent Romantic imagination a competing version of perception, inseparable from the body and the material world. This materialist version of perception challenges the much revered transcendent imagination constructed both by Romantic poets such as Wordsworth, Coleridge, Percy Bysshe Shelley, and John Keats and also by decades of Romantic scholars. As William Galperin observes, critics have characterized the male Romantic poets as "virtually united in their suspicions regarding the world viewed as against a world of imagination" (19–20).[3] W. J. T. Mitchell offers William Blake as an exception to the Romantic poets' commitment to "'imagination'" as "a power of consciousness that transcends

---

    2   See Richardson's "Romanticism and the Body" for a helpful analysis of this emerging research area, including an overview of major scholarly contributions.

    3   The Romantic-era commitment to internal vision, evident in philosophy and in poetry, figured also in the recurring trope of blindness. See Edward Larrissy's *The Blind and Blindness in Literature of the Romantic Period*.

mere visualization" (49). Idealism and the related transcendent imagination replace the "mirror" with the "lamp" (as in M. H. Abrams's influential formulation), the "eye" with the poetic "I" (Galperin 31). *Seeing Suffering* identifies and explores the theory that the subjective "I" is dependent upon the physicality and physiology of the individual "eye," thus highlighting the Romantic-era writers' awareness of the radical physicality of perception, the commingling of mind and body with the world outside. If some Romantic-era writers attempt to transcend the visual world, those who are always already thought of as bodies—women—might instead explore the potential of this connection between the individual physiology of perception and their particular imaginations.

As the physiological question of how one sees became central in conversations about perception, several Romantic-era social movements raised questions about how we might perceive the suffering of others. Diane Long Hoeveler notes that a "fascination with suffering ... permeated the texts produced during the Romantic era" ("Secularization" 113), perhaps most graphically in the gothic novel. The literary recreation of torture, living interment, and other forms of suffering dramatized and displaced the extremities of immanent suffering brought to the public's attention by debates about the abolition of slavery, about animal rights, and about the lives of the poor. Activists detailed the physical suffering of slaves and of animals to argue that these groups deserved basic rights and protections. This book's attention to suffering and to the social relationships it shapes and is shaped by builds on Alan Bewell's inspiring *Romanticism and Colonial Disease*. Bewell argues for the ways in which the "new disease reality" of colonialism shaped Romantic-era ideas about foreign bodies and lands (17). Focusing on the exchange of diseases that took place between British colonizers and indigenous populations, Bewell examines the connections between the physical and the cultural in what Mary Louise Pratt describes in *Imperial Eyes* as "contact zones." Bewell's investigation of physical suffering conjures new understandings of geography and global relations. As we reconstruct the ways in which the British understood their world in the late eighteenth century, we inevitably reconsider the ways in which they experienced subjectivity. Thus, how one sees, suffers, and is perceived to be suffering reconstituted the Romantic-era sense of the subject—that is, both the boundaries of what we might call the integrated self and this self's unique perspective. The women writers I discuss in this book—Mary Wollstonecraft, Charlotte Smith, and Mary Shelley—deploy body-based ideas about vision and suffering to assert themselves as creative subjects within patriarchal culture. They rely on a physical, embodied mode of seeing in order to represent the marked nature of illness, the therapeutic importance of the viewer's location, and the invisibility of particular forms of suffering. In addition, they invent narrative forms designed to make the social causes of suffering culturally visible.

The Materiality of Vision

Romantic-era medical theories of vision both reinforce the philosophy of subjective perception and ground it in physical structures. Historian Luke Davidson argues that in this period "[t]he eye came to be understood, by both specialists and nonspecialists, as the quintessential organ, both in its healthy and morbid states" (325). In particular, new understandings of the physiology of the eye, the theory of color vision, and the exploration of the eye's pathology (or "morbid anatomy") together added a crucial physical dimension to philosophical debates about perception. In turn, the earlier philosophical interest in vision helped raise "eye doctors" from the status of itinerant quacks to culturally legitimate specialists during the late eighteenth century (Davidson 329). Previously regarded in optics as a passive participant in the transmission of light and images to the brain, the eye was increasingly thought of as a changing physiological entity upon which individual vision depended. Young, dubbed the "father of physiologic optics," explained in his work *On the Mechanism of the Eye* (1801) that the eye is able to accommodate its focus for near and far objects because the ciliary muscles attached to the lens change the shape of the lens, and thus alter its focal length (Sherman 4). In addition, Young measured the edge of the "blind spot" in the eye (that is, the location of the optic nerve), offered a groundbreaking description of astigmatism based on his own eyes, and mapped the borders of the human visual field by explaining the difference in the character of central and peripheral vision (Arrington 112). This research into the physiology of the eye represented a major conceptual shift: "Whereas the camera model posited an eye that was monocular, disembodied and therefore static, timeless and universal, the physiological model of the eye was imbedded in the density of the binocular body and therefore subject to physiological and pathological fluctuations as well as to fluctuations in time and space" (Brownlee 3–4). The act of seeing was understood to be dependent upon individual variations in the anatomical characteristics and physiological function of the eye, as well as upon the particular and fluctuating circumstances of the viewer's environment.

A renewed interest in color blindness and color vision at the end of the eighteenth century dovetails with this physiologically based, subjective understanding of vision. According to medical historian Paul D. Sherman, the subject of color blindness was virtually ignored between Robert Boyle's description of the condition in 1688 and a series of case studies published at the end of the eighteenth century. Joseph Huddert penned the "first published account of genuine cases of color blindness" in the *Philosophical Transactions* in 1777 (Sherman 119). Additional case studies appeared in 1778, 1779, 1781, and 1792 in various publications, including the *Encyclopedia Britannica*. The most influential of this series was John Dalton's 1794 description of his own color blindness (Sherman 117–26). These reports of color blindness inspired Young to elaborate a scientific theory of color vision that described the relationship between the retina and the sensation of three basic colors through the vibration of light—the basis for current understandings of rods and cones (Gorin 59–60). This research on color blindness emphasized that what one sees is dependent upon the particularities of one's own body. Furthermore, in the case studies, the only evidence of what colors the subject sees is his or her own description of the visual field. Johann Wolfgang von Goethe, like Dalton, based his largely discredited but influential *Theory of Colors* (1810) entirely on his subjective visual experience. The complete reliance of these case studies on the narrated experience of the color-blind person demonstrates the culture's focus on the subjective and embodied nature of vision.

In addition to these developments in theories of vision, newly emergent pathologies in Europe brought attention to the eye at the turn of the century. The

1798 outbreak of trachoma, or the "Egyptian ophthalmia," in Britain increased the demand for knowledgeable practitioners of "eye medicine," and led to the establishment of hospitals devoted especially to the treatment of eyes: first the Royal Infirmary for Diseases of the Eye in 1805, and then the London Eye Infirmary three months later (Davidson 314–16).[4] At least eleven cities in England established their own eye hospitals within the next twenty years (Gorin 71–72). As the Egyptian ophthalmia became epidemic, "eye hospitals were opened, textbooks were written, and ophthalmology became more specialized and increasingly professionalized" (Albert and Edwards 155). In short, "more attention was paid to eye disorders and to those who treated them" (Albert and Edwards 155). Wardrop, one of the most influential in a new wave of eye doctors, composed *Essays on the Morbid Anatomy of the Human Eye* (1808), the first major treatise on the eye's pathology (McGrew and McGrew 231). Wardrop argued that, rather than affect the entire body or the eye as a whole, disease affects specific anatomical structures within the eye (Albert and Edwards 148). He classified eye diseases according to the tissue in the eye that was affected; for example, rather than use the general term "ophthalmia," he referred to "conjunctivitis" to describe inflammation in the conjunctiva tissue (Gorin 73). In addition to creating a more anatomically based nomenclature for eye disease, Wardrop decried the disjuncture between anatomy and physiology, recommending instead that they be considered always in relation to each other: "A knowledge of the qualities of the different parts of which our organs are composed, must afford the surest means of acquiring information concerning the functions of these organs, and of becoming acquainted with the changes which they undergo in disease" (xxi). Thus, within just a few decades, theories of vision became focused on the physiology of an individual's eye; the perception of abnormalities in vision, such as color blindness, became dependent on the individual's narration of them; and the nomenclature of eye disease became more closely linked to specific anatomical structures.

This notion of individual, body-based perception reverberates through Romantic-era literature. The dependence of vision upon individual physiology is captured in Blake's eloquent description of subjective vision: "Every body does not see alike ... As a man is, So he Sees. As the eye is formed, such are its Powers" (702). Significantly, "[e]very *body*" sees "as he is" and "as the eye is formed"; thus, vision and subjectivity are embodied and linked through the unique physiology of an individual's eye. Similarly, Wordsworth equates subjectivity with what and how one sees. For example, the formative "spots of time" he relates in *The Two-Part Prelude* (1799) are moments of startling visual apprehension that develop the poet's sense of self (I.288). Rowing on the lake at night, the young Wordsworth suddenly apprehends "a huge Cliff" that seems to "[uprear] its head" with "voluntary power," and then appears to pursue Wordsworth as he rows away in his boat (I.108). The sublimity of the cliff's sudden emergence depends on Wordsworth's subjective vision of it, a vision that changes as his boat moves in the water. The creation and effect of the image are intertwined with the viewer's physical circumstances. Wordsworth recalls,

---

4 See also Rosen, whom Davidson credits with noting the connection between the outbreak of the Egyptian ophthalmia and the development of ophthalmology as a specialization in the early nineteenth century.

"After I had seen / That spectacle, for many days my brain / Worked with a dim and undetermined sense / Of unknown modes of being" (I.119–22). This sublime visual experience conveys to the young Wordsworth a powerful sense of his own subjectivity. The visible world, which is available to us through our own particular physiology, in turn shapes our subjectivity: "Thus day by day my sympathies increased / And thus the common range of visible things / Grew dear to me" (II.215–16). In these passages, Wordsworth portrays subjectivity and vision as mutually constitutive.

For a wide range of writers, the eye signifies both cognitive function and sensibility. The artist Edward Dayes equates seeing with rational thought in his guide to drawing, noting how "the curious and ever-restless eye of the artist *comprehends* more, at one view, than the common observer will notice in an age" (257, my emphasis). And, yet, even as the eye serves as a metonym for the rational process, the eye is also the gateway of emotional and physical sensibility. Physician Arthur Edmondston claims:

> There is no organ in the body on which impressions can be made more easily than on the eye. From its acute sensibility, and the peculiar delicacy of its structure, there subsists an almost immediate communication between it and every surrounding object; and agents, which are perfectly innoxious when applied to the other parts, cannot approach the eye for an instant, without deranging its functions. (104)

Emphasizing the eye's physical embodiment of sensibility, Edmondston also uses a word more commonly associated with the intellect—"derangement"—to describe its pathology. The eye is essential to perception and thus to feeling in the economy of sensibility, and yet it is also the embodiment of (potentially deranged) intellectual activity. Describing the eye's "acute sensibility" and "the immediate communication between it and every surrounding object," Edmondston also illustrates the intense vulnerability these affective and perceptive powers imply (104). "Agents" that do not harm any other part of the body "cannot approach the eye for an instant, without deranging its functions" (104). The eye allows seeing subjects to differentiate between self and world through the visual images it forms and thus helps construct the "I-you" boundaries that are crucial to identity. In Edmondston's formulation, the eye is the organ most likely not only to express suffering (as in tears), but also to suffer pain itself. Thus, the eye's acute sensitivity to external agents situates it as a marker of the subject's formative boundaries. To summarize, three major shifts in medicine contributed to the culture's understanding of vision as material and subjective: the focus on physiology rather than optics, the reliance on individual accounts of seeing to explore color blindness, and the anatomical specificity used in the diagnosis and naming of eye diseases. Concurrently, some poets equated subjectivity with what and how one sees, while artists and physicians portrayed the eyes as the seat of rational thought and the gateway of feeling.

Social Movements

At the same historical moment that vision was increasingly understood as both powerful and contingent upon the individual subject's body, social movements concerned with the suffering of slaves and animals focused on connections among vision, suffering, and subjectivity. Between 1770 and 1840, British citizens, law makers, and writers argued with increasing passion for the abolition of slavery and for legal restrictions on cruelty to animals. In this moment of cultural watershed, the currents of debate about suffering overlap, intertwine, and compete with one another.[5] A brief review of the legislative history of both movements, although representing only the most pragmatic and public outcomes of these debates, offers a sense of the degree to which people were talking about embodied suffering in the late eighteenth century. The 1772 Mansfield Judgment, in which William Murray, Lord Mansfield ruled that a slave brought to England by a Virginia planter be freed, sparked in the popular imagination the notion that British soil should be free from slavery (Lee 11). However, while slavery was, in effect, not permitted in Britain, it took more than thirty years of debate and many failed bills for Parliament to pass a law in 1807 that officially ended Britain's involvement in the slave trade. Finally, the 1833 Abolition Act mandated the gradual emancipation of slaves in the British West Indian colonies.

In the Romantic era, the average British citizen would have heard about the suffering of slaves on a frequent basis. The abolitionist movement, Debbie Lee observes, coincided with the rise of print culture, and thus the details of Parliamentary debates and of various court cases were more available to the reading public than they were in previous eras (25–28). In addition to the Acts described above, Parliament hotly debated other issues related to the abolition of slavery, including the relocation of free blacks from London and Nova Scotia to Sierra Leone (H. Thomas 1–4). Also finding its way into print, court cases such as the *Zong,* in which a slave ship's captain chose to throw nearly one hundred ill Africans overboard during the Middle Passage in hopes of obtaining recompense for his loss of "property" from insurance, "brand[ed] the brutality of slavery on the British consciousness" (Lee 12). Church-going British citizens would have encountered ideas about suffering under slavery each Sunday, as clergy of almost every denomination proclaimed from the pulpit their abolitionist or pro-slavery viewpoints based on Biblical evidence.[6] In addition, writers such as Anna Letitia Barbauld, Ottobah Cugoano, William Cowper, Amelia Opie, Mary Prince, and Robert Southey wrote literature designed to increase British citizens' sympathy for the suffering of slaves, while radicals boycotted products made by slave labor in the colonies.

In many eighteenth-century minds, the movement to abolish slavery was linked with the animal rights movement because some of the same people were active in both causes, and because abolition and animal rights activists shared assumptions about suffering. Animal rights activist and abolitionist Susanna Watts published a periodical to promote the end of both slavery and animal abuse entitled *The Humming Bird*

---

5   Perkins, Ferguson, and K. Thomas point out that the concern for animal suffering at times reinforces and at times obscures concern for the suffering of slaves, the poor, and others. As Thomas explains, "a concern for animal welfare could be an alternative to charity rather than a form of it" (185), and that both the "campaign against animal cruelty" and "the anti-slavery movement of the late eighteenth and early nineteenth centuries [could be seen] as a means of diverting radical energies away from the miseries of the English working class" (187).

6   See H. Thomas (29–47) for an explanation of particular denominations' perspectives on slavery.

(1825), which invited submissions "devoted to the cause of suffering animals as well as to that of suffering men" (qtd. in Ferguson 55). Major abolitionists, such as William Wilberforce, Thomas Clarkson, and Thomas Erskine, also actively promoted animal rights legislation. During the same period of time that they debated the abolition of slavery and the slave trade, Members of Parliament considered several bills to prevent cruelty to animals, including Sir William Pulteney's 1800 unsuccessful proposal to the House of Commons to end bull-baiting and Erskine's 1809 bill to punish the abuse of horses, mares, asses, and oxen (Perkins 18). In response to the failure of Erskine's bill, outraged citizens in Liverpool established the first Society for the Suppression and Prevention of Wanton Cruelty to Animals (Ferguson 30). Following twenty years of failed animal rights bills such as these, the 1822 "Act to Prevent the Cruel and Improper Treatment of Cattle"—which protected oxen, sheep, cattle, and horses—was the first proposal to become law. Parliamentarians continued to present bills designed to protect other animals, such as dogs and cats, well into the Victorian era. In addition, the Society for the Prevention of Cruelty to Animals, whose founding members included Wilberforce, was established in London in 1824 and was endorsed as a Royal Society by Queen Victoria in 1840 (Perkins 19).[7]

The Romantic-era animal rights movement sought to shift the focus away from the use-value of animals to an awareness of animals as sensitive and suffering creatures. The cult of "tender-heartedness" in the eighteenth century and the later current of utilitarian thought, Keith Thomas argues, encouraged behaviors that would reduce suffering: "[A]lthough its main implications were for the human species, whether slaves, children, the criminal or the insane, its relevance to animals was inescapable" (175). This focus on relieving the suffering of animals occurred during the same period in which literature—particularly, but not exclusively, children's literature—portrayed animals with characteristics of human subjectivity, such as names and voices.[8] David Perkins asserts that in Romantic-era literature, "it became common to present animals as individuals, each with its unique character and life history" (3). I cite just a few of the many literary works that feature anthropomorphized animals in Romantic era: Anna Letitia Barbauld's "The Mouse's Petition" (1773), Sarah Trimmer's robin family in *Fabulous Histories* (1786), Robert Burns's "To a Mouse" (1786), Maria Edgeworth's "The Little Dog Trusty" from *Early Lessons* (1801), William Roscoe's *The Butterfly's Ball and the Grasshopper's Feast* (1807), and Lady Catherine Dorset's *The Peacock "At Home"* (1807). If the Parliamentary debates sought to protect animals against cruelty, the literature of the period imagined animals as emotional, intelligent, and vulnerable to pain.

While many discursive strategies were employed in both the abolitionist and animal protection movements—for example, the assertion of the natural rights of all living creatures, and the Christian-based concern that cruelty to humans and animals would morally corrupt the oppressor—I wish to emphasize the argument

---

    7   However, as Batra observes, these advances in the protection of animals reflect a class bias. They are "largely confined to checks on cruelty by the lower classes. Middle- and upper-class treatment of animals (especially in "huntin', shootin', and fishin'") were entirely ignored" (113).

    8   See Perkins and Ferguson for extended analyses of the relationship between the depiction of animals in literature and the anticruelty movement.

based on suffering. Perkins describes the overlapping portrayal of the suffering of animals and people: "In many Romantic poems animals are fellow sufferers with human beings ... . [T]he shared sense of subjection to accident, sickness, pain, and death was naturally a ground of sympathy" (937). The focus on suffering necessarily shifted the conversation from concern about economics or ethics to sympathy with the perspectives of the oppressed in both movements. In the early pages of *The History of the Rise, Progress and Accomplishment of the Abolition of the African Slave Trade* (1808), Clarkson explains the challenge of representing the enormity of human suffering caused by the slave trade:

> Where shall I find words to express properly [the slaves'] sorrow, as arising from the reflection of being parted for ever from their friends, their relatives, and their country? Where shall I find language to paint in appropriate colors the horror of mind brought on by thoughts of their future unknown destination, of which they can augur nothing but misery from all that they have yet seen? How shall I make known their situation, while laboring under painful disease, or while struggling in the suffocating holds of their prisons, like animals inclosed in an exhausted receiver? How shall I describe their feelings as exposed to all the personal indignities, which lawless appetite or brutal passion may suggest? How shall I exhibit their sufferings as determining to refuse sustenance and die, or as resolving to break their chains, and, disdaining to live as slaves, to punish their oppressors? How shall I give an idea of their agony, when under various punishments and tortures for their reputed crimes? Indeed every part of this subject defies my powers ... in the words of a celebrated member of Parliament, ... "Never was there so much human suffering condensed in so small a space." (I.19)

Clarkson struggles to "paint [the suffering of slaves] in appropriate colors," that is, to offer visual evidence of their torment. Clarkson traveled extensively and, as Lee explains, relied on a range of strategies to convince Britons of the suffering caused by the slave trade: "Not only did Clarkson submit facts and figures, numbers and dimensions, and stories of ill treatment, he brought in actual iron instruments used on slave ships: handcuffs, leg shackles, thumbscrews, speculums for force-feeding slaves who would rather die" (15). Elaine Scarry observes that instruments of torture make pain "visible to those outside the person's body" (28). Displaying shackles and other tools of the slave trade as empirical evidence, Clarkson attempted to illustrate the physical pain of bondage to people who would never feel it. Rather than lecture the public about ethics or morality, Clarkson chose to make the slaves' suffering visible to the English.

Similarly, in his *A Letter on the Abolition of the Slave Trade* (1807), Wilberforce charges his readers to rely on their imaginative vision to apprehend the progression of a fictional slave's torment:

> *See* our wretched family or individual arriving at the destined port, and then call to mind the abominations of the sale of a negro cargo. *See* the wretched individual or family exposed naked like brutes, and the same methods taken as with their fellow brutes, to ascertain whether or not their limbs and members are perfect. *See* them forced to jump or dance, to prove their agility; or, still more affecting, *see* them afraid, each lest the other only should be bought by some particular purchaser, and therefore displaying their agility, while their hearts are wrung with anguish in order to induce the buyer to take them both. (342–43, my emphasis)

Even after offering 340 pages of damning information about the practice of slavery, Wilberforce finds it necessary to employ fiction to induce his readers to "see"—that is, to bear witness and feel sympathy for—the emotional and physical suffering of slaves sold at market.

Likewise, eighteenth-century animal rights activists foregrounded the suffering of animals. Keith Thomas attributes the increased interest in animal suffering to "a new mode of thinking": "[It] was the feelings of the suffering object which mattered, not its intelligence or moral capacity" (176). Attention to the suffering of animals represented a major change in discussions about the brute insensitivity of animals and disputes about their intelligence. In 1789, Jeremy Bentham famously countered Descartes' influential 1637 argument that human superiority to animals was evident in the existence of our souls and in our ability to speak. Descartes insisted that because animals could not speak, they could not reason and thus were of a different order than humans and had no right to or need of protection. In his *Introduction to the Principles of Morals and Legislation*, Bentham challenges this view of animals, questioning the "insuperable line" Descartes draws:

> Is it the faculty of reason, or, perhaps, the faculty of discourse? But a full-grown horse or dog, is beyond comparison a more rational, as well as a more conversable animal, than an infant of a day, or a week, or even a month, old. But suppose the case were otherwise, what would it avail? The question is not, Can they *reason*? nor, Can they *talk*? but, Can they suffer? (282–83)

For Bentham and animal rights activists of the early nineteenth century, the suffering of animals proved their connection to humanity and thus their right to be protected. As Perkins phrases it: "Though age-old, the suffering of animals at the hands of humans gradually became visible, so to speak, in the course of the eighteenth century" (13).

Seeing Suffering

The attention to seeing suffering that permeated the abolitionist and animal rights movements also pervaded educational and medical discourse.[9] For Jean-Jacques Rousseau, learning to bear suffering and learning to see the suffering of others were essential elements in the education of a human being, and thus foundational in the creation of an ideal society. He asserts in *Emile* (1762) that "To suffer is the first thing [Emile] ought to learn and the first thing he will most need to know" (78). Emile must gradually inure himself to suffering, beginning by "bearing slight pains

---

9   John Wesley, founder of the Methodist church, further exemplifies the late-eighteenth-century belief in the power of visually witnessing suffering. In his sermons and in Charles Wesley's hymns, the brothers "[present] the sight of Christ's suffering as having a profound transformative power, at the heart of Christian experience" (Cruickshank 311). The Wesleys thought that seeing the suffering of their savior would produce a strong emotional response in members of their church that would, in turn, lead to a spiritual awakening. Joanna Cruickshank argues that "Wesley's portrayal of spiritual change ... relies not only on association between emotional and spiritual responses, but also on a fundamental association between the experience of sight and these responses" (324).

without terror" so that he might learn "to bear [the] great pains" that are simply part of human experience. Emile is also directed to observe the suffering of others—especially the poor and the sick—in order to learn compassion. Allan Bloom explains the significance of this component of Emile's education:

> Prior to Rousseau, men believed that their claim on civil society had to be based on an accounting of what they contributed to it. After Rousseau, a claim based not on a positive quality but on a lack became legitimate for the first time. This he introduced as a counterpoise to a society based on Locke's teaching, which has no category for the miserable other than that of the idle and the quarrelsome. The recognition of our sameness and our common vulnerability dampens the harsh competitiveness and egotism of egalitarian political orders. Rousseau takes advantage of the tendency to compassion resulting from equality, and uses it, rather than self-interest, as the glue binding men together. (18–19)

In this reading of Rousseau, human beings know one another—that is to say, we begin to understand one another's subjectivity—through our common suffering.

However, as Bentham argues, the way in which one sees the sufferer—categorically or individually—affects the viewer's ability to respond sympathetically. Linking the plight of animals with that of slaves, Bentham observes:

> The French have already discovered that the blackness of the skin is no reason why a human being should be abandoned without redress to the caprice of a tormentor. It may come one day to be recognized, that the number of legs, the villosity of the skin, or the termination of the *os sacrum*, are reasons equally insufficient for abandoning a sensitive being to the same fate. (283)

Bentham acknowledges how the marked nature of "othered" human bodies ("the blackness of the skin") or of animal bodies ("the number of legs") allows viewers to distance themselves from or "abandon" other "sensitive beings." The dominant, white viewer (in the case of slaves) or human viewer (in the case of animals) cannot or will not see past the physical evidence of difference to perceive a subject who suffers.

Romantic-era theoretical claims about subjective, embodied vision, then, were made against cultural practices of seeing the "other" categorically rather than individually.[10] The popularity of physiognomy and phrenology, as well as the proliferation of diagnostic portraits of the mentally ill, institutionalized the culture's interest in the visible evidence of suffering.[11] Within this practice of "seeing the insane," Sander Gilman identifies a tension between definitions of fixed facial structures versus moveable expressions, as well as between illustrations of "types" versus portraits of individuals. Johann Caspar Lavater's *Physiognomische Fragmente* (1774–78) was first published in England in 1789 and included a number of plates

---

10 Richardson notes: "Romantic-era theorists of the body saw it as remarkably malleable and subject to cultural fashions—changing patterns of diet and of hygiene, transformations in living conditions, work, and exercise—yet the Romantic era also saw a remarkable expansion of interest in biological universals" ("Romanticism and the Body" 8).

11 See Hall for a discussion of phrenology and Romanticism.

illustrating the physiognomy of mental illness.[12] Focusing primarily on the fixed aspects of physiognomy, Lavater identified generalizable facial features indicating idiocy, cretinism, melancholia, mania, and other conditions (Gilman 62–65). In contrast, in his *A Treatise on Insanity* (1801), Phillipe Pinel noted both the physical structure and the facial expressions of the insane in order to make "limited inferences" from individual cases; however, Gilman notes, while Pinel "centers his attention on the particularities of a single patient, implicit in his analysis is the application of the methodology of diagnosis to similar cases" (72, 76). Taking Pinel's interest in individual suffering a step further, his student Jean Etienne Dominique Esquirol published the *Dictionary of Medical Sciences* (1812–22) with plates illustrating "specific cases rather than typical images of categories of insanity" (Gilman 76). Even within the attempt to represent individual sufferers, however, the goal is still to diagnose, to observe aspects of a "specimen" of suffering and then apply that knowledge to other specimens. The eyes of the patient were often read within the diagnostic structure, yet the gaze with power radiated from the physician or reader onto the patient.

These examples of diagnostic seeing illustrate that when the object of vision is a person rather than a thing, the visual field is potentially charged with hierarchical difference, including gender difference, the focus of this study. Jacqueline Labbe argues in *Romantic Visualities*: "The mechanics of opposition that reveal themselves in gendered visualities are especially strong during the late eighteenth century ... . In a culture based on visuals, on perception, how does one escape, manipulate, or negotiate—or accept—the power of the eye?" (35). Women and others marked by difference were thought of more often as bodies than as reciprocally perceptual beings and thus struggled not only to escape visual objectification, but also to become seeing subjects. Citing just one example of this dynamic, Elizabeth Bohls points out the difficulty women had in occupying the role of viewer in scenic tourism, in which "aesthetic distance ... reinforces the social distance between the aesthetic subject and the 'Vulgar,'" a body-based category that included women (13).

Similarly, the man of sensibility's affective responses to the suffering of the poor, the insane, and the women he encounters direct the reader's attention less to these sufferers than to the male viewers' own capacity to feel. Laurence Sterne's Yorick in *A Sentimental Journey* (1768) and Henry Mackenzie's Harley in *The Man of Feeling* (1771), for example, observe suffering figures in their travels in order to shed tears and thus demonstrate their own depth of emotion. In a variation on this mode of seeing suffering sentimentally, the narrators of Wordsworth's poems observe "betrayed women, beggars, maniacs, discharged soldiers, and decrepit old men," yet the narrators respond with calm contemplation rather than with tears (Averill 10). In this economy of sensibility—whether it leads to the male viewer's tears or rumination—women's suffering is valued differently than is men's. In response to this construction of suffering, the works of Wollstonecraft, Frances Burney, and Ann Radcliffe are "[c]rowded with outrageous and rigidly gendered contests over the dignity of meaningful suffering" (Johnson 14). Citing an emblematic example of this

---

12 See Tytler for references to Lavater in Romantic-era fiction and Erle for a discussion of the effect of Lavater's illustrated work on reading character.

struggle within the economy of sensibility, Claudia Johnson argues that the moment the decaying body in *The Mysteries of Udolpho* (1794) is revealed to be male rather than female, "it underscores in ludicrously graphic terms ... a competition over the site of legitimate suffering" (96). Emily St. Aubert's misrecognition of the corpse as that of a woman "dramatizes the necessity of establishing the priority of male suffering and the presumption of female pathology: men, in other words, are the ones who really suffer, and to perceive that women suffer is to be imagining things" (Johnson 97). The problem the novel presents, Johnson argues, is the difficulty of articulating women's suffering "within the discourse of male sentimentality, where men occupy the site of legitimate suffering" (97). Thus, the attempt to see women's suffering constitutes a complex field of vision—the overlapping and sometimes clashing gaze of the one whose vision defines, marks, or sympathizes with the sufferer and the gaze of the sufferer herself—both what she sees and how her visual activity appears to others.

In this context, the conceptualization of vision as embodied in a specific individual became an effective tool with which women might break through the assumptions limiting the culture's ability to see both their suffering and their talent. Donna Haraway's feminist analysis of embodied vision resonates with the Romantic-era interest in the physiology of perception. Haraway asserts that "all eyes, including our own organic ones, are active perceptual systems, building in translations and specific ways of seeing" (190). Haraway's conception of "the embodied nature of all vision" is the foundation of her theory of visuality, which challenges traditional Western claims for the pure objectivity and transcendent vision of the disembodied viewer (188). To see is to express the self, and yet the embodied nature of seeing dismantles the hierarchy between the looking subject and the one seen. Specific, subjective, physically located, the viewer can no longer claim objective and omniscient vision.

Romantic-era interest in embodied vision opens up space for disempowered groups such as women to understand their cultural invisibility to be contingent upon individual perceptions. In *Letters Written in France* (1790), Helen Maria Williams compares French revolutionary women to "secret springs in mechanism ... which, though invisible," shape social movements (72):

> The women have certainly had a considerable share in the French revolution: for, whatever the imperious lords of the creation may fancy, the most important events which take place in this world depend a little on our influence; and we often act in human affairs like those secret springs in mechanism, by which, though invisible, great movements are regulated. (72)

Although Williams's use of the word "invisible" seems from the vantage point of the twenty-first century to be rather commonplace, in the context of the late-eighteenth-century conception of subjective vision, invisibility emerges as a tool for negotiating the fraught relationship between gender and cultural authority. To say, then, that a woman is invisible, or to feel invisible as a woman, is not a sign that a woman is ineffective, but is rather an indication that the "imperious lords" misperceive her as inconsequential. Williams uses invisibility to express succinctly women's generally unperceived effectiveness in public life and discourse. Invisibility, then, serves as a metaphor for unacknowledged talent and thus for cultural disempowerment.

However, when chosen by women, invisibility can offer a refuge, a kind of rogue freedom, an escape from the constraining gaze of patriarchal culture. Like Williams, Wollstonecraft, Smith, and Mary Shelley take advantage of the balance in power implied in embodied vision in order both to dismantle the objectifying male gaze and also to be taken seriously as viewers and creative subjects themselves.

A major component of this study, the concept of embodied vision, highlights the ways in which the seeing subject and the object of vision interact. Kaja Silverman's *World Spectators* posits that the viewer and the objects seen come in to being together: "Creatures and things invite us to answer their appeal in a manner which, although fully responsive to their formal co-ordinates, is absolutely particular to ourselves" (22). Thus, the materiality of the object is as important as is the materiality of the seeing subject's vision. Each having only a partial view, seeing subjects in this model work toward a collective vision of phenomenal forms rather than, as Plato would have it, transcendence of the phenomenal world (Silverman 2). Visibility, in Silverman's terms, depends "upon a confluence of the phenomenal, the psychic, the specular, and the social" (3). Because embodied vision is always partial, the most accurate or ethical vision is collaborative. In this study, the exploration of how one sees suffering will almost always involve not just the exchange between the seeing subject and the person seen, but rather repeated and revised reciprocal looking that is shaped by emotional and social contexts: "[T]he relationship between ourselves and the world should not be thought of in terms of cause and effect; we do not first embrace our 'thereness,' and then care for others. Rather we become ourselves by caring for others" (Silverman 24). To see another's suffering is to "become ourselves;" to have one's own suffering come into the view of another is to feel our subjectivity validated.

In the chapters that follow, I address two major questions: How do women authors portray embodied vision to claim literary authority and to express the conditions that make creativity possible? And, how do women writers' experiments in literary form make visible previously unseen suffering? In my analysis of novels, poetry, travel writing, and children's literature, I argue that Wollstonecraft, Smith, and Mary Shelley explore the stakes of being visible or marked as women in their culture, yet invisible or disempowered as authors.[13] Their innovations in literary form push against and perhaps at moments overcome the constraints placed on women's expression of both creativity and suffering—constraints that ultimately limit cultural perceptions of their subjectivity. Writing about the AIDS crisis, David Morris argues, "An understanding that suffering is always social allows us to recognize the implicit narratives and speech genres that shape our individual experience. It allows us to create new genres and new plots to replace narratives that prove harmful or inadequate" (215–16). The three writers I discuss in this book each experimented with narrative form in order to express the connections between the individual experience of suffering and its social context, causes, or ramifications. With her innovative mixing of the English and Italian sonnet and her focus on the speaker's subjective experience in nature, Smith sought in the *Elegiac Sonnets* (1784–97) to express her own melancholia and in so doing ignited

---

13 Because Percy Bysshe Shelley was called "Shelley," I will use Mary Shelley's full name throughout the book to avoid confusion.

the Romantic sonnet revival. Mary Shelley's *Frankenstein* (1816), a meditation on the culture's inability to see and sympathize with the suffering of those marked by difference, is an originating text in the genre of science fiction. Wollstonecraft's *Letters from Norway* (1796), hailed by critics as a major experiment in form, mingles the political and the personal in a manner that her daughter Mary Shelley develops further in *Rambles in Germany and Italy* (1845).[14] In her poetry, botanical references, and innovative set of framed novellas *Letters of a Solitary Wanderer* (1800–1802), Smith offers a model for a new language that might communicate both what is individual and what is generalizable about the experience of suffering. Finally, Smith and Wollstonecraft draw on the episodic form of children's literature to invent a new narrative form—the fictional ethnography—a collection of verbal portraits that situates individual suffering within its social context.

Part 1, *Illness*, examines the effect of illness constructions on women's literary authority and creative power. Chapter 1 traces a shift in medical characterizations of melancholia—from an association with both feeling and intellect, to an association with just intellect—that I argue significantly affected society's ability to see women as producers of meaningful literature in the Romantic era. Smith leverages her culture's interest in the individual physiology of vision, in color vision, and in eyes as the embodiment of both feeling and intellect to revise this medical model. Furthermore, by foregrounding the suffering body also as a seeing body in the *Elegiac Sonnets*, she revises the cult of sensibility's focus on the sympathizing subject's one-way looking at the suffering object. In short, Smith attempts to make her illness visible, without rendering her poetic talent—cast as her own ability to see, to reason, and to feel—invisible.

Chapter 2 shifts the discussion of illness and creative vision from melancholia to eye disease. By referencing eye disease in *Frankenstein* and by creating parallels between Victor's scientific vision and her own dream vision, Mary Shelley examines what it means to create when one is marked by gender or ethnic difference. I contextualize the repulsion that Victor feels when the creature looks back at him through watery, yellow eyes within the history of the "Egyptian ophthalmia," a gruesome and ultimately blinding illness brought home by British soldiers fighting in the alliance against Napoleon in Egypt. In addition to creating a demand for the development of ophthalmology as a specialty, this epidemic revealed in physical terms the culture's fear of difference. Mary Shelley demonstrates that when difference takes on the threat of contagion, it destroys the sympathetic connections that make narrative possible. The resulting cultural invisibility—that is, the state in which being marked makes one's own experience of self difficult to convey to others—differs greatly from the freedom from scrutiny that a more positive form of invisibility offers. Like Smith, Mary Shelley suggests that being held in a sympathetic gaze encourages creativity; Victor, for example, basks in Walton's loving gaze as he relays the narrative that Walton records in letters to his sister. However, when one cannot find a sympathetic gaze, Mary Shelley recommends invisibility as a productive creative space.

---

14 Angela D. Jones's assessment is representative: "[T]he travelogue form, licens[es] Wollstonecraft to roam philosophically as much as she does literally, all the while blurring boundaries between personal and descriptive modes" (209).

Part 2, *Healing*, argues that women writers articulate models of seeing therapeutically that move the individual from a sense of isolated suffering to forms of healing social interaction or expression. Chapter 3 reconsiders the gendered aspects of two important topics in Romantic scholarship—travel writing and landscape aesthetics—in terms of a rich body of medical literature on health travel. Medical treatises by Romantic-period physicians assert that the motion, exercise, and change of scenery inherent in traveling helped to heal a number of illnesses. At the end of the eighteenth century, literary texts and travel guides depict viewing the picturesque landscape in particular as a critical feature of health travel. I argue that conventions of picturesque aesthetics such as variety, novelty, and balance parallel the characteristics of travel extolled by medical writers. The twenty-five letters of Wollstonecraft's travel narrative, *Letters from Norway*, mingle the discourses of health travel and picturesque tourism, thus revealing that Wollstonecraft's trip was neither solely an effort to complete Gilbert Imlay's business nor just an opportunity to explore Scandinavian culture, but also an attempt to heal her emotional pain and melancholia while traveling through—and viewing—picturesque and sublime landscapes. Reinforcing medical understandings of the eyes as the seat of rationality and feeling, Wollstonecraft revises the conventions of landscape aesthetics, projecting onto the landscape her own intense rational ability and emotional depth. She reconceptualizes "the frame" in the picturesque aesthetic, turning what was essentially a distancing technique into the projection of a therapeutic, maternal embrace. In return, she experiences moments of healing in the landscape's sheltering, maternal love.

Chapter 4 returns to Smith, who asserts in her poetry and novels that the only reliable therapy for her melancholia is seeing nature scientifically, that is, botanizing. Smith's reliance on botanizing as therapy seems to follow both the general medical advice of Romantic-era physicians such as Robert Whytt and William Buchan that melancholics engage in outdoor activities, as well as the specific recommendation by Thomas Trotter that young girls botanize to prevent nervous illnesses. Yet Smith goes beyond these medical recommendations to portray the major activities of scientific botany—collecting, naming, and contextualizing—as a model for a language of suffering. The language that Smith proposes has the power to create a new field of visibility in which not only individual suffering but also the social patterns which underlie that suffering become visible and can be named.

Chapter 5 argues that Mary Shelley's travel narrative, *Rambles in Germany and Italy*, which describes her attempt to restore her mental and physical health in Germany's spas and Italy's salubrious climate, is both trauma narrative and political argument. Mary Shelley includes in *Rambles* accounts of two types of treatment she explored on these trips—the institutional medicine she encountered in her visits to Germany's spas and the salutary landscape she observed both at the spas and while traveling. Ultimately Mary Shelley, like her mother, champions the balm derived from viewing the picturesque landscape over the prescriptive spa regimen. In short, she decides it is more beneficial for her health to gaze at the landscape than it is to be caught in the medical gaze. And yet while she refers to "novelty," one of the major conventions of picturesque travel, the scenes that capture Mary Shelley's attention are deeply imbued with memory and loss. Returning to Italy for the first time in the twenty years after the loss of her husband and four children, Mary Shelley sees the outline of her traumatic past written on the landscape through which she travels and in the art she views. Aligning individual pain with social suffering, she conveys her hopes for the success of the Italian Risorgimento to the reader by offering public scenes of anguish and courage that, like her own life experiences, are written on the land.

The third section, *Social Justice*, delineates the ways in which Smith and Wollstonecraft train others to see suffering. I argue that the experimental, fictional form they developed, which I call *fictional ethnography*, focuses attention on the social context of suffering. Wollstonecraft's *Original Stories* (1788) and Smith's children's work *Rural Walks* (1795), the subject of chapter 6, portray the relationship between illness and poverty in late-eighteenth-century England through interactions between charitably minded teachers and the impoverished ill. While eighteenth-century didactic literature commonly taught gentry children how "best" to offer charity to the poor, Wollstonecraft and Smith direct readers' attention not to the act of charity but to the lives of the poor. Their multiple portraits of poor people voice a biting critique of England's efforts to distinguish between the "deserving" and "undeserving" poor. Developing three major aspects of late-eighteenth-century didactic children's literature—the mother-teacher figure, the portrayal of learning as experiential and dialogic, and the episodic, narrative structure—Wollstonecraft and Smith transform their children's books into fictional ethnographies of the poor. Their books expose the social structures underlying poverty and teach children to see these structures. In addition, Smith's fictional ethnography educates children about political reform and institutional relief for the poor.

Mary Wollstonecraft's unfinished novel, *The Wrongs of Woman* (1798), the subject of chapter 7, encodes her experience with gender oppression in approximately twenty-seven fictional portraits of women of various classes. All of the portrayed women struggle to survive within the structure of English marriage law, which allows men to abuse, rob, rape, and neglect their wives. Just as I argue that Wollstonecraft's and Smith's children's literature be taken seriously for its intervention into the problem of poverty, so I suggest that Wollstonecraft's novel of social criticism be interpreted as an extension of children's literature. While it certainly shares the goals of the Jacobin novel, Wollstonecraft's formal innovation—an innovation driven by the difficulty of expressing women's suffering in the language of the father—is based on the narrative structure of didactic children's literature. The novel unfolds as a dialogue in the asylum that becomes an ethnography compiled by two teacher figures—Maria and Jemima. In addition to revising the Jacobin novel, Wollstonecraft identifies the limits of the sentimental novel. She exposes the ways in which sentimental seeing forestalls social action, and she teaches her readers to see the social context of suffering instead. With her final fictional ethnography, Wollstonecraft urges women to recognize their common vulnerability and mutual dependence.

PART 1
Illness

Chapter 1

Melancholia and the Poetics of Visibility: Charlotte Smith's *Elegiac Sonnets*

"Every body does not see alike ... As a man is, So he Sees.
As the eye is formed, such are its Powers."

William Blake

In the five *Elegiac Sonnets* (1784–97) devoted to the suicide of the melancholic hero of Goethe's *The Sorrows of Young Werther* (1774), Charlotte Smith speaks in Werther's voice, recreating the man of sensibility's experience with terminal love melancholia. The five sonnets depict Werther's suicidal longing as a series of visual tableaux, as a complex matrix of looking and being seen. Werther first describes himself "lingering" around Charlotte's house, "haunt[ing] the scene where all [his] treasure lies" (Sonnet 21, ll. 5–6). Readers then witness Werther's love-sick wandering in the woods, where he flees to "hide [his] sorrow and [his] tears" (Sonnet 22, l. 2). We watch him gazing at the North Star which, he opines, has shone on Charlotte. We follow him as he chooses his grave site, where he imagines Charlotte weeping over his tombstone. Finally, we are privy to his fantasy that Charlotte will picture the "worms" that will "feed on [his] devoted heart, / where even [her] image shall be found no more" (Sonnet 25, ll. 11–12). As readers of Smith's sonnets, we not only watch Werther's wandering body perform suffering, but also view his complex internal world of imagined looking and loss. We see him suffer; we see him imagining that he sees Charlotte suffering from grief; we see him imagining that he sees Charlotte picturing the worms that will eat his "devoted" heart. And finally, we see him imagining that she will understand the loss of his love in visual terms; she will see her image erased from his worm-eaten heart.

I begin with a description of this visual complexity to introduce Smith's major strategies for making women's melancholic suffering visible in not just these, but in all ninety-two of the *Elegiac Sonnets*. First, Smith employs her culture's interest in vision to mediate late-eighteenth-century gendered definitions of the relationship between emotion and reason, and thus gendered definitions of melancholia—a topic I explain at some length in the first sections of this chapter. In the Werther sonnets, to which I will return, Smith inhabits Werther's excessive emotion; she cross-dresses as the man of sensibility in order to claim the public expression of emotional pain for women. This cross-dressing speaker, the female poet in the male icon's clothing, invites readers to compare cultural norms for men's and women's emotional expressivity. As she re-appropriates from Goethe the discourse of loss and longing, Smith modifies the German poet's version of melancholia, offering her readers not only a portrait of sensibility, but also a glimpse of the balancing rationality that might have saved Werther. Second, Smith asks readers to "see" the suffering body—in some cases her own, but more often the bodies of characters suffering from melancholia—in order to bring attention to the materiality of suffering and to portray sufferers also as seers. In the Werther sonnets, for example, she offers Werther's wandering body to readers' view while she simultaneously draws our attention to Werther's own field of vision. By re-envisioning the relationship between melancholic thought and feeling and by emphasizing the melancholic's seen and seeing body, in the *Elegiac Sonnets* Smith challenges late-eighteenth-century norms for emotional expression, particularly those established by the cult of sensibility.

With her depiction of women's melancholic suffering, Smith also claims literary authority. She wishes, that is, to make visible both her suffering and her poetic talent. At the end of the eighteenth century, a male author's expression of melancholia signified a literary genius based in suffering, rational power, and linguistic facility. The frequent portrayal of melancholia—especially in poetry—made the condition, as Guinn Batten points out, almost synonymous with British Romantic literature for the generations that followed (10).[1] One might cite, in addition to the compelling suicide of Werther, the dark suffering of Lord Byron's brooding and psychically tortured Manfred, and the unalleviated despair expressed in Percy Bysshe Shelley's "Stanzas Written in Dejection, Near Naples." More emblematic than these of Romantic melancholia, though, is the ultimately redeeming melancholia of William Wordsworth's *The Prelude*, Samuel Taylor Coleridge's "Dejection: An Ode," and John Keats's "Ode on Melancholy." This Romantic-era preoccupation with melancholia derived from the literature of earlier centuries, including Aristotle's description of male, melancholic genius in his *Problems* and Marcilio Ficino's elaboration on the subject in *On Life* (1489). The figure of the male melancholic, Juliana Schiesari argues, was useful for transforming loss into masculine cultural power (29). Robert Burton's elaborate verbal performance in *Anatomy of Melancholy* (1621), for example, demonstrates that the cultural power associated with melancholic suffering is specifically linked to the production of language. In the midst of a Romantic-era struggle between male and female authors for dominance of the British literary marketplace, portraying oneself as melancholic was one way to signal literary genius.[2]

Although the association between male melancholia and male literary genius was longstanding, a female author's claim of melancholic genius was complicated by the deeply gendered solutions emerging to address the "problem" of sensibility in late-eighteenth-century British culture. Smith acknowledges her culture's celebration of male melancholic genius in *Conversations Introducing Poetry* (1804), one of six books she wrote for children. The teacher figure Mrs. Talbot informs her son George that men of genius, especially poets, are prone to melancholia:

> It has been observed, George, that almost all men of genius have a disposition to indulge melancholy and gloomy ideas; and in reading our most celebrated poets, we have evidence that it is so. (*WCS* 13:193)

---

1   Batten observes that the terms "melancholia" and "Romanticism" have been so closely associated that only one book-length study of Romantic melancholy—Eleanor Sickles's *The Gloomy Egoist* (1932)—preceded Batten's analysis of Romantic melancholy and commodity culture in the works of male Romantic poets.

2   For a detailed description of this phenomenon of gendered competition in the literary marketplace, see especially Marlon Ross.

Although Smith shares a tendency toward melancholy with these "men of genius," her gender presents an impediment to making her literary talent visible. It is significant, as Schiesari observes, that Burton and other male melancholics who describe their condition grant that women may also suffer from the illness, but assert that women display none of the genius associated with it (15). In fact, according to Burton, many female melancholics (specifically "maides, nunnes, and widows") "cannot tell how to expresse themselves in wordes, or how it holds them, what ailes them, you cannot understand them, or well tell what to make of their sayings" (I: 414–15). By identifying nuns, maids, and widows as those whom melancholia renders inarticulate, Burton suggests that without an intimate connection to a man, a woman who suffers literally makes no sense. The incomprehensibility that Burton assigns to the expression of women's melancholia was refigured in the 1780s and 90s as "hysteria," a condition attributed to women's ungovernable bodies and overindulgence in sensibility. At the same cultural moment, the definition of melancholia underwent a major shift, becoming more firmly identified with rational ability than with feeling. To claim the connection between melancholia and literary genius for women, then, Smith wrestled with her culture's gendered conceptions of rationality and sensibility. Rather than embrace the exclusive connection between rationality and melancholia emerging in the 1780s, Smith invoked a mid-eighteenth-century formulation of the condition that attributed to the melancholic both rational agility and acute sensibility. Emphasizing the embodied nature of melancholic suffering—by refusing to separate body and mind, by drawing the reader's attention to the bodies of melancholic wanderers, and by employing her culture's interest in embodied vision—Smith challenges the late-eighteenth-century portrayal of the male melancholic as a purely rational, nearly bodiless figure.

The Problem of Sensibility

To understand the intervention that a portrayal of embodied melancholic vision makes on behalf of women writers, one must first explore the history of gendered definitions of melancholia—always contingent on understandings of the relationship between the body and mind. The significance of Smith's claim that emotion might support rather than undermine the poet's rational command of language—or, put differently, that sensibility and rationality are interdependent—is best understood in the context of the redefinition of melancholia in late-eighteenth-century literary and medical texts. In the introduction to her anthology, *The Nature of Melancholy from Aristotle to Kristeva* (2000), Jennifer Radden asserts, "the man of melancholy in Romantic writing was, like the suffering Werther, all feeling, all sensibility" (30). While the equation of melancholia and sensibility would seem to hold for Werther and for a legion of Byronic heroes, a shift in the medical definition of melancholia worked to counter the self-destructive strain of feeling associated with Wertherian melancholia. This discomfort with sensibility in the 1780s and 90s and the resulting shift in definitions of the illness melancholia significantly affected society's ability to see women as producers of meaningful literature.

To delineate the effect that the "problem" of sensibility had on Romantic-era literary and medical discourse about nervous illnesses, we must look back to early- and mid-eighteenth-century literary and medical profiles of melancholia, which did not yet exclude sensibility. Prior to 1780, melancholia and sensibility had a close relationship; the person of sensibility—that is, the person of great sensory perception and intuition—was thought to have an increased capacity for the Lockean brand of rational thought that leads to moral reflection. Sensibility was synonymous with great feeling, refinement, and femininity, but was still assumed to coexist with rational thought in a single mind, especially in a melancholic one. Early- to mid-century poems such as James Thomson's *The Seasons* (1726–30), Edward Young's "Night Thoughts" (1742), Thomas Warton's "The Pleasures of Melancholy" (1745), and Thomas Gray's "Elegy Written in a Country Churchyard" (1751) popularized the connections among melancholia, solitary pensiveness, and sensibility. For example, in *Autumn*, from *The Seasons*, Thomson characterizes philosophic melancholy as literary inspiration:

> He comes! he comes! in every breeze the Power
> Of Philosophic Melancholy comes!
> His near approach the sudden-started tear,
> The glowing cheek, the mild dejected air,
> The softened feature, and the beating heart,
> Pierced deep with many a virtuous pang, declare.
> O'er all the soul his sacred influence breathes;
> Inflames imagination; through the breast
> Infuses every tenderness; and far
> Beyond the dim earth exalts the swelling thought. (ll. 1004–13)

In Thomson's portrayal, philosophic melancholy not only affects the rational, creative mind, but also refines the poet's sensibility. Although Thomson's metonyms for the poet are gendered in correspondence to sensibility and rationality (the feminine "breast" and the masculine "swelling" of thought), this melancholic poet contains both. The passage continues to intermingle the two qualities:

> Ten thousand fleet ideas; such
> As never mingled with the vulgar dream,
> Crowd fast into the mind's creative eye.
> As fast the corresponding passions rise,
> As varied, and as high ... (ll. 1014–18)

Thomson demonstrates that philosophic melancholy inspires both rational thought, "ten thousand fleet ideas," and also sensibility, or "the corresponding passions." In mid-eighteenth-century literature, these qualities were companion aspects of literary genius. Also worth noting is Thomson's portrayal of the physical "symptoms" of melancholia: "the sudden-started tear, / The glowing cheek, the mild dejected air, / The softened feature" (ll. 1006–8). Like the physical manifestation of sensibility in tears and blushes—a topic I address in the final section of this chapter—melancholia in Thomson's poem is visibly apprehensible.

By the 1780s and 90s, the cult of sensibility became associated with the French Revolution, a trend, Janet Todd argues, that was largely due to reports from English radicals in France. For example, Helen Maria Williams reported the downfall of the monarchy and the initial Jacobin triumph in terms of domestic sensibility (Todd *Sensibility* 131). The subsequent Jacobin terror, then, implicated sensibility as encouraging an obsession with self-indulgent feelings that overlooked rationally based justice. The man of sensibility, immensely popular just decades before, for example in Laurence Sterne's *A Sentimental Journey* (1768) and Henry Mackenzie's *Man of Feeling* (1771), suddenly became an effete embarrassment, and fear surfaced that over-refined sensibility would emasculate men and corrupt women (Todd *Sensibility* 131). Thus, the post-French Revolution "problem" of where to locate emotion emerged. The terms under which the general cultural acceptance of sensibility disintegrated were both political and gendered. As Chris Jones argues, "criticism of [sensibility in] the 1790s was not predominantly aesthetic, but political, social, and moral" (4). In a complementary interpretation of this "crisis over sensibility," G. J. Barker-Benfield suggests that debates about sensibility turned around conceptions of the "natural" order of the sexes (360). I argue that in an attempt to save the long-standing profile of the English melancholic genius, the culture characterized sensibility and rational thought, once seen as partners in creating human knowledge, as gendered and oppositional. As I will demonstrate, medical discourse played a critical role in this realignment of sensibility and rationality.

Mid-eighteenth-century medical texts, like literary texts of the period, portrayed the origin of melancholia as a combination of rational intelligence and refined sensibility. The physician George Cheyne, who claimed nervous illness as distinctly English in his influential treatise *The English Malady* (1733), describes nervous illnesses as affecting those who "are quick, prompt, and passionate; are all of weak Nerves; have a great deal of Sensibility; are quick Thinkers, feel Pleasure and Pain the most readily, and are of most lively Imagination" (105). Cheyne does not regard sensibility and rational thought as oppositional; rather, the English Malady most afflicts people who are "quick Thinkers" *and* "have a great deal of Sensibility" (105). Two years later, the Dutch physician Herman Boerhaave describes the causes of melancholia as, among other things, "A violent Exercise of the Mind; the dwelling Night and Day mostly upon one and the same Object; a constant Wakefulness; great Motions of the Mind, whether of Joy or Sorrow; great and laborious Motions of the Body much repeated ..." (176). Boerhaave's description of causes includes an obsessive studiousness, but it also emphasizes strong emotions such as joy or sorrow, as well as physical exertion. Both physicians depict the body—its weak nerves or its overexertion—as contributing to the melancholic state.

A crucial shift in these definitions occurred in the late eighteenth century, when medical literature began to exhibit a pronounced focus on the melancholic's rational capabilities. This shift excluded sensibility from the realm of melancholic genius and placed it in an oppositional and feminine category. Women's perception, in turn, became associated with sensibility and was pathologized in terms of the emerging nervous illness, hysteria.[3] Indeed, the categories "hypochondria" and "hysteria," both of which Cheyne used in 1733 to describe an advanced melancholia characterized by "fits" or near seizures, became important tools for making this gendered distinction in the 1790s.[4]

---

3   Helpful studies of literature and hysteria include Ender, Logan, and Showalter.

4   Although in his general description of "the English malady," Cheyne does not distinguish between hysteria and hypochondria, as Barker-Benfield points out, in Cheyne's eighteen case studies he does assign "hysterical fits" to women and "epileptick," "nervous," or "hypochondriacal fits" to men (Barker-Benfield 25).

Unlike Cheyne, William Buchan, author of the most widely used eighteenth- and nineteenth-century home health guide, *Domestic Medicine* (16th ed. 1798), draws a gendered line between melancholia/hypochondria and hysteria, associating the first two conditions with men and masculine activities, and the third with women and feminine activities. Although Buchan describes hypochondria as less "violent" (acute) and more "permanent" (chronic) than melancholia, this distinction is not nearly as significant as are the characteristics these two masculine disorders share. According to Buchan, melancholia is caused by "intense application to study" or "intense thinking" (*Domestic* 420, 427), and hypochondria is induced by "long and serious attention to abstruse subjects" (*Domestic* 453). Buchan identifies the population most likely to suffer from hypochondria as "[m]en of a melancholy temperament, whose minds are capable of great attentions, and whose passions are not easily moved" (*Domestic* 453). He suggests that men suffer from melancholia and hypochondria, then, for two reasons: first, their rational intellect and ability to concentrate predispose them to the illness, and second, they choose to devote themselves to a level of study characterized by abstract reflection and solitude. Both the perceived origin of the illness and its manifestation naturalize rationality as a male characteristic.

Just as they attribute male nervous illnesses to intelligence, medical writers attribute the female nervous illness hysteria to an essentialized body—women's "nature," sexual characteristics, reproductive processes, or inactive lifestyle—to anything, that is, except the rational mind. Buchan ascribes the onset of hysteria to physical irritation and emotional excess:

> Women of a delicate habit, whose stomach and intestines are relaxed, and whose nervous system is extremely sensible, are most subject to hysteric complaints. In such persons a hysteric fit as it is called may be brought on by an irritation of the nerves of the stomach or intestines, by wind, by acrid humour, or the like. A sudden suppression of the menses often gives rise to hysteric fits. They may likewise be excited by violent passions or affections of the mind, as fear, grief, anger, or great disappointments. (*Domestic* 447)

In this model of nervous disorders, too much thinking pushes a highly rational man into melancholia/hypochondria, while too much emotion pushes a woman of refined sensibility into hysteria.[5] Late-eighteenth-century medical texts, then, reassign characteristics of the mid-century medical definition of melancholia according to gender: melancholic men inherit the association with rationality, while "nervous" females inherit the association with extreme emotion and the body.

The physician Thomas Trotter's work *A View of the Nervous Temperament* (1812), notable for its emphasis on the social circumstances of the patient, specifically identifies "Literary Men" as the primary group affected by melancholia. Trotter's account of the behavior of literary men is extensive:

---

5   The medical treatise *Observations on the Nature, Causes, and Cure of Those Disorders, Which Have Commonly Been Called Nervous, Hypochondriac, or Hysteric* (1797) by the physician Robert Whytt, to which most other writers dealing with nervous illness refer, offers a nearly identical account of the gendered nature of these illnesses.

The philosopher and man of letters, who devote most of their time to study, must lead a sedentary life ... . The mind itself, by pursuing one train of thought, and poring too long over the same subject, becomes torpid to external agents: and an undue mental exertion seems to subtract from the body much of that stimulation which ... belongs to emotion and passion ... . Hence the numerous instances of dyspepsia, hypochondriasis and melancholia, in the literary character. (36–38)

Like Buchan, Trotter suggests that melancholic literary men think rationally to the exclusion of emotion and passion. This association between male melancholia and genius had been common in western culture for centuries, beginning perhaps with Aristotle's account of the melancholic tendencies shared by great intellectuals and heroes. Indeed, in their focus on "literary men," Buchan and Trotter do not differ much from earlier writers such as Bernard Mandeville, who described melancholia as "the Disease of the Learned" (95). The exclusion of sensibility—and thus the elision of the body—marks the crucial difference between the late-eighteenth-century depiction of the male melancholic genius and its forbears.

Revising gendered medical and cultural definitions of melancholia in her poetry, Smith invents a model for expressing emotion and suffering that had an enormous influence on what we now call Romantic poetry. Most notably, Smith's argument that one must temper sensibility with rational reflection informs Wordsworth's struggle to integrate emotion into poetry judiciously. For example, Wordsworth famously asserts in the "Preface to *Lyrical Ballads*" that poetry "takes its origin from emotion recollected in tranquillity" (756). Poems of value, he argues, are produced by a "man who, being possessed of more than usual organic sensibility had also thought long and deeply" (744–45). Whereas Smith portrays the necessity of balancing passion and reflection, Wordsworth's "Poet is chiefly distinguished from other men by a greater promptness to think and feel without immediate external excitement" (753). Wordsworth agrees with Smith that poetry should emerge from a feeling mind, yet he attempts to naturalize this tendency in the implicitly male poet. This "true" poet has "an ability of conjuring up in himself passions, which are indeed far from being the same as those produced by real events ..." (751). Filtered through the poet's rational mind, passion acquires rather than loses poetic power. Thus, by inserting this step of contemplation into a poet's reaction to passion, Wordsworth saves the poet from the fate of the effeminate man of sensibility. Both Smith and Wordsworth temper emotion with reason; Smith, however, portrays the intellect as a factor that deepens, rather than ameliorates, suffering.

Because she refused to separate rational thought and emotion, Smith had to maneuver carefully through rhetoric supporting and denouncing sensibility in the period. She worked to distinguish her representation of emotion both from the essentializing association between sensibility and hysteria, and also from the strain of self-serving male melancholic sensibility that was under attack in the 1790s. In her 1797 preface to the *Elegiac Sonnets*, Smith distances herself from the false emotional performance that characterized the cult of sensibility:

That these [sonnets] are gloomy, none will surely have a right to complain; for I never engaged they should be gay. But I am unhappily exempt from the suspicion of *feigning* sorrow for an opportunity of shewing the pathos with which it can be described. (11, original emphasis)

Though her "gloomy" sonnets heavily reference the tradition of poetic melancholy, in the preface Smith attempts to distinguish herself from those writers who "[feign] sorrow" simply to highlight their great artistic sensibility and verbal dexterity. The teacher in Smith's *Conversations Introducing Poetry* (1804) continues her instruction about "men of genius," especially "our most celebrated poets" who "have a disposition to indulge melancholy and gloomy ideas," criticizing those who, in contrast, pretend to suffer from melancholia:

> If, however, a certain degree of melancholy is supposed to be the accompaniment of genius, there is no species of affectation more absurd and disgusting, than pretending to be absent, "melancholy and gentlemanlike"—an air which is often assumed by solemn coxcombs, who, while they would fain have it mistaken for a symptom of superior intellect, make it the cloak of supercilious pride, and pompous stupidity. (*WCS* 13:197)

According to Smith, these pretenders feign melancholia in order to claim superior intellect; in so doing, they make real suffering and authentic genius more difficult to see. True melancholics feel sympathetic sensibility and pursue intellectual study, while those who "*fancy* themselves affected with pensive poetical dejection" "have *no sensibility* but for themselves, and *no study* but how to make themselves of importance" (*WCS* 13:197–98, my emphasis). Contrasting legitimate emotion with sham displays of feeling, Smith seeks to make her melancholic suffering visible.

Authentic Suffering

As Smith attempted to contrast her authentic suffering with the man of sensibility's affectation, a tension arose between her publicly expressed troubles and the creation of a melancholic mood in her poetry. In her letters and in the prefaces to her novels and poetry, Smith describes the coalescence of financial difficulty and maternal grief that cause her melancholia.[6] Having grown up in a genteel family, she experienced a radical change in socioeconomic position after she was forced at age 15 to marry Benjamin Smith. During the 23 years they lived together, Benjamin Smith squandered his wife's money and failed to support their twelve children.[7] Twenty years into the marriage, Smith began her writing career, composing the *Elegiac Sonnets* while she stayed with her husband in debtors' prison. In spite of disabling chronic rheumatism and severe bouts of melancholia, which she terms "extreme depression of spirit," Smith continued to write at a furious pace, and with good reason (*Elegiac Sonnets* 7). When the Smiths separated in 1787, she became the sole provider for eight children between the ages of two and seventeen (Turner 36).[8] Although her father-in-law bequeathed a trust fund to his grandchildren, Smith never received the money for them and spent her life in a relentless battle with the trust fund's custodians. In

---

6   In addition to Smith's letters and prefaces, consult Fletcher for biographical information.

7   For a more complete description of this marriage, see Stanton ("Charlotte Smith and 'Mr. Monstroso'").

8   For a detailed account of Smith's financial situation, including both expenses and income, see Stanton ("Charlotte Smith's Literary Business").

addition, seven of Smith's twelve children died in her lifetime. The most devastating loss seems to have been the death of her daughter Anna Augusta in 1795. In a letter she wrote to Joseph Cooper Walker five years after this daughter's death, Smith expresses her awareness of the toll grief has taken on her physical and mental health: "[T]he regret and anguish I have now felt five years for the loss of my loveliest and most deserving child, is slowly undermining not only my frame but the few powers of mind I possess'd" (*CLCS* 339). Smith's literature and letters reveal that this grief did not abate before her own death in 1806.

With a few important exceptions, Smith confines her specific description of these troubles to the prefaces of the ten editions of the *Elegiac Sonnets* (and to the prefaces of her novels), allowing the sonnets themselves to cultivate a melancholic mood rather than detail her individual circumstances. For the most part, this compartmentalization seems to have been effective. In her lifetime, Smith was widely praised for her portrayal of subjective poetic melancholy. Smith's sonnets led the way in shifting the focus of British contemplative melancholic poetry from a preoccupation with the transitory nature of life to an interest in the speaker's own state of mind. The majority of Smith's reviewers embrace her depiction of the melancholic mind, praising—as *The Monthly Review* does—"the elegant writer's gloomy cast of thought" (458). Even the prickly Reverend Richard Polwhele expresses high regard for Smith's depiction of melancholic feelings: "The Sonnets of Charlotte Smith, have a pensiveness peculiarly their own. It is not ... the gloomy melancholy of Gray ... . It is a strain of wild, yet softened sorrow, that breathes a romantic air" (18). In his introduction to William Lisle Bowles's *Sonnets* (1796), Coleridge hails Smith's representation of depressive moods in her sonnets as a major literary innovation. Based on Smith's poetry, Coleridge asserts, "In a Sonnet then we require a developement of some lonely feeling, by whatever cause it may have been excited; but those Sonnets appear to me the most exquisite, in which moral Sentiments, Affections, or Feelings, are deduced from, and associated with, the scenery of Nature" (1139). Coleridge praises Smith's portrayal of nature's capacity to educate the emotions.

However, in his celebration of the melancholic sonnet developed by Smith, Coleridge quickly tosses out of consideration "whatever cause [by which the lonely feeling] may have been excited" (1139). The critical success of the *Elegiac Sonnets*, then, rested in part on Smith's recasting and depersonalizing the individual experience of melancholia into the interaction of the melancholic mind with Nature. Yet the multiple prefaces detailing her troubles, which Sarah Zimmerman terms "an on-going plot ... a serialized autobiographical narrative," were published alongside these melancholic sonnets (60). In the 1792 preface, Smith refers to the relentless battle to wrestle her children's inheritance from the trustees of her father-in-law's estate. She asks, "Can the *effect* [of melancholia] cease, while the *cause* remains?" (5, original emphasis). Referencing this "cause" again in 1797, she tells her readers, "The injuries I have so long suffered under are not mitigated; the aggressors are not removed; but however soon they may be disarmed of their power ... they can neither give back to the maimed the possession of health, or [sic] restore the dead" (9). Each volume of the *Elegiac Sonnets* offered readers what Daniel E. White has described as a "dual structure": both the "real" autobiographical story of Smith's melancholia in the prefaces and the idealized representation of these feelings in the sonnets (65). By restricting the details of her individual troubles to the prose and expressing a more generalized melancholic mood in the poetry, Smith manages both to claim the feelings she expresses as authentic—thus distinguishing herself from the man of sensibility—and also to exhibit her impressive poetic facility.

In several instances, however, this boundary between autobiography and poetry does not hold.[9] Stuart Curran points out, "the six sonnets impelled by the death of her favorite daughter ... represent a grief untransmuted from its actual sources in her experience" ("Charlotte Smith and British Romanticism" 72–73). Although they are only six of ninety-two, the sonnets that invoke her daughter's death with quiet references to "the form / I loved," or "that form adored," remind readers that Smith's melancholia in all the sonnets has its source in authentic feeling (Sonnet 89, ll. 11–12; Sonnet 91, l. 9). The struggle between experience and art enacted by this "dual structure" demonstrates to readers that Smith's literary facility is not founded upon superficial emotion. However, as Jacqueline Labbe convincingly argues, even authenticity can be performed: "Smith's own insistence on her sincerity has resulted in a picture of her poetry as unmediated, as emanating from the genuine distresses and woes of Smith herself" (*Charlotte Smith* 91–92). Accepting Labbe's point as a caveat, I argue that Smith's particular mode of performing authentic suffering—with a focus on inconsolability and on the body—nonetheless challenges the gendered boundaries of acceptable emotional expression.

Although she restricts specific descriptions of the causes of her suffering to the prefaces and footnotes, in the sonnets Smith presents her suffering as unrelenting. If, with her "dual structure," Smith responds to the challenge of claiming authentic melancholy in the cult of sensibility's wake, her insistent expression of suffering challenges the cultural value placed on women's fortitude in the eighteenth century. Women's suffering, as Claudia Johnson argues, was valued differently than was male suffering at the end of the century. In his enormously popular *An Enquiry into the Duties of the Female Sex* (1791), Thomas Gisborne praises men for their courage in battle, and women for their fortitude "in bearing the vicissitudes of fortune, in exchanging wealth for penury," and especially for "supporting the languor and acuteness of disease" (20). He extols women's "firmness, composure and resignation, under tedious and painful trials" (20). In essence, Gisborne praises men for bravery, women for enduring ill health and financial stress. Jan Fergus compellingly argues that characters in Romantic-era literature—such as the whining Mary Musgrove and the stoical Anne Elliot in Jane Austen's *Persuasion*—teach us that women were rewarded for silence rather than for expression in the face of suffering: Austen "interrogate[s] the way the expression of suffering seems to be admirable or legitimate in men, excessive or comical or otherwise illegitimate in women" (Fergus 79). By identifying the causes and expressing the severity of her suffering, Smith radically challenges the premium placed on women's fortitude.

---

9   Zimmerman argues that Smith blurs the line between autobiography and fiction to keep her readers interested in her literary productions. Similarly, Labbe ("Selling") argues that Smith told her sad story in the prefaces in order to elicit readers' sympathy and thus sell her poetry.

In a move that, at first, would seem to please Gisborne and other proponents of women's stoical suffering, two of Smith's ninety-two *Elegiac Sonnets* directly invoke fortitude. In Sonnet 47, "To Fancy," Smith grieves the early scenes of her life "which shew'd the beauteous rather than the true!" (l. 4). Looking at the "sad grave of murder'd Happiness," Smith resigns herself to be "to my wayward destiny subdued: / Nor seek perfection with a poet's eye, / Nor suffer anguish with a poet's heart!" (ll. 8, 10, 12–14). Although she promises to subdue her feelings, she notes a cost; she will no longer feel "with a poet's heart" or see "with a poet's eye." Fortitude requires her to relinquish both painful feelings and artistic judgment. Fortitude is, then, unacceptable to Smith. In Sonnet 35, "To Fortitude," Smith expresses hope that

> Strengthn'd by thee [fortitude], this heart shall cease to melt
> O'er ills that poor Humanity must bear;
> Nor friends estranged, or ties dissolved be felt
> To leave regret, and fruitless anguish there. (ll. 9–12)

Fortitude promises to numb the pain both of her own suffering and also of sympathetic feelings for "poor Humanity's" suffering. In contrast to the resignation of feeling these lines call for, the final couplet sarcastically suggests that if fortitude subdues her awareness of loss, her sympathy for others, and the expression of pain, it might as well guide her to death: "And when at length it [this heart] heaves its latest sigh, / Thou and mild Hope shall teach me how to die!" (ll. 13–14). First acknowledging the value her culture places on women's fortitude, Smith subsequently decries the sacrifices this suppression of grief requires, abandoning all reference to fortitude in the other ninety sonnets.

In fact, although one would assume that sonnets entitled "elegiac" would depict feelings of profound loss that modulate into acceptance, Smith's expression of suffering remains insistently unmitigated in the sonnets. There is, for example, no moral lesson to be derived from, no peace to be made with the loss of her favorite child Anna Augusta.[10] Judith Hawley remarks that Smith "violates the genre of the elegy with her refusal to accept an aesthetic consolation" (188). Similarly, Kathryn Pratt notes that Smith's speaker "emerges from her poetic visions to find her suffering unalleviated" (563). In Sonnet 5, "To the South Downs," Smith quotes the phrase, "your turf, your flowers among," from Gray's "Ode on a Distant Prospect of Eton College" to emphasize the authentic and unrelenting quality of her melancholia:

> Ah! hills belov'd—*your turf, your flowers* remain;
> But can they peace to this sad breast restore;
> For one poor moment soothe the sense of pain,
> And teach a breaking heart to throb no more? (ll. 1–8, my emphasis)

Seeing childhood scenes again creates a contrast between childhood happiness and adult despair. In Gray's "Ode," the childhood scene brings a moment of relief from sadness: "I feel the gales, that from ye blow, / A momentary bliss bestow"

---

10 See Sonnets 65, 74, 78, 89, 90 and 91.

(Gray, ll. 15–16). Although the reference suggests that such childhood scenes might offer Smith the kind of healing they offer Gray, in Smith's sonnet the scenes do not relieve the poet's incurable despair. She states clearly in the final line: "There's no oblivion—but in death alone!" (l. 14). Smith refuses to offer readers evidence of consolation, refuses to contain her grief within the bounds of fortitude.

How then does Smith escape categorization as the inarticulate female mourner imagined by Burton? In contrast to Burton's notion that extreme emotion undermines women's command of language, Smith attributes her rational poetic talent to the suffering that deep feeling invokes. Jerome McGann's comment about the relationship between knowledge and sorrow in *The Poetics of Sensibility* underscores Smith's linkage of rationality with suffering: "The wisdom of Ecclesiastes, that Knowledge increaseth Sorrow, centres the imaginations of sensibility and sentiment, which made an important addition to that wisdom by reversing its terms" (7). Sorrow, in Smith's poetry, increases knowledge and poetic prowess. The first sonnet in the collection links poetic achievement with relentless emotional pain. "The partial muse" (l. 1) honors the poet's talent by "weav[ing] fantastic garlands for [her] head" (l. 4). However, the muse also "[r]eserves the thorn to fester in the heart" (l. 8). This image of pressing the thorn into the poet's heart alludes to the nightingale's song, that is, to the expression of women's suffering (13n). In the preface to the sixth edition of the *Elegiac Sonnets*, Smith reports that a friend has said of her poems, "Toujours Rossignols, toujours des chansons tristes" ("Always nightingales, always sad songs"). Smith replies, "It was unaffected sorrow drew [the sonnets] forth: I wrote mournfully because I was unhappy—And I have unfortunately no reason yet, though nine years have since elapsed, to *change my tone*" (5, original emphasis). Whether Smith imagined the nightingale as Procne, the sister who killed her son to revenge herself on her husband, or Philomela, the sister this husband raped, she voices melancholic feelings that result from circumstances particular to women— maternal grief and violence against women under patriarchal law.

And yet, Smith claims, this suffering enhances her poetic talent: "Ah! then, how dear the Muse's favors cost, / If those paint sorrow best—who feel it most!" (ll. 13–14). Smith emphasizes the poet's capacity for deep feeling and also claims for the poet the rational aesthetic judgment associated with painting. As I mention in the introduction, the artist Edward Dayes asserts in 1801 that drawing trains the mind to think clearly by educating the eye to see: "[T]he curious and ever-restless eye of the artist *comprehends* more, at one view, than the common observer will notice in an age" (257, my emphasis). "It is not too much to say," he insists, "that drawing opens the mind more than years devoted to the acquiring of languages, or the mere learning of words: it teaches [one] to think" (258). Dayes suggests that the training of the eye involved in drawing strengthens intellectual ability in the way that learning language does. In asserting that "those paint sorrow best—who feel it most," Smith invokes her culture's interest in visuality to locate rational aesthetic judgment and command of language in emotion.

Additionally, Smith adapts one of Alexander Pope's most famous lines as the final line of her sonnet in order to challenge his claim on women's emotion. In the last lines of *Eloisa to Abelard*, Pope has Eloisa attest to his poetic talent: "The well-sung woes will soothe my pensive ghost; / He best can paint 'em, who shall feel 'em most" (ll. 365–66). Pope's lines complacently silence Eloisa's pain by attributing her consolation to his own ability to sing her woes well, thus proclaiming in the heroic couplet his own triumphant union of rationally disciplined poetic art with sensibility and melancholy. In ventriloquizing Pope at the end of her own sonnet, Smith rejects the easy consolation of his lines. Rather than emphasize her ability to console others with her poetry, Smith notes "how dear the Muse's favors cost" the poet who feels acutely her own pain (l. 13).[11]

Ventriloquizing, Suicide, Insomnia

Ventriloquizing other poets, as she does Pope, is one of three major strategies Smith employs in the *Elegiac Sonnets* to emphasize the melancholic's combination of emotion and reason.[12] In addition to ventriloquizing, Smith evaluates romantic versus philosophical suicide, and refers to symptoms of melancholia such as insomnia. She depicts the melancholic as a person of great feeling and impressive intellect, a portrait of the sufferer that draws on the mid-century medical model of the condition, but incorporates from the Wertherian model of melancholia the quality of inconsolability. Furthermore, she presents the melancholic body not as a problem to be transcended as Pope does—abandoning Eloisa's body in his last lines and substituting his own disembodied suffering—but as evidence of authentic suffering.

Smith portrays her own ability to think rationally in the midst of great emotion by ventriloquizing well-respected male authors, projecting her own thoughts and feelings through the bodies of their texts, or through their characters. In a moment in which women poets were experiencing a reification of gender norms that precluded the expression of suffering, Smith moves easily between male and female voices, thus calling for the dismantling of gendered constraints on emotional expression and emphasizing the need for rational thought. Writers whose words Smith relies upon to express grief, despair, and the desire for death include (among others) Goethe, Pope, Milton, Shakespeare, Gray, and Rousseau. Curran notes that in thirty-six of her ninety-two sonnets, Smith speaks through the texts of other authors ("Charlotte Smith and British Romanticism" 72). In Sonnet 90, "To Oblivion," for example, Smith slightly alters the words of three male authors to express grief for her daughter and the desire for death. Smith is careful to place quotation marks around these lines:

> I only ask exemption from the pain
> Of knowing "*such things were*"—and are no more;
> Of dwelling on the hours for ever fled,

---

11 The layering of speakers in this sonnet—Smith speaks through Pope, who speaks through Eloisa—demonstrates nicely Labbe's argument that in "none of these poems is the 'I' plainly feminine" (*Charlotte Smith* 102).

12 Almost every scholar studying these sonnets comments on Smith's ventriloquizing, most notably Kathryn Pratt and Judith Hawley. My use of the term "ventriloquize," first suggested to me by Jeanne Moskal and also used by Stuart Curran, revises E. E. Bostetter's argument that Romantic poets Wordsworth, Coleridge, Keats, Shelley, and Byron saw themselves as the mouthpieces through which truth spoke (Bostetter 4), and instead posits ventriloquizing as a multi-layered performance.

And heartless, helpless, hopeless to deplore
"Pale misery living, joy and pleasure dead:"
While dragging thus unwish'd a length of days,
"Death seems prepared to strike, yet still delays." (ll. 8–14, my emphasis)

In her footnotes, Smith identifies the authors of the second two quotations—respectively, Sir Brook Boothby, author of the sonnet sequence *Sorrows Sacred to the Memory of Penelope* (1796), and Thomas Warton, author of "The Pleasures of Melancholy"—drawing attention to the fact that she quotes by providing the original lines for readers. Although the first quotation, "such things were," refers to the death of her daughter Anna Augusta, Smith relies on Shakespeare's words from *Macbeth* (Curran 77n) to translate the specific cause of grief into a more general expression of mood. The emotions conveyed in this sonnet are overwhelming—she describes herself as "heartless, helpless, hopeless"—yet by quoting other authors to convey those emotions, Smith highlights her intellect.

In other words, Smith's ventriloquizing demonstrates to her readers that in moments of intense suffering, the poet's rational mind is fully engaged. In fact, Smith's footnotes highlight her extensive literary knowledge. Some include the precise poetic reference and others just the author's name, an inconsistency that might reflect Smith's difficult circumstances—she was often away from her library during her frequent moves to alleviate financial and health problems and to hide from her estranged husband. However, this inconsistency also suggests that Smith spontaneously thought of references as she wrote, and thus highlights her impressive command of the English literary corpus. With her ventriloquizing technique, Smith expresses extreme despair, yet she processes her emotions through a reflective mind that is well acquainted with the great works of English literature. Furthermore, as Adela Pinch argues in her study of epistemologies of emotion, *Strange Fits of Passion*, when Smith quotes another poet, she "is in the odd position of sympathizing with her own feelings, of being feeling's object and subject" (63). In this sense, Smith becomes both sufferer and witness to suffering, or as I suggest below, both sufferer and seer. Simultaneously occupying the position of sufferer and witness to suffering, the speaker retains control of her subjectivity, rather than surrendering the interpretation and ownership of her emotional experience to, for example, a man of sensibility such as Yorick or Harley.

Smith validates the combination of melancholic feeling and reflection also by engaging with her culture's discussion of romantic versus philosophical suicide. This discussion occurred in the midst of rising numbers of suicides in the upper classes in England,[13] and essentially imagined the consequences of pursuing a life at either one of two extremes: a life guided wholly by one's emotions or a life guided

---

13 A remarkable number of aristocrats committed suicide in the second half of the eighteenth century, a trend that Minois attributes more to "gambling debts and debauchery" rather than to their claim of philosophical suicide (262). Drawing a great deal of public attention to suicide, twenty-one members of Parliament died at their own hands in the eighteenth century (Minois 263). In addition, in the increasingly homophobic late-eighteenth-century culture, other public figures such as the British foreign minister Lord Castlereagh killed themselves, preferring suicide to blackmail or public exposure (Crompton 301–6).

wholly by one's rational mind. David Hume and others wrote treatises justifying suicide as a rational choice, while the public simultaneously developed a cult-like fascination with suicide motivated by emotion, most emblematically the suicide of Goethe's heart-broken Werther. In 1783, the year before Smith published the *Elegiac Sonnets*, Hume's name appeared for the first time on his philosophical defense of suicide, *Essays on Suicide and the Immortality of the Soul*, precipitating a heated debate in literary magazines about the significance of one's rationale in determining the morality of one's suicide. Philosophical suicide was thought to be the result of a deep consideration of one's life, and, although punishable as a crime, was justifiable to some in its dispassion and in its connection to "the Enlightenment idea that the rational man has a sovereign liberty that permits him to leave life when it becomes burdensome" (Minois 264). As with philosophical suicide, the interest in romantic suicide, or the suicide of the lover, reached a high pitch just as Smith began the *Elegiac Sonnets*, a trend indicated in part by the multiple translations of *The Sorrows of Young Werther* published in England between 1779 and 1799. Based wholly in feeling, romantic suicide could be attributed to madness, and thus was not punishable by the state.[14] Sidestepping the legal issues in her portrayal of suicide, Smith tempers one justification of suicide with the other in order to emphasize both the intellectual and the emotional components of melancholic suffering.

In the Werther sonnets, Smith speaks in the male sufferer's voice to claim authentic emotion for women and to argue that the man of sensibility lacks the rational understanding that gives suffering value. In rewriting Goethe, Smith joined over a dozen women writers—including Jane Austen, Amelia Pickering, Mary Robinson, and Anna Seward—who, writing tributes to Werther between 1785 and 1805, explore the benefits and costs of cultivating sensibility (Conger 21). In her study of women writers' responses to Werther in this period, Sydney McMillen Conger associates Smith's sonnets with other 1780s women's literature that expresses noncritical admiration for Werther. While I agree with Conger that Smith celebrates Werther's depth of feeling, I find Smith's representation of sensibility to be much more revisionist than Conger allows. Far from simply indulging in a dangerous association with suicidal sensibility in these sonnets, Smith challenges what Schiesari describes as "the male appropriation of a 'feminine' position under the guise of 'sensitivity' or 'nostalgia' or 'loss'" (29). While Smith, as Conger suggests, takes pleasure in Werther's excessive sensibility, she merges her poetic voice with Werther's in order to reclaim emotion from the man of sensibility. In addition, and more crucially for this argument, Smith's representation of Werther's thought process tempers the celebration of sensibility to make a revisionist

---

14 In legal terms, a suicide connected with insanity, categorized as *non compos mentis*, carried with it no penalties, while a deliberate, premeditated suicide, categorized as *felos de se*, was punishable with religious restrictions on the burial of the body, a punishment in effect until 1823, and with the Crown's seizure of all property, which lasted until 1870 (Newman 686). However, in the late eighteenth century, the practice of punishing suicide was decreasing; generally suicides were declared the result of *non compos mentis*, a verdict often obtained through bribery (Minois 263).

argument for the critical role of reason, even melancholic reason, in achieving an understanding of suffering.[15]

The first in the series, Sonnet 21, "Supposed to be written by Werther," distinguishes between contemplative melancholia and love melancholia, associating the latter with madness. With the phrase "Like the poor maniac" (l. 5), Smith refers to an episode in *The Sorrows of Young Werther* in which the hero observes a lunatic. Smith's footnote provides us with the passage from Goethe: "'Is this the destiny of man? Is he only happy before he possesses his reason, or after he has lost it?'" Smith quotes Goethe to claim rational thinking as an essential part of the unhappy, yet intellectually productive and self-aware, state of melancholia. Smith's Werther, though, is enslaved by Passion, and is thus unwilling and unable to listen to reason: "I hurry forward, Passion's helpless slave! / And scorning Reason's mild and sober light, / Pursue the path that leads me to the grave!" (ll. 10–12). Reasonable reflection, the melancholic quality Smith holds so dear, has the power to keep Werther from suicide. In Sonnet 23, "By the same. To the North Star," Smith repeats this point. Full of despair and pining for Charlotte, Smith's Werther cries, "So o'er my soul short rays of reason fly, / Then fade:—and leave me to despair, and die!" (ll. 13–14). Reason stands between Werther's desire for death and his actual suicide. When sensibility takes away that reason, death ensues. Even, or perhaps especially, at the extreme end of melancholia, Smith insists on the value of rational thought.

Smith's ventriloquizing of another literary character, however—Shakespeare's Lady Constance from *King John*—suggests that her primary concern is not to recommend rational thought as an antidote to suicide, but rather to demonstrate that authentic melancholia is based in rational thought and in deep emotion. In Sonnet 6, "To Hope," Smith asks Hope to visit her: "O Hope! thou soother sweet of human woes! / How shall I lure thee to my haunts forlorn?" (ll. 1–2). But Hope flies by "and will not hear" (l. 8). After Hope has deserted her, Smith quotes Lady Constance to invoke inevitable death: "Come then, '*pale Misery's love!*' be thou my cure, / And I will bless thee, who, tho' slow, art sure" (ll. 13–14, my emphasis). In her grief for her son Arthur's imprisonment, Lady Constance courts death, imploring: "Misery's love, / O, come to me!" (3.4.35–36). Smith quotes this line to express her own maternal grief. She places Shakespeare's phrase in quotation marks and footnotes the reference to draw the reader's attention to her source. And, if the reader knows the play, he or she will remember that Lady Constance situates her suicidal thoughts in reason, not in madness. Shortly after uttering the quoted phrase, Lady Constance responds to Cardinal Pandulph's accusation that she suffers from madness, not sorrow:

> I am not mad, I would to heaven I were!
> For then 'tis like I should forget myself.
> O, if I could, what grief should I forget!
> ...

---

15 McGann's argument that "sensibility emphasizes the mind in the body" elucidates Smith's achievement in these sonnets (7). Indeed, Smith's poetics offer a third option to the contrast McGann draws between the Della Cruscan poets' emphasis on the ephemeral and material, and Wordworth's poetry of "sincerity" (McGann 75–79). Smith focuses on both the particular materiality of experience, while she cultivates a tone of sincerity that Wordsworth would emulate.

For, being not mad, but sensible of grief,
My reasonable part produces reason
How I may be deliver'd of these woes,
And teaches me to kill or hang myself.
...
I am not mad; too well, too well I feel
The different plague of each calamity.
(Shakespeare *King John* 3.4.48–50, 53–56, 59–60)

Whereas madness would obliterate Lady Constance's suffering, her sane awareness of grief increases its pain. In full command of her senses, she reasons that suicide will provide relief. Lady Constance's suicidal wish is poignant precisely because both her deeply felt grief and also her rational contemplation of that suffering recommend that she end her life. In invoking this example of maternal grief, Smith relies on both the content of the reference and also her ventriloquizing technique to emphasize that suffering involves both feeling and reason.

Smith grounds this abstract assertion that suffering calls upon emotion and thought in her bodily experience of insomnia, a commonly recognized symptom of melancholia from which she suffered. With her depiction of insomnia, Smith offers readers her wakeful body and mind as evidence of both emotional pain and rational cogitation.[16] In Sonnet 32, "To melancholy. Written on the banks of the Arun, October 1785," Smith's poet-speaker sits by the river on an autumn evening feeling alone and melancholy, her only company the "strange sounds" and "mournful melodies" (ll. 7–8). The speaker is awake because she struggles to soothe her "pensive visionary mind" (l. 14). She longs for companionship, imagining that she might meet the melancholic poet Thomas Otway beside the river "and hear his deep sighs swell the sadden'd wind" (l. 11). In this sonnet, Smith highlights the melancholic poet's intense desire for companionship as well as her impressive, though painful, mental activity. The speaker's wakeful body offers physical proof of a melancholic mind that will not turn itself off, that is, bodily evidence of rationality.

In Sonnet 74, "The winter night," Smith combines the three techniques I have identified—ventriloquizing, exploring suicide, and referring to insomnia—to make her suffering visible. The speaker cannot sleep because she is grieving for her daughter:

'Sleep, that knits up the ravell'd sleeve of care,'
Forsakes me, while the chill and sullen blast,
As my sad soul recalls its sorrows past,
Seems like a summons, bidding me prepare
For the last sleep of death ... (ll. 1–5)

---

16 Smith biographer Rufus Paul Turner reports that from 1797 on Smith frequently wrote poems during the nights she suffered insomnia, including "Evening" which appears in the posthumous volume *Beachy Head* (81). Coleridge includes in his 1796 sonnet anthology two of Smith's sonnets that describe insomnia: "I love thee mournful sober-suited night," and "In this tumultuous Sphere for thee unfit" (also titled "To night" and "To tranquillity" in the *Elegiac Sonnets* where they are numbered 39 and 41, respectively).

Quoting from Shakespeare's *Macbeth*, Smith simultaneously refers to her wakeful rumination and demonstrates her knowledge of English literature. She depicts herself as both sufferer and witness to suffering with this quotation. Furthermore, the passage merges the material body and the immateriality of the soul/mind. Smith embeds the line "the sad soul recalls its sorrow past" in a reference to a physical sensation: "while the chill and sullen blast ... seems like a summons." The physical response to the cold—"chill"—along with the emotional/intellectual recollection of sorrow together create the summons to death.

Just as Smith depicts the coalescence of body and mind, she blurs the distinction between a desire for sleep and a desire for death. Smith does not fear "the last sleep of death," but rather welcomes it, just as she would welcome ordinary sleep on this cold night:

> But wherefore fear existence such as mine,
> To change for long and undisturb'd repose?
> Ah! when this suffering being I resign,
> And o'er my miseries the tomb shall close,
> By her, whose loss in anguish I deplore,
> I shall be laid, and feel that loss no more! (ll. 9–14)

The "sleep of death" would grant Smith "undisturb'd repose," or relief from the mental disturbance of melancholic pain. Death would reunite her with her daughter in the grave, allowing her to "feel that loss no more." This connection between sleep and death builds tension between, on the one hand, the rational mind that cannot stop thinking in order to escape into sleep, and, on the other hand, deeply felt, nearly suicidal emotions. Foregrounding her suffering, wakeful body with references to insomnia, Smith further emphasizes her physicality by wishing to place her body beside Anna Augusta's in the grave. The speaker resigns her "suffering being" and imagines that "o'er my miseries the tomb shall close." In these lines, the body becomes the speaker's misery and is interred. Thus even as Smith insists on her rational ability in the midst of great pain, she emphasizes also the materiality of her suffering body.

The Sufferer as Seer

Given the efforts of medical writers such as Buchan and Trotter to depict the male melancholic genius as a wholly rational, nearly bodiless figure, Smith's emphasis on the body in her references to insomnia and in her focus on vision has risks. In contrast, the payoff of separating melancholic genius from an association with the body is enormous. Transcending the body means escaping the threat of being marked, or of being defined negatively by one's "natural" physical characteristics. Instead, Smith insists first on honoring her own individual vision, and second on foregrounding, rather than transcending, her seeing and suffering body in her poetry. While the male melancholic could abandon his body in order to claim the power associated with transcendent melancholic vision, a woman melancholic such as Smith, always caught in the essentialist woman-*as*-body formulation, could not choose to transcend the body, but might use the embodiment of her suffering to her advantage.

Smith's focus on the melancholic's eyes in the *Elegiac Sonnets* collapses the cult of sensibility's gap between sympathetic seer and sufferer, between the viewing subject and the object of his gaze. Eyes in the sonnets somaticize the combination of emotion and reason so crucial to claiming literary authority for women writers. Building on the cult of sensibility's tradition of displaying physical signs of great feeling, especially tears and blushes, Smith expresses the poet's depth of emotion with weeping eyes. Some of her epithets for the poet's eyes include: the "imploring eye of woe" (Sonnet 9, l. 8), the "streaming eye" (Sonnet 11, l. 14), "swimming eyes" (Sonnet 23, l. 1), "weary eyes" (Sonnet 54, l. 13), "ever-streaming eyes" (Sonnet 68, l. 2), "tired, and tear-swoln eyes" (Sonnet 79, l. 5), "eyes suffused with tears" (Sonnet 68, l. 14), "eyes, that only wake to weep" (Sonnet 66, l. 14), and "eyes that turn reluctant from the day" (Sonnet 90, l. 2). Todd observes that the literature of sensibility offers "a kind of pedagogy of seeing and of the physical reaction that this seeing should produce, clarifying when uncontrolled sobs or a single tear should be the rule" (*Sensibility* 4). The literature of sensibility trains one both how to see particular kinds of suffering and how to be seen sympathizing with this suffering. However, while the man of sensibility wishes both to see sympathetically and to be seen sympathizing, the (often female) sufferer is seen but does not see. In her revision of this tradition, Smith offers teary eyes as proof of the great suffering that leads to poetic vision and presents the way those suffering eyes see as evidence of the female poet's rational thought.

Giving the sufferer the power to look, Smith describes loss as a change in the visual field—a movement from light to darkness, from color to blankness—that she and her speakers feel and consider intellectually. As I explain in the introductory chapter, a new understanding of ocular physiology's influence on visual perception offered a physical metaphor for subjectivity in the late eighteenth century. The dependence of vision upon individual physiology supports a Berkeleyian understanding of perception, captured in William Blake's eloquent description of subjective vision: "Every body does not see alike ... As a man is, So he Sees. As the eye is formed, such are its Powers" (702). By giving her sufferers the power to look, Smith balances her solicitation of sympathy with her insistence on an actively perceiving, if suffering, subjectivity. Smith depicts lost happiness as a fading vision in the "poet's eye" (Sonnet 32, l. 6; Sonnet 47, l. 13). In the final sonnet in the collection, Smith depicts her memory of past happiness as a fading painting:

> ... so frail, so fair,
> Are the fond visions of thy early day,
> Till tyrant Passion, and corrosive care,
> Bid all thy fairy colours fade away! (Sonnet 92, ll. 9–12).

What fades in these delicately fair and fond visions are the "fairy colours." In Sonnet 63, "The gossamer," she compares the hope she felt early in life to a fragile and "glittering" web blown down by the wind: "—So, evanescent, fade / Bright views that Youth with sanguine heart believes" (ll. 10–11). Smith laments the "visions bright and warm" of her childhood home, which are "obscured for ever" (ll. 7, 9): "My fate / Nor hope nor joy illumines—Nor for me / Return those rosy hours which here I used to *see*!" (ll. 13–14, my emphasis). Portraying happiness as a colorful—

fairy-coloured, "bright," "glittering," "rosy"—vision, Smith affirms the subjective nature of visual perception. Smith's references to color and loss of color occur in the midst of surging interest in color blindness in England, reflected in a series of case studies published in scientific, philosophical, and popular venues between 1777 and 1794, culminating in Thomas Young's theory of color vision, an argument fully articulated in his 1801 *On the Mechanism of the Eye*. These case studies, described in my introductory chapter, depended on the color blind person's subjective description of abnormal vision, thus demonstrating the individual, physiological nature of visual perception.

Using color as a metaphor for the subjective perception of happiness, Smith invokes lack of color to describe despair. When the colorful vision of happiness disappears, what remains is "blank" (connoting, among other things, whiteness, as in the French "blanc"). In Sonnet 53, "The Laplander," Smith contrasts the laplander's waiting for the light during the long winter with the waiting of "the sufferer" who "O'er the *blank void* [the waste of joyless life] he looks with hopeless pain; / For him those beams of heaven shall never shine again" (ll. 13–14, my emphasis). Without light, there is no color; without joy, the world is a "blank void." Similarly, in Sonnet 58, "The glow-worm," Smith observes that like the death of the glow-worm, "So turn the world's bright joys to cold and blank disgust" (ll. 4). Once again, Smith places light ("bright joys") and lack of color ("blank disgust") in opposition. Yet the word "blank" also connotes an absence of meaning or interest. Comparing herself to "the unhappy exile" in Sonnet 43, Smith suggests that he "perhaps may know / Such heartless pain, such *blank despair* as mine" (ll. 7–8, my emphasis). The exile, confined alone on an island, is tortured by the illusion of hope, which arrives visually: "And, if a flattering cloud appears to show / The fancied semblance of a distant sail, / Then melts away—anew his spirits fail" (ll. 9–11). If hope presents itself as a visual image, despair is the absence of that image. Smith expresses this connection between despair and the inability to see hope in her lament that she will never again see Anna Augusta's form: the sun "Shines not for me—for never more the form / I loved—so fondly loved, shall bless my sight" (Sonnet 89, ll. 11–12). Similarly, in *The Prelude*, Wordsworth uses the word "blank" to describe both darkness and desertion: "in my thoughts there was a *darkness*, / Call it solitude or *blank desertion*" (I:394–95, 1850, my emphasis). Such usage figures despair as both absence of color and absence of companionship. Longing for Anna's company, Smith wishes neither to touch her daughter nor to hear her voice, but rather *to see her form*.

Although the sufferer's vision is profoundly influenced by emotion, Smith also depicts the sufferer's ability to look as evidence of rationality. With her sometimes condescending comparisons between the poet figure and working class and insane characters, Smith attributes differences in vision to differences in intellect. In Sonnet 9 she compares the shepherd's gaze with her own: "Blest is yon shepherd, on the turf reclined, / Who on the varied clouds which float above / Lies idly gazing" with a "vacant mind" (ll. 1–3). Unlike her

> *he* has never felt the pangs that move
> Th' indignant spirit, when with selfish pride,
> Friends, on whose faith the trusting heart rely'd,
> Unkindly shun th' imploring eye of woe! (ll. 5–8, original emphasis)

He can gaze "idly," rather than with the "imploring eye of woe," because his mind remains "vacant" and his trusting heart has not been betrayed. In other words, he does not possess the poet's acute reason and has not suffered the same kind of loss as she has. The woodman, similarly described in Sonnet 54, is oppressed with toil, but naps or shuts his eyes. The poet envies his sleep as an escape from care: "Would I could taste, like this unthinking hind, / A sweet forgetfulness of human care, / Till the last sleep these weary eyes shall close" (ll. 11–13). With eyes shut, the woodman is "unthinking"; his lack of vision signifies his lack of rational function during sleep. The weeping eyes that populate Smith's sonnets demonstrate the poet's desire for sympathy; the change in visual field demonstrates her subjectivity and depth of feeling. Additionally, the comparison between "unthinking" eyes and "thinking" eyes demonstrates her rational poetic perception. Reason deepens feeling, and thus deepens suffering. In Smith's portrayal of suffering, the cult of sensibility's object of sympathy and sympathizing onlooker are contained in one body; indeed, the capacity to emote and the ability to analyze emerge from the same bodily organ.

Smith further collapses the gap between sufferer and seer—between the body of the sufferer and the eyes that see him—with her portrayal of a series of melancholic wanderers in the *Elegiac Sonnets*. These wanderers—including a maniac, a shipwrecked mariner, a pilgrim, a Laplander waiting for the sun, an exile, and the poet herself—challenge readers to see the melancholic body not just as an abject object of pity, but as a creative being who looks and therefore has agency. In the illustration that accompanies Sonnet 70, "On being cautioned against walking on an headland overlooking the sea, because it was frequented by a maniac," Smith works to complicate the distinction between sufferer and seer (Figure 1). At first glance, the maniac, the "solitary wretch" in the foreground of the plate, seems the clearest sufferer, while the speaker trails behind observing him on the cliff. Yet both the illustration and the text emphasize not just the speaker's, but also the sufferer's, ability to see. In the plate, the maniac's heavy eyebrows darken and exaggerate his eyes. The sonnet explains that he visually assesses—"with wild and hollow eyes"—the cliff as a potential location for a suicidal jump (l. 3). The speaker looks sympathetically at the maniac, seeing both her own pain and his. She compares her suffering to the maniac's, noting that unlike him, she retains a painful awareness of the "depth" and "duration" of her "woe" (l. 14). Smith chooses to place the following lines beneath the engraving: "In moody sadness, on the giddy brink, / I see [or 'view' in the caption] him more with envy than with fear;" (ll. 9–10). Labbe observes that the speaker in this illustration looks more like Smith than does any other woman depicted in the plates accompanying the *Elegiac Sonnets* (*Charlotte Smith* 15). Smith, then, depicts herself observing another sufferer even as she offers the image of her own suffering body to readers' view.

Similarly combining seer with sufferer, another of Smith's speakers compares herself to a shipwrecked mariner. She looks out over the ocean from high on the rocks, a powerful vantage point from which Smith's despairing speakers frequently gaze:

Already shipwreck'd by the storms of Fate,
Like the poor Mariner, methinks, I stand,
Cast on a rock; who *sees* the distant land
From whence no succour comes—or comes too late.

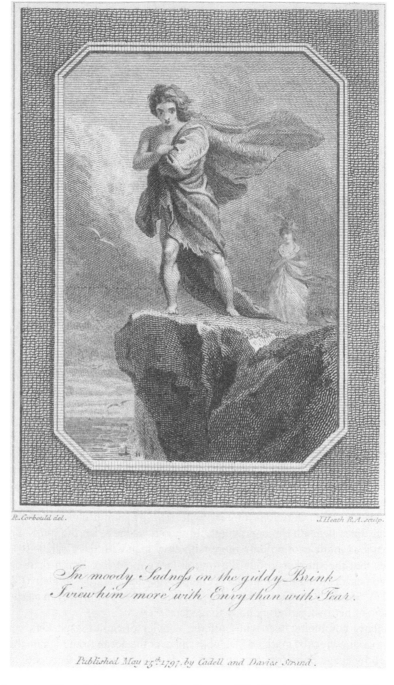

R.Corbould del.   J.Heath R.A.sculp.

*In moody Sadness on the giddy Brink
I view him more with Envy than with Fear.*

Published May 15th 1797, by Cadell and Davies Strand.

Fig. 1.   The plate accompanying Sonnet 70. *Elegiac Sonnets*, **1800, vol. 2**

Faint and more faint are heard his feeble cries,
'Till in the rising tide the exhausted sufferer dies.
(Sonnet 12, ll. 9–14, my emphasis)

The speaker not only imagines seeing the mariner despairing on the rock, but also imagines him looking at "the distant land / From whence no succour comes" (ll. 11–12). His despairing body, like the speaker's, is also an actively perceiving body. In Sonnet 52, the poet compares herself to a pilgrim wandering the cliffs over the sea:

Faltering and sad the unhappy Pilgrim

....

Journeys alone, along the giddy height
Of these steep cliffs; and as the sun's last ray
Fades in the west, *sees*, from the rocky verge,
Dark tempest scowling ...
(Sonnet 52, ll. 1, 4–7, my emphasis)

Smith emphasizes the pilgrim's ability to see or understand rationally his own suffering, externalized here as the ominous "dark tempest scowling." Just as the pilgrim teeters dangerously above the waves, seeing only a storm in the fading light, the poet wanders a rough path, seeing no comfort in the darkness left by the fading of "Friendship's cheering radiance":

... So, with heart oppress'd,
Alone, reluctant, desolate, and slow,
By Friendship's cheering radiance now unblest,
Along Life's rudest path I seem to go;
Nor *see* where yet the anxious heart may rest
(ll. 9–13, my emphasis)

Smith foregrounds the suffering body, thus increasing the reader's understanding of isolation that perhaps both causes and accompanies melancholia. Consistently placing these wandering bodies on steep cliffs above the ocean, Smith paints a picture of the precariousness inherent in a life of despair—it teeters always near disaster, especially when "unblest" by "Friendship's cheering radiance."

Smith's repeated presentation of the sufferer as both wanderer and seer expresses the desire to retain one's subjectivity while finding a home in someone else's sympathetic gaze. In contrast to the portrait of the male melancholic literary genius composing alone in his study, Smith's vision of female melancholic genius depends on a sympathetic interaction with another person. Indeed, second to "tear suffused eyes," the eyes that populate the *Elegiac Sonnets* in greatest number are lover's eyes. The speaker in her sonnets "From Petrarch" longs to see and be seen by Laura's eyes (Sonnet 15, ll. 6–7, 13–14). In a sonnet written to a friend on her anniversary, Smith expresses her wish that her friend's married love continue: "And still, with ray serene, shall those blue eyes / Enchant the husband, and attach the friend" (Sonnet 20, ll. 7–8). Eyes can thus anchor a sympathetic attachment between individuals. In the last of Smith's five sonnets written in the voice of Werther, the speaker expresses the wish that only Charlotte's teary eyes, not "common eyes," behold his grave (Sonnet 24, l. 4). Similarly, the speaker in Sonnet 38, longing for Emmeline, wishes in his dreams "to see; / Tears of fond pity fill thy soften'd eyes" (ll. 6–7). The desire to be seen is a plea for sympathetic human connection in the midst of suffering. Smith figures despair as a lack of, and hope as the possibility of, a sympathetic connection.

Although she populates her sonnets with suffering and seeing bodies, the poet also at times voices a strong desire to hide her body. If foregrounding the body expresses the hope for sympathy, hiding the body expresses the pain of being fixed in an unsympathetic gaze. The character Walsingham (in one of the *Elegiac Sonnets* republished from Smith's novel *Montalbert*) declares his intention to hide in the forest "from a World I wish to shun;" (Sonnet 67, l. 10). Likewise, Smith's Werther cries out, "O Solitude! To thy sequester'd vale / I come to hide my sorrows and my tears" (Sonnet 17, ll. 1–2). In some cases, this need to retreat from the world, to hide the suffering body, is crucial for preserving creative energy. In Sonnet 7, the speaker speculates that the absent nightingale, or the "The sweet poet of the woods!" (l. 1), hides silently among the trees: "And shepherd girls from eyes profane shall hide / The gentle bird, who sings of pity best" (ll. 11–12). Protected by young women from "eyes profane," the bird who sings of women's suffering takes refuge in the woods, resting and preparing to sing again. This retreat from the unsympathetic gaze makes possible her continued expression. The speaker in "To the goddess of botany" seeks to elude "the view / of Violence and Fraud" and with the goddess of botany "Find shelter; where my tired, tear-swoln eyes ... might rest" (ll. 1–2, 5, 8). Like the nightingale hiding from "eyes profane," the speaker finds her creative energy sapped by "the view / of Violence and Fraud." This desire to hide from the hostile gaze—a topic I take up at length in chapters 2 and 5—highlights the risks of exposing one's bodily suffering in the search for sympathy, and reveals the creative benefit of being held in a sympathetic gaze.

Offering an example of the kind of sympathy, or exchange of looks, for which she longs, Smith names the moon the "Pale eye of evening" (Sonnet 62, l. 11). This eye in the night sky sympathizes with the poet, seems to look back at her and understand her pain. In a sonnet that expresses hope for comfort, the poet, wandering alone gazing at the moon, identifies herself as a "Poor wearied pilgrim—in this toiling scene" (Sonnet 4, l. 14):

> Alone and pensive, I delight to stray,
> And *watch* thy [the moon's] shadow trembling in the stream,
> Or *mark* the floating clouds that cross thy way.
> And while I *gaze*, thy mild and placid light
> Sheds a soft calm upon my troubled breast
> (ll. 2–6, my emphasis)

The poet emphasizes her own vision—she watches, marks, and gazes at a world that is emotionally responsive (the moon's shadow trembles), and shapes her emotions (the mild and placid moon sheds calm). Sympathy in this formulation is multi-directional, reflected back and forth among several bodies. The moon reflects the sun's light, transferring the glow of daytime to the nighttime side of the world. The water of the stream on which the poet gazes reflects this light again, with a sympathetic trembling that embodies the speaker's mood. Finally, the moon reflects back the poet's gaze in the ultimate statement of sympathy; the poet "gazes" and the moon's "mild and placid light / Sheds a soft calm upon my troubled breast" (ll. 5–6). Thus, the moon's traditional depiction as representative of the feminine and the intuitive coalesces with Smith's focus on its ability to reflect the light of reason.[17] Smith proposes this combination—emotion, reason, mutual sympathy—as essential components for women's creative genius, and especially for women's literary expression of suffering. Lamenting the pain of isolation inherent in despair, Smith calls again and again for company, for a sympathetic viewer, for a social context. She seeks not Romantic solitude, but sociability. She seeks, that is, to move beyond the Keatsian "sole self" not to transcendence, but to a sympathetic world (1.72).

Smith draws on her culture's interest in visuality both to demonstrate the authenticity of her individual suffering and also to overcome gendered restrictions on expressing melancholia. In the *Elegiac Sonnets*, Smith invokes vision's associations with subjectivity, sensibility, and rational thought in order to negotiate the challenges of claiming melancholia as a woman in her cultural moment. Repeatedly depicting both the "streaming eye" of sensibility and the more rational "poet's eye," Smith insists on the interplay of sensibility and rationality in the female melancholic poet. Even as she argues for a new model of expressing melancholic suffering, Smith calls attention to the irony of making one's suffering visible by presenting readers with melancholic speakers whose bodies alternatively appear and disappear. Women poets who display characteristics of melancholia to make their suffering visible might be erased as overly emotional (and thus not comprehensible) or as overly rational (and thus unnaturally masculine). Smith leverages potentially detrimental connections between women's bodies and nervous illness to her advantage by placing descriptions of the physical symptoms of melancholia, such as insomnia, alongside the blushes and sighs of sensibility. By presenting the body as a vehicle of authentic melancholic symptoms, rather than as the cause of nervous illness, Smith seeks to make her rational ability, her deep feeling, her poetic talent, and her suffering visible.

But, as is well known, some of her reviewers could not see past Smith's female body to her mind. In spite of her careful attempts to maneuver around the negative association between sensibility and hysteria, several of Smith's reviewers categorize her poetic voice as a mourning or hysteric voice. *The Critical Review* praises the second volume of the *Elegiac Sonnets* for being more cheerful than Smith's previous poetry, but in doing so, the reviewer characterizes the preceding editions as "whining production[s]":

> Poor Charlotte! still weeping and wailing, and gnashing thy poetical teeth! Will thy most melancholy Muse never part with her fables? Believe us old critics, whose 'heyday in the blood is tame,'—even for us thou hast wailed too much. Are there always to be clouds upon thy horizon? Not a beam of sunshine to break through the dismal gloom? ... In sooth, we have had so much lamentation, that we are tempted to cry out ... 'Oh! 'tis so moving, we can read no more.' (149)

This critic registers his impatience with Smith's relentlessness of complaint, her refusal to be consoled. Both the positive and dismissive comments focus on the

---

17 Lokke argues that the vantage point of the moon represents a position of detachment that is empowering to Smith.

reviewers' feelings about Smith's troubles, and thus reveal the limits of sensibility as "an ethic of care" (Gilligan 62–63).[18] By characterizing Smith's melancholic poetry as a hysterical, nonverbal "lamentation," and offering readers an image of Smith "weeping and wailing, and gnashing [her] poetical teeth," the reviewer undercuts Smith's command of language, denying her access to the symbolic realm. The reviewer's description of Smith's melancholia alludes to the biblical sufferings of the damned, a portrait of the writer that contrasts sharply with the image of the melancholic artist as a divinely gifted translator between the gods and humans. Although Smith repeatedly emphasizes the rational and emotional components of her suffering, some reviewers read her expression of melancholia as a symptom of hysteria rather than of productive genius. It is not surprising, then, that although Wordsworth and Smith both present readers with a balance of emotion and reason, it is Wordsworth's emotion recollected in tranquility rather than Smith's unyielding expression of suffering that prevailed in the literature.

Nonetheless, Smith's efforts in her poetry to balance emotion and intellect—to temper the excess of sensibility inherent in Wertherism and the obsessive rationality celebrated in 1790s medical texts—led her to paint a new portrait of melancholic genius for the culture. If, as Schiesari claims, "the historical boundaries of a great age of melancholia ... are coterminous with the historic rise and demise of 'the subject' as the organizing principle of knowledge and power" (2), then what is at stake in Smith's representation of melancholia is the claim for subjecthood. Labbe convincingly argues that Smith uses poetry to "map aspects of the self," specifically "aspects of the social self ... that society uses to define and contain women" (*Charlotte Smith* 8). I would add that in addition to outlining the social restrictions on women's expression, Smith also imagines a sympathetic world in which women's genius can flourish. By focusing on the body and particularly on vision, by making her melancholic wanderers both the lookers and the looked-at, Smith cultivates sympathy for women's suffering without denying women agency.

Most crucially, Smith's formulation of the embodied melancholic seer/sufferer differs sharply from the tradition of male melancholic transcendence of the body.[19] Donna Haraway describes the politics of transcendent vision, of separating the ability to see from the possibility of being seen as "the gaze that mythically inscribes all the marked bodies, that makes the unmarked category claim the power to see and not be seen, to represent while escaping representation" (188). Smith's insistence on what Haraway terms "the embodied nature of all vision"—a theory of visuality that challenges traditional western claims for the pure objectivity and transcendent

---

18 Anne K. Mellor similarly invokes Gilligan in order to argue in "A Novel of Their Own" that women novelists of the Romantic era "insist on the primacy of the family or the community and their attendant practical responsibilities over the individual" (330).

19 In contrast to Wordsworth's escapist version of transcendence, Kari E. Lokke argues, Smith presents transcendence as providing "potentially emancipatory distance and detachment" from the "male-dominated economic and political struggles of her time" (86). It becomes for Smith "a vehicle through which to represent with utmost clarity, detachment, and compassion the precise contours of the contemporary political landscape" (Lokke 87). Lokke calls for a redefinition of the way we define "transcendence"; I would argue that thinking about vision as always embodied accomplishes the same end.

vision of the disembodied viewer—answers a particular challenge faced by women (188). In her analysis of Simone de Beauvior's writing, Genevieve Lloyd explains this challenge, arguing that "'transcendence,' in its origins, is a transcendence of the feminine" (101):

> Male transcendence ... is different from ... female transcendence ... . It is breaking away from a zone which for the male, remains intact—from what is for him the realm of particularity and merely natural feelings. For the female, in contrast, there is no such realm which she can both leave and leave intact. (101)

Rosemary Tong elaborates Lloyd's position: "To accept the ideal of transcendence as liberating places the feminist in a paradox rooted in the existentialist opposition between the looker and the looked-at, between self and other" (Tong 190). If the woman transcends the body into seer, then she obliterates herself as the one seen. If one considers this irony within the dynamics of sensibility, transcending the body means trading the potential for receiving another's sympathy—dependent on the visibility of suffering—for power. To reverse this formulation, a woman might accept the role of object of sympathy, but at the risk of losing the power to look, tantamount to losing her subjectivity.

Smith wants both to gain sympathy for her suffering and also to preserve her rational, actively perceptive subjectivity. Seeing the dangers of embracing either the profile of the melancholic emerging from the cult of sensibility, or the 1780s and 90s characterization of the rational melancholic genius, Smith insists instead on a melancholia rooted in the deep feeling and reflection derived from lived experience. As I argue in the chapters that follow, Mary Wollstonecraft and Mary Shelley, like Smith, suggest that creative genius emerges from sympathy rather than from solitude. This focus on the social context of creativity and the social causes of suffering ultimately challenges the longstanding model of the solitary Romantic genius, opening up new ways of thinking about the relationships among health, vision, and justice in the Romantic era.

Chapter 2

Contagion, Sympathy, Invisibility: Mary Shelley's *Frankenstein*

"The monstrous is ... never based on more than a shift in perception."
Roland Barthes

"[I]n quarters where we can never be rightly known, we take
pleasure, I think, in being consummately ignored."
Charlotte Brontë

Mary Shelley famously describes the inspiration for her novel *Frankenstein* as a vision. After days of being unable to "think of a story" to contribute to the writing contest proposed by Lord Byron for the group assembled at the Villa Diodati in the summer of 1816, Mary Shelley retired to her room alone (*WMS* 1:178). As she lay in bed after midnight, her imagination directed her to see the scene that was to become the genesis of her novel:

> My imagination, unbidden, possessed and guided me, gifting the successive images that arose in my mind with a vividness far beyond the usual bounds of reverie. *I saw*—with shut eyes, but acute mental vision,—*I saw* the pale student of unhallowed arts kneeling beside the thing he had put together. *I saw* the hideous phantasm of a man stretched out ... (*WMS* 1:179, my emphasis)

In this moment of intense creation—a profoundly visual experience—Mary Shelley herself remains alone and ungazed upon, seeing but not seen. In the introduction to *Frankenstein*, a novel replete with references to eyes and to looking, Mary Shelley suggests that invisibility has its benefits. Thirty-five years later, Charlotte Brontë's stubbornly unreadable character Lucy Snowe would explain, "[I]n quarters where we can never be rightly known, we take pleasure ... in being consummately ignored" (109). Like Lucy, Mary Shelley posits physical invisibility—a retreat from the public eye—as preferable to cultural invisibility—the culture's inability to see an individual's suffering and subjectivity.

Mary Shelley's celebration of the visionary's invisibility would seem to contrast with Charlotte Smith's wish to be held in a sympathetic gaze, yet the two writers both wish to escape judgmental eyes in order to write. While Smith voices the occasional desire to hide her body from the hostile glare of "Violence and Fraud," she primarily devotes herself to imagining a sympathetic world in which women's suffering and talent can be seen. Mary Shelley expresses less faith than does Smith in the human ability to look beyond gender or ethnicity in order to sympathize, and thus focuses on the advantages of hiding the body, on invisibility. Although the creature, for example, expresses his deep desire "to see [the De Lacey family's] sweet looks turned toward [him] with affection" and expresses his need for "kindness and sympathy," his physical appearance prevents him from receiving this level of acceptance; he is happiest when he is not seen (*WMS* 1:99). As one reviewer's characterization of Charlotte Smith's melancholic sonnets as "whining" demonstrates, creative expression is limited when one's audience perceives one as an "other"—woman, daughter, monster. To explore the reasons that the "sweet looks" or sympathetic gazes are less likely to turn toward those whose bodies mark them as the subjugated "other," Mary Shelley invokes the history of the contagious eye disease ophthalmia in her novel.

This gruesome and ultimately blinding illness, brought home by soldiers fighting in the alliance against Napoleon in Egypt, continued to rage in England and France while Mary Shelley wrote *Frankenstein*. The "Egyptian ophthalmia," as it became known, provided an embodied example of the fear that contact with alterity would destroy one's identity. This fear of contagion limits the viewer's ability to see both suffering and individual subjectivity in "the other." In *Frankenstein*, Mary Shelley suggests that those marked by physical difference can overcome the cult of sensibility's dependence on the visual apprehension of suffering by removing themselves from this economy, by moving from sight to hearing, from visibility to invisibility. When the visual evidence of difference is put aside, sympathy is possible. However, just as sensibility was a fraught emotional mode for Smith in the 1780s and 90s, sympathy was a thorny category for Mary Shelley twenty years later. At once nurturing and threatening to creativity, associated with both healing and contagion, sympathy, Mary Shelley suggests, is nonetheless crucial for narrative expression.

In her exploration of narrative and sympathetic vision, Mary Shelley emphasizes the physicality of her characters' eyeballs. Most prominent, of course, are the eyes that elicit the least sympathy—the creature's yellow, watery eyes, which I discuss at length below. However, Mary Shelley draws the reader's attention to other characters' eyes as well, especially Victor's. As he recounts his creation of the monster to Robert Walton, Victor notes, "my eyes swim with the remembrance" (*WMS* 1:37). He recalls that his "eyeballs were starting from their sockets" as he assembled the creature's body parts (*WMS* 1:38). Describing Victor to his sister, Walton focuses on Victor's eyes as well: "I never saw a more interesting creature: his eyes have generally an expression of wildness, and even madness" (*WMS* 1:17). Similarly, when Henry Clerval arrives in Ingolstadt, he assesses Victor's well-being by looking at his eyes. Victor reports that Henry "saw a wildness in my eyes for which he could not account" (*WMS* 1:43). Informed by the tenets of physiognomy, Walton and Henry sympathetically assess Victor's state of mind by looking.[1] So often scrutinized by his concerned friends, Victor is haunted by a nightmarish vision of gazing eyes after he is acquitted of Henry's death:

---

1   In her introduction to *Frankenstein*, Betty T. Bennett notes: "The repeated emphasis on the interpretation of facial expression probably derives from [Mary Shelley's] awareness of the systems of the Swiss physiognomist J. C. Lavater and of the phrenologist F. J. Gall" (*WMS* 1:xciv).

I saw around me nothing but a dense and frightful darkness, penetrated by no light but the glimmer of two eyes that glared upon me. Sometimes they were the expressive eyes of Henry, languishing in death, the dark orbs nearly covered by the lids, and the long black lashes that fringed them; sometimes it was the watery clouded eyes of the monster, as I first saw them in my chamber at Ingolstadt. (*WMS* 1:140)

Alternatively emanating from the creature's diseased eyes and Henry's "expressive eyes," this penetrating glare flips between the moment the creature looks at Victor (the inception of the disastrous chain of events) and one of the most distressing of these events (the death of Henry). Victor imagines these eyes in terms of their physical detail—Henry's "dark orbs" and "long black lashes," and the creature's "watery clouded eyes." He sees Henry's eyes "languishing in death" and the creature's eyes opening for the first time. Formally acquitted of Henry's murder, Victor nonetheless seems to understand his role in both Henry's and the creature's suffering by envisioning their eyes as they looked at these crucial moments.

Victor's horrified response to the moment of animation, the most dramatic moment of othering in the novel, is largely cast in terms of the creature's unusual eyes. Although Victor describes the creature he has painstakingly assembled as if he were seeing him for the first time, there are in fact only two aspects of the creature Victor would not have observed in his laboratory—the creature's body moving and his eyes looking. When the creature opens his eyes and looks back, Victor immediately shifts from seeing him as a creature to seeing him as a monster. As Roland Barthes asserts "The monstrous is ... never based on more than a shift in perception" (15). Victor's awareness of the creature's status as an independent being causes this shift:

I saw the dull yellow eye of the creature open; it breathed hard, and a convulsive motion agitated its limbs. How can I describe my emotions at this catastrophe, or how delineate the wretch whom with such infinite pains and care I had endeavoured to form? His limbs were in proportion, and I had selected his features as beautiful. Beautiful!—Great God! His yellow skin scarcely covered the work of muscles and arteries beneath; his hair was of a lustrous black, and flowing; his teeth of a pearly whiteness; but these luxuriances only formed a more horrid contrast with *his watery eyes that seemed almost of the same colour as the dun white sockets in which they were set*, his shriveled complexion and straight black lips. (*WMS* 1:39–40, my emphasis)

The creature's sentience is apparent to Victor when his "dull yellow eye" opens; Mary Shelley thus signifies the creature's subjectivity through his ability to see. In the moment that he views the creature as a whole being rather than as assembled pieces, Victor apprehends the creature's otherness.

In the frontispiece to the 1831 edition of the novel depicting this moment, both the creature's eyes and Victor's eyes glow (Figure 2). With this illustration, Mary Shelley highlights the importance of both Victor's and the creature's perception. As he sees the creature's eyes, Victor realizes that the creature can see him, an understanding that becomes horrifying when he later wakes from a nightmare under the creature's gaze: "I beheld the wretch ... . He held up the curtain of the bed; and his eyes, if eyes they may be called, were fixed on me" (*WMS* 1:40). In this later scene, he and the creature have switched places; Victor lies down while the creature looks over him expectantly. In both scenes, Victor fixates on the creature's eyes, horrifying in their watery yellowness. The creature's eyes, more than any other feature, mark him not just as other, but as a threatening other in Victor's mind.

The creature's black flowing hair, yellow skin, and large frame have inspired critics to identify him as a racially other, and potentially revengeful, child of a negligent empire: a Mongolian (Mellor "*Frankenstein*"), a West Indian slave (Ball, Malchow), a Bengali (Lew), or an Anglo-Indian (Neff). Elizabeth Bohls acknowledges the multi-referentiality of the creature's physical difference. The creature, she suggests, is "an amalgam of everything that [the British] were not. His looming shadow on the periphery of civilized life interweaves concrete categories of cultural exclusion" ("Standards" 34). These readings convincingly assert that Mary Shelley interrogates the consequences of imperial desire for both the colonizer and the colonized, and they cite the creature's ethnically suggestive physical characteristics as well as the mutually enslaving power dynamic between Victor and his creature to support this argument.[2] I claim that the repulsion that Victor feels when he sees the creature look back at him with a "dull yellow eye," with his "watery clouded eyes," enacts a particular kind of othering expressed in terms of the physicality of the eye (*WMS* 1:39–40). The creature's eyes implore Victor for sympathetic communication, yet their diseased appearance prevents Victor from looking at his creature compassionately. Yellow, watery eyes were symptomatic of several systemic diseases, including yellow fever. However, *Frankenstein* so abounds with allusions to vision and blindness that the yellow, watery eyes suggest a more direct reference to eye disease in particular.

Contagion

The two most likely early-nineteenth-century medical explanations for the creature's yellow, watery eyes would be the noncontagious condition epiphora and the highly contagious disease ophthalmia. The differing significance of these two illnesses captures the tension between how the creature sees himself and how others see him. Epiphora, or "the watery eye," much discussed in early-nineteenth-century medical literature, was caused, as the physician James Ware asserts in 1792, "either by a more copious secretion of tears than the puncta Lacrymalia are able to absorb; or ... by an obstruction in the lachrymal canal" (*Chirurugical* 1–2). In other words, either the individual suffering from "the watery eye" makes more tears than can be absorbed or s/he has blocked tear ducts. Ware presented case studies to the Medical Society of London in 1790 in order to promote the treatment he espoused for the watery eye: flushing the duct with water via a syringe. He does not blame the patients whose cases he describes, including a "lady in Great Russell Street," "a lieutenant in his majesty's navy," "a clergyman from Bristol," and "a young woman in Basinghall Street," for their condition; for example, he does not attribute their watery eyes to poor hygiene or other behaviors (*Chirurugical* 10–19). If the creature, in keeping with this range of respectable people, is literally afflicted with the watery eye, or epiphora, then his "watery eyes" serve as physical evidence of his connection to

---

2   In addition to those by the scholars named above, consult articles by the following for discussions of Mary Shelley's critique of empire and orientalism: Gayatri Spivak, Zohreh T. Sullivan, and Donald Bush.

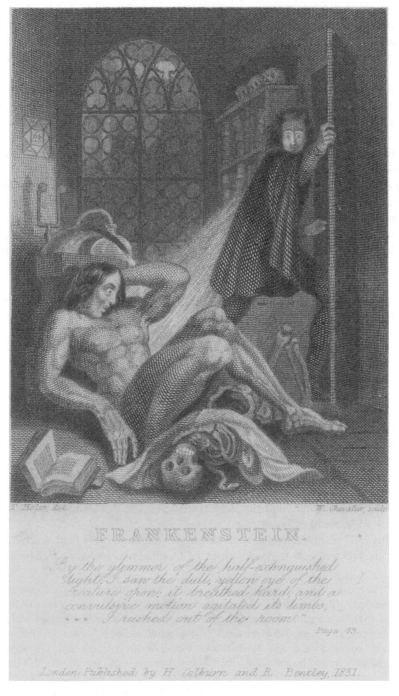

Fig. 2. **Frontispiece by W. Chevalier.** ***Frankenstein*, 1831**

humanity, a connection that corresponds to his more abstract human qualities such as his desire for companionship, his capacity for sympathy, and his ability to express himself. Since one possible cause of the epiphora was excess tears, the creature's watery eyes also indicate his capacity for depth of emotion, his vulnerability, and his ability to sympathize with others' pain.

This humanizing illness contrasts with the so-called Egyptian ophthalmia, a contagious eye disease that figures the creature as a threatening other. As I explain below, ophthalmia was initially thought to be endemic to Egypt, the illness of another people in the eyes of the British. Once it was discovered to be contagious also to Europeans—becoming, in fact, epidemic in England—the disease served as evidence that contact with ethnic others was threatening to one's health. If the creature's watery eyes are symptomatic of epiphora, Mary Shelley presents the reader with physical evidence of the creature's affective capacity. Yet this potential reading of the creature's body exists in tension with the contagious, and much more threatening Egyptian ophthalmia. Mary Shelley found a model for racial and ethnic othering and a means for expressing fear of contagion in the widespread outbreak of Egyptian ophthalmia during the Napoleonic Wars. Her reference to ophthalmia served as a physical metaphor for the fear of difference that shuts down sympathetic communication, a metaphor made more powerful by the real presence of the epidemic in British lives. This health crisis persisted in England from the time the author was four until many years after the publication of her first novel.

From their initial invasion of Egypt in 1798, Napoleon's troops, and the British troops fighting in the alliance against them between 1801 and 1804, contracted the "Egyptian ophthalmia" in great numbers. The symptoms of Egyptian ophthalmia were yellow eyes and a purulent discharge, accompanied by a gritty feeling and intense pain in the eye. The infection could rupture the cornea, causing blindness. The illustration from John Vetch's medical treatise on the subject depicts the progression of the disease: the eruption of granules on the conjunctiva, the clouding of the eye with opaque scar tissue, and finally the rupturing of the cornea (Figure 3).[3] A surgeon treating the French army in Egypt estimated in a pamphlet published in 1806 that two-thirds of the 32,000 French soldiers fighting in Egypt were afflicted by Fall 1798 (Wagemans and van Bijsterveld 139). The British army experienced a similarly widespread outbreak.

In his 1807 pamphlet, Vetch notes that in a battalion of more than seven hundred men, "six hundred and thirty-six cases of Ophthalmia, including relapses, were

---

3   The cause of Egyptian ophthalmia, also called "trachoma" or "granular conjunctivitis," was identified in the late 1950s as the microorganism *Chlamydia trachomatis* (Albert and Edwards 154). In the early nineteenth century, three diseases were unwittingly included in the clinical category "Egyptian ophthalmia": the infection caused by *Chlamydia trachomatis*, gonorrheal conjunctivitis, and Koch-Weeks conjunctivitis (Albert and Edwards 155). Although easily treated by antibiotics, the *Chlamydia trachomatis* infection is still prevalent in sub-Saharan Africa, the Middle East, Central Asia, Southeast Asia, and in impoverished areas of Latin America and Australia. The World Health Organization has identified it as the world's leading cause of preventable blindness (Zingeser). The current trachoma epidemic is a striking current example of the interdependence of poverty and illness that Charlotte Smith addresses in *Rural Walks* (see chapter 6).

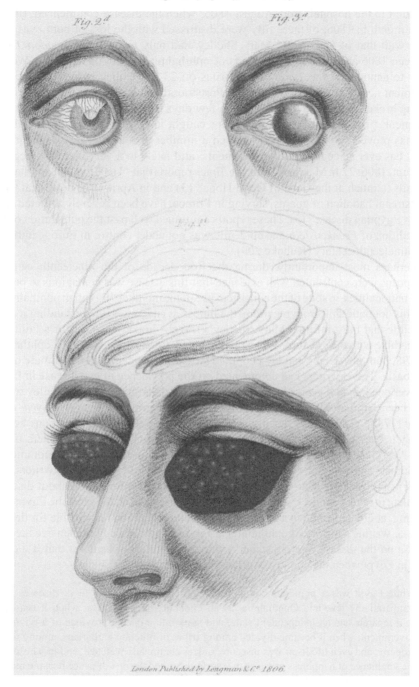

Fig. 3.   John Vetch, *An account of the ophthalmia which has appeared in England since the return of the British Army from Egypt*, 1807

admitted to the hospital, from August 1805, when the disease commenced, till the same month in 1806; of these fifty were dismissed with the loss of both eyes, and forty with that of one" (69).[4] Mary Shelley had only to open the *London Times* between 1806 and 1816 to find reports of ophthalmia's effect on soldiers. "We are sorry to announce," the *Times* editor writes on 23 September 1806, "that the 89th Regiment ... have been disembarked at Portsmouth, on account of the Ophthalmia having broken out among the men" (3). A few days later the *Times* offers a summary statement: "The disorder which our troops caught in Egypt, called the ophthalmia, and has proved so fatal in depriving such a number of brave fellows of their eye-sight, has ever since infected our regiments, and lately to a very alarming degree" (26 Sept. 1806: 2). In March of 1808, the *Times* reports that "The Egyptian ophthalmia prevails ... much at the Cape of Good Hope" (3) and in April 1816 notes that "The Coldstream battalion of guards, serving in France, have been severely afflicted with ... this Egyptian disease" (3). These reports continued well past the publication of the first edition of *Frankenstein*; the epidemic was not under control in Europe until the mid-nineteenth century (Kuhnke 209).

Perhaps most importantly, during the first decade of the nineteenth century, Europeans were confronted with evidence that this disease was contagious to people of all nationalities, in spite of the consistent use of the moniker "Egyptian ophthalmia." It is this dramatic shift from regarding the illness as endemic to understanding it as an epidemic that most informs Mary Shelley's novel—in particular Victor's failure to sympathize with the creature. When the European troops first contracted ophthalmia in 1798, both physicians and lay people regarded it as endemic to the climate of the Nile basin. Travel writers had commented on the prevalence of eye disease in Egypt for over one hundred years. An avid reader of travel narratives, Mary Shelley would have been familiar with these accounts. For example, in his *Voyage in Syrie et en Egypt* (1788), Constantin-François Volney notes that many of the Egyptians he met had their eyes bandaged (Wagemans and van Bijsterveld 138). The writers of the 1762 *New General History of the World* confirm that the eye disease is so common in Egypt that "some travellers call it the land of the blind" (5:173). Travel writers, and the British physicians who relied on their narratives for information about diseases prevalent in other countries, speculated variously that the heat, the sand, the Egyptians' clothing, and/or a decline in agricultural production might be responsible for the eye disease. Writing a history of ophthalmia in Egypt as part of a comprehensive medical treatise on the disease, the physician Arthur Edmondston speculates that it did not exist in Egypt when the country was independent and powerful:

> While Egypt was a populous country, and agriculture flourished in it, diseases were comparatively few, and Ophthalmia, as an endemic, unknown. But when it ceased to be a separate and an independent state, and sunk into a distant province of a tyrannical government; when it became divided among tribes of illiterate barbarians, among whom property, and even life itself was insecure, unless continually watched, and in whose eyes the semblance of happiness was a crime, agriculture and the arts of peace became matters of but secondary consideration. (67)

---

4   R. M. Feibel characterizes Vetch's efforts to educate the public about the contagious nature of ophthalmia and his recommendations for prevention and treatment of the disease as "major milestones in the history of ophthalmology" (128).

It is perhaps impossible to ascertain, with any degree of precision, the period when Ophthalmia first became so widely prevalent in Egypt; but it is highly probable, that its occurrence was in some measure connected with the final subjugation of that country by the Turks ... . Idleness and the indulgence in depraved habits rendered the frame obnoxious to general disease; and the constant use of the turban, enjoined by the rigid tenets of the Koran among all ranks, weakened and exposed the eyes directly to the action of every exciting cause of Ophthalmia. (71)

Although it is true that local circumstances such as access to water and the prevalence of flies did contribute to the spread of the disease, this account of the Egyptian endemic also conveys the sense that when the "right people" hold political power, a country experiences immunity from disease. Such a theory reflects the fantasy that difference will protect those in power, indeed that physical evidence of difference stabilizes hierarchical structures.

Wanting to feel protected from the illness, British physicians and the British public assumed that ophthalmia would not survive an attempt to invade the British Isles. However, this fantasy of protection was soon shattered in England. Edmondston describes the spread of ophthalmia to Europe: "Though annually fatal to the sight of multitudes in [Egypt], it was scarcely known in Europe by name, until the lust of universal domination carried to Alexandria the arms of Bonaparte" (62). In an 1806 letter to the editor of the *London Times*, the physician James Ware warns the public that the illness is not endemic to Egypt:

The violence of the inflammation of the eyes, to which the natives of Egypt are subject, is well known; and the melancholy proofs we have had of its tendency to destroy vision, as evidenced by the great numbers of soldiers who returned to England ... in a state of total blindness, must unavoidably give pain to every one who reflects upon them. The general opinion has hitherto been, that the Ophthalmia ... was confined to Egypt, and was dependent on such local circumstances as rendered other countries secure from its influence. (11 August 1806: 2)

The rapid spread of the illness within Britain, these "melancholy proofs" of its existence (i.e., the increasing number of British soldiers blinded by ophthalmia), quickly taught the public that British citizenship did not protect them from this so-called Egyptian illness. As Edmondston notes, the illusion of immunity actually fueled the epidemic:

Multitudes of soldiers, on their arrival in England from Egypt, laboured under Ophthalmia ... . Intimate and frequent intercourse naturally took place between them and persons in perfect health; cleanliness ... was here disregarded, *for the disease was considered local and uninfectious.* Owing to these circumstances, Ophthalmia appeared at the same time in the most distant parts of Great Britain; and that peculiar modification of it is now familiar to almost every medical practitioner. (47, my emphasis)

Within a year of the initial outbreak, even the most rural practitioner in Britain had encountered the Egyptian ophthalmia.

The history of this illness illustrates two major perceptions of difference. The endemic model of disease ultimately affirms the stability of difference in a way that suggests containment within the borders of ethnic or other identity, a model that reflects what Alan Bewell describes as "the fallacy of 'colonial geography,' which assumes that disease is 'natural' or 'the norm' elsewhere" (312). The endemic model, in other words, offers physical evidence of otherness and often of inferiority. In contrast, the epidemic model of disease presents a picture of contagion in which national borders, ethnicity, and other forms of difference are permeable. To be at the top of the hierarchy is not to be protected. An epidemic—uncontained difference that threatens to spread—is potentially infectious to those in power.

Once the medical community and the public realized that ophthalmia was a boundary-crossing epidemic, rather than a condition endemic to Egypt, they became deeply interested in learning how the disease was transmitted. Responding to the spread of contagious disease in the colonial "contact zone"—including smallpox in the American colonies, yellow fever in the West Indies, and the world-wide cholera epidemic which began in 1817—the authors of early-nineteenth-century medical treatises explored the nature of contagion.[5] Joseph Adams, secretary to the medical society of London and a member of the London College of Physicians, notes in 1809 that "contagion is a term so frequently brought into use, and discussed with so much ease, that one might think its laws were to be ascertained with the same certainty as the solution of a mathematical problem" (10). However, the "ablest practitioners of the present day," he observes, dispute "whether the yellow fever of the West Indies and the Americas, the influenza, and even the plague, are contagious" (10). Similarly, in his treatise on ophthalmia, Edmondston describes the contentious debate about contagion:

> Much has been written on the subject of epidemic and contagious diseases, and many attempts have been made to ascertain the limits of each ... . The plague and the yellow fever, those great destroyers of the human race, are considered by one set of physicians as dangerous and contagious, and by another set as harmless endemics of the countries where they prevail. (60)

Both physicians and the public so vehemently questioned the contagious nature of ophthalmia that physicians like Edmondston were moved to write treatises proving that the disease was transmitted through physical contact and not caused merely by local circumstances.

The shift from thinking about ophthalmia as endemic to Egypt to understanding its universally contagious nature inspired hyperbolic descriptions of the illness, and, I argue, influenced Mary Shelley's depiction of the creature's threatening otherness. An anonymous 1808 pamphlet testifies to the impact the illness had on the British imagination and sense of security: "Egyptian Ophthalmia was a disease, from the terrors of which no person could feel secure" (*Identities Ascertained* iv). The author terms the illness "a disease, that from the military has been transported to

---

5   The concept "contact zones," from Mary Louise Pratt's groundbreaking book *Imperial Eyes: Travel Writing and Transculturation*, is very useful for discussions of disease and empire, though Pratt herself does not address the transmission of disease. Alan Bewell, however, develops this concept in his eloquent introduction to *Romanticism and Colonial Disease*. For a late-eighteenth-century monograph on the transmission of disease, see James Carmichael Smyth's *The Effect of the Nitrous Vapour, etc.*

private life, and is regarded with universal apprehension" (3–4). The disease was not simply something to avoid, but something that inspired "terror" and "universal apprehension," language that resonates with Victor's fears about the creature's destructive influence. Just as the Egyptian ophthalmia was "transported" from the military "to private life," so the destructive effects of Victor's laboratory experiment are transported into the private sphere of his family and friends.

The transition Victor makes from imagining that he is creating a worshipful species to imagining that he is creating a predatory species mirrors the transition from endemic to epidemic understandings of eye disease. Initially, Victor assumes that his creation will amplify rather than threaten his own power. Hard at work in his laboratory, he rhapsodizes about his future relationship with the creature and its offspring: "A new species would bless me as its creator and source; many happy and excellent natures would owe their being to me. No father could claim the gratitude of his child so completely as I should deserve theirs" (*WMS* 1:37). He conceptualizes the creature as a different species; he imagines the creature will become "many happy and excellent" creatures; and he fantasizes that this species will worship him. In short, he imagines difference as endemic, hierarchical, and thus nonthreatening. However, when Victor considers creating a female creature, he begins to regard difference as potentially epidemic, rather than endemic: "Even if they were to leave Europe, and inhabit the deserts of the new world, yet one of the first results of those sympathies for which the daemon thirsted would be children, and a race of devils would be propagated upon the earth, who might make the very existence of the species of man a condition precarious and full of terror" (*WMS* 1:128). Victor's description of the "terror" a race of creatures might incite certainly alludes to the Reign of Terror, but also reflects the culturally available discourse of contagious difference.

The crucial distinction between Victor's initial fantasy about the creature and his later fear of him, between his understanding of difference first as endemic and then as epidemic, results from the creature's desire for sympathy, a desire conveyed only after the creature opens his eyes. Although it is not only Victor who is horrified by the creature's appearance, Victor is the only character who focuses on the creature's watery, yellow eyes. Walton and the De Lacey family comment on the creature's large stature and hideous face, but not specifically on his eyes. Although Walton makes frequent observations about Victor's eyes, when he first views the creature, he notes the creature's face only in general terms: "Never did I behold a vision so horrible as his face, of such loathsome, yet appalling hideousness" (*WMS* 1:167). The creature's diseased eyes, then, are Victor's metonymic fantasy. Victor's obsession with the creature's eyes expresses the scientist's sudden apprehension of the creature's otherness, specifically his ethnic otherness and more generally his otherness as an independent being who seeks sympathy from his creator.

The contrast between Victor's unique obsession with the creature's watery eyes and other characters' responses to his general hideousness demonstrates Victor's fear of sympathizing with such difference. Other scholars have characterized Victor's refusal to create a female creature as symptomatic of his fear of female sexuality, or as a reflection of Mary Shelley's own ambivalence about the female body's reproductive power.[6] However, it is significant that as he pieces together the

---

6 See Mellor ("Possessing Nature" 224–25), and Hoeveler ("Fantasy" 20–21).

body of the creature, Victor already envisions the species multiplying, and feels no horror. It is certainly plausible that Victor simply does not expect reproduction to involve a female until the creature requests a companion. After all, he created the male creature on his own and perhaps imagined the species multiplying in other ways. It is also true, though, that between the time he assembled the first creature in his lab and the moment of his refusal to create a second, Victor becomes aware that the creature is a separate being and that he "thirsts" for "those sympathies" intrinsic in a parent's, friend's, or partner's love (*WMS* 1:128). While he assembles the creature in his lab, Victor's scientific gaze protects him from sympathizing, but the moment the creature looks back at him, Victor fears that his supposed objectivity will be contaminated with feeling. Sympathy invites a level of identification between self and other that dissolves the illusion of stable, hierarchical, endemic difference. Sympathy, then, can lead to contagion; yet, as I explain below, sympathy also makes narrative possible.

Sympathy

In her invocation of contagion and sympathy, Mary Shelley explores the human interactions that encourage and support creative expression. Romantic-era medical sources argue both that sympathy can spread contagion and also that disease and deformity can destroy individuals' sympathetic responses to one another. The theory of sympathetic contagion explains Victor's anxious reaction to the deformed creature's plea for compassion. In late-eighteenth-century medical treatises, "sympathy" referred to the physiological effects of similarity between individuals. Janis McLarren Caldwell explains that eighteenth-century "theorists of physiologic sympathy," such as David Hume, David Hartley, and George Cheyne, also believed in "social sympathy, or the literal transmission of sympathy from body to body" (263–64). While these theorists intended to establish physiological and social sympathy as "a foundation for moral behavior," Caldwell points out that "fears of social contamination inevitably arose" (265). The medical theory of sympathetic contagion reflects this fear of social contamination. The physician Robert Whytt observes that "there is a wonderful sympathy between the nervous systems of different persons, whence various motions and morbid symptoms are often transferred from one to another, without any corporeal contact or infection" (*The Works* 583). According to this theory, the transmission of symptoms required proximity but not actual contact between individuals with similar nervous systems. Thus, when these individuals looked into each other's eyes, one might feel the other's symptoms. Also prevalent was the hypothesis that not just symptoms but also disease itself could be transferred by looking at someone with a similar nervous system. In his 1806 treatise on ophthalmia, Edmondston argues that ophthalmia is conducted by physical contact; however, he first works to dispel popular and long-standing perceptions that eye disease could be contracted not through touch, but simply by looking sympathetically. For example, Edmondston observes that in Aristotle's assertion "when one person gazes on the eye of another labouring under Ophthalmia, the former is also seized with it," Aristotle "confound[ed] the idea of contagion with the power of imitation" (3). Likewise, Edmondston notes, Plutarch assumed that disease was passed by sympathy (5). Edmonston reports that Boerhaave also believed that "Ophthalmia may be contracted by the simple inspection of the eyes of a person labouring under it, yet his object is to show that such an effect is the result of a sympathetic action," rather than physical contact (8). There is, according to Edmonston, a long tradition of confusing the transfer of disease by contact with its transfer through sympathy. In this formulation, the eyes are both the literal site of disease and the means for transmitting it sympathetically. Thus, if Victor looks into the creature's diseased eyes and sympathizes with him, he risks acknowledging similarity. Sympathy will destroy the boundary between himself and the monster. If, as the model of sympathetic contagion suggests, the monster's difference/disease is catching to those with similar nervous systems, then the discovery that he sympathizes with the creature will force Victor to see the monstrous in himself.

Several eighteenth-century physicians argue against the possibility of sympathetic contagion, focusing instead on the alienating effect of disease and deformity. They posit that, unlike sympathy between organs (a popular model in the period), sympathy between individuals requires voluntary participation, therefore making contraction of disease by this means unlikely.[7] Edmonston explains:

> [W]e cannot sympathize with objects of horror or disgust, and such I conceive disease to be under any form. There is an insuperable repugnance in human nature to every species of corporeal pain; and we never behold a disease in another person, without a self-congratulation at our own exemption, and a hope that we may escape it altogether. If this view be correct, it does not appear that Ophthalmia can be propagated by sympathy. (107)

Edmondston does not accept the theory of sympathetic contagion, because he believes that illness inspires negative responses that challenge the emotional connection between individuals. Like other physicians, Edmondston emphasizes contagious disease's power to threaten compassionate interactions among people. In an 1814 treatise, Adams describes the social effects of contagion: "[T]he uncertainty in which it [is] involved ... has often ... stifled the feelings of consanguinity, friendship, and love" (v). The fear of contagion that one feels when observing the diseased body of another obstructs sympathy, and, for Mary Shelley, becomes a metaphor for the difficulty of sympathizing with the narratives of those who are marked by difference. When one's narrative finds no sympathetic audience, one becomes culturally invisible.

In narrative terms, sympathetic contagion is body-based persuasion, dependent upon the mutually sympathetic nervous systems of the speaker and the audience. In contrast, an alienating deformity prevents the speaker from cultivating sympathy

---

7   Edmondston explains that sympathy between two organs of an individual body differs from sympathy between two people: "Sympathy in a medical sense, strictly speaking, means the communication of painful or pleasureable sensation from one organ to another of the same body. Thus the uterus sympathizes with the mammae, the head with the stomach, or, in other words, the one is affected by impressions made upon the other ... . In a more general sense, sympathy implies the quality of being affected by the affection of another, or a participation in the pains and pleasures of another" (106).

and thus from persuading his audience of anything but his otherness. In an attempt to gain sympathy, the creature tries to tell his life story to the De Lacey father and to Victor. Although he does manage to express himself to both men, he ultimately fails to obtain their compassion. Unlike his creature, Victor does not even venture to share his shameful story of creation to the court at Justine's trial, or even to the seemingly more sympathetic listeners Elizabeth and Henry, although the lives of all three friends depend upon their knowing about the creature. Victor does, however, manage to relay the story (except its core scientific secret) to both Walton and the magistrate in Geneva. In contrast, Walton writes a complete (we assume) account of all these stories in his letters to his sister Margaret. What conditions make telling these tales possible? What conditions prevent the narrators from talking or writing?

In responding to these questions, I will pay special attention to the ways in which characters use their eyes to communicate sympathy to one another and to express their own desire for a sympathetic audience. Most movingly, the creature longs for a friend—yet his physical appearance prevents humans from gazing lovingly on him, making friendship impossible. His failure to find a sympathetic audience, at least in person, reflects Edmondston's and Adams's claims that disease—here physical deformity and the more metaphorical contagion of difference—obstructs sympathetic connection. The creature comes closest to obtaining sympathy from the De Laceys, the exiled French family who unknowingly educate the creature as he observes them from the hovel outside their cottage in Germany. The creature uses the language of vision to express both his growing affection for the family and his desire for their acceptance: "The more *I saw* of them [the cottagers], the greater became my desire to claim their protection and kindness; my heart yearned to be known and loved by these amiable creatures: *to see their sweet looks turned toward me with affection*, was the utmost limit of my ambition" (*WMS* 1:99, my emphasis). Significantly, the creature has the best chance of receiving sympathy from the blind De Lacey father. Knowing that the father will not discern his otherness, will not be frightened by the potential contagion of this difference, the creature hopes to find in him a sympathetic listener and friend. He describes to the old man the way in which prejudice blinds others to his essential goodness: "I have a good disposition; my life has been hitherto blameless, and, in some degree, beneficial; but a fatal prejudice *clouds their eyes*, and where *they ought to see* a feeling and kind friend, they behold only a detestable monster" (*WMS* 1:100, my emphasis). The creature locates the failure of vision (and thus sympathy) in the eyes of those who reject him, not in his own vision or aspect. This observation becomes painfully actualized at his most vulnerable moment of self-disclosure to the old man. The return of the sighted members of the De Lacey family violently interrupts the creature's narrative, dashing his dream of acceptance. The creature becomes culturally invisible because those around him cannot see past his immediate appearance to apprehend his ability to be "a feeling and kind friend." With this interaction, Mary Shelley suggests that blindness to the physical evidence of difference is crucial for sympathetic communication to take place.

Indeed, when the creature seeks his creator's compassion, he exhorts Victor to listen to him rather than to look at him: "How can I move thee? Will no entreaties cause thee to turn a *favorable eye* upon thy creature, who implores thy goodness and compassion?" (*WMS* 1:75, my emphasis). If Victor does not see his creature with "a favorable eye," the creature despairs of being able to persuade him with conversation. Because not being seen seems a better option than being seen unfavorably, the creature appeals to Victor's hearing rather than vision[8]: "Let your compassion be moved, and do not disdain me. *Listen* to my tale: when you have heard that, abandon or commiserate me, as you shall judge that I deserve. But *hear* me" (*WMS* 1:75, my emphasis). Victor refuses, lamenting both the creature's ability to see and his own apprehension of the creature's difference: "Cursed be the day, abhorred devil, in which you first saw light! .... Begone! Relieve me from the sight of your detested form" (*WMS* 1:75). Victor describes the creature's reply: "'Thus I relieve thee, my creator,' he said, and placed his hated hands before my eyes, which I flung from me with violence; 'thus I take from thee a sight which you abhor. Still thou canst listen to me, and grant me thy compassion'" (*WMS* 1:75). The creature hopes that by covering Victor's eyes, by temporarily removing Victor's ability to perceive physical difference, he will be able to relay his narrative, and ultimately gain Victor's sympathy. Victor at first responds with a degree of compassion to his creature's request to create a companion, but then becomes repulsed by the creature's appearance: "His words had a strange effect upon me. I compassionated him, and sometimes felt a wish to console him; but when I looked upon him, when I saw the filthy mass that moved and talked, my heart sickened, and my feelings were altered to those of horror and hatred" (*WMS* 1:110). The creature's desire for sympathy drives his creative expression. In the end, however, the creature's narrative fails to transcend physical difference. The creature's deformity so severely marks him that his suffering becomes invisible to Victor.

Victor's response to the creature's desire for a companion invokes both the model of the alienating effects of deformity and the competing theory of sympathetic contagion. Acutely aware that his physical difference impedes others' ability to sympathize with him, the creature importunes Victor for a companion creature with whom he might share a sympathetic bond: "I demand a creature of another sex, but as hideous as myself .... It is true, we shall be monsters, cut off from all the world; but on that account we shall be more attached to one another .... Let me see that I excite the sympathy of some existing thing; do not deny me my request!" (*WMS* 1:109). In short, he asks for a companion who will see in him similarity rather than difference. And, ironically, it is this problem of sameness and difference around which Victor's decision turns. He becomes afraid that the creature's desire for sympathy will lead him to reproduce, that sympathy from another creature will spread the contagion of his difference. Yet, Victor is also afraid that sympathy will fail, that ultimately the reflection of the creature's ugliness in a female partner will overwhelm the potential pleasures of identification: "They might even hate each other; the creature who already lived loathed his own deformity, and might he not conceive a greater abhorrence for it when it came before his eyes in the female form?" (*WMS* 1:128). Deformity, as in Edmondston's view, will obstruct the couple's sympathetic connection. Likewise, Victor fears that the "bride" will

---

8   Elizabeth Bohls argues that Mary Shelley's "formal innovation," the combination of the creature's "horrific appearance and riveting speech," reveals that his ugliness is not absolute, but constructed by European aesthetic standards ("Standards" 34).

reject the creature and seek a human mate instead, prompting the grieving creature to lash out against humankind. Refused a companion, the creature's only real hope for a sympathetic audience is one with which he has no direct contact—readers of the novel.

In contrast with the creature, Victor tells his tale under the watchful and sympathetic eye of Walton. Walton yearns for a friend who reflects his own ambitions and intellectual abilities. Expressing this desire in terms of vision, Walton writes to his sister Margaret, even before he meets Victor: "I desire the company of a man who could sympathize with me; whose eyes would reply to mine" (*WMS* 1:13). Walton looks for a kind of double in his potential friend. In his essay on the "highly complex continuum of male-male sympathies" in *Frankenstein*, Eric Daffron points out that in the discourse of physiognomy, doubling was rooted in sympathy (418). Johann Caspar Lavater describes in his *Essays on Physiognomy* the signs indicating that one has found his double: "The ardour of his eyes will nurture thine, and the gentleness of his voice will temper thy too piercing tones. His love will shine on thy countenance, and his image will appear in thee. Thou wilt become what he is, and yet remain what thou art. Affection will make qualities in him visible to thee which never could be seen by an uninterested eye" (3:151). When they meet, Walton immediately feels himself in sympathy with Victor and expresses this identification and compassion in the loving way that he watches the ailing Victor's face and eyes: "I sat watching the wan countenance of my friend ..." (*WMS* 1:163). "I sat by his bed watching him; his eyes were closed, and I thought he slept ..." (*WMS* 1:165). By highlighting both Walton's loving look and Victor's visual activity, these passages express the potential for deep sympathy between the two men.

Walton's sympathetic gaze, a gaze that commingles desire for Victor's friendship and compassion for Victor's suffering, makes it possible for Victor to narrate his story. Walton watches him lovingly, focusing especially on Victor's eyes, as he tells the tale: "Sometimes, seized with sudden agony, he could not continue his tale; at others, his voice broken, yet piercing, uttered with difficulty the words so replete with agony. His fine and lovely eyes were now lighted up with indignation, now subdued to downcast sorrow, and quenched in infinite wretchedness" (*WMS* 1:159). It is not only the sympathetic gaze that makes Victor's narration possible, but also the similarity between Walton and Victor. If sympathy alone made his narration possible, Victor would have told the story to both Henry and Elizabeth, the friends who also look on Victor with sympathetic gazes. Under Henry's watchful eye, Victor regains his health in Ingolstadt; Elizabeth bestows upon the broken Victor "soft looks of compassion" with "her ever-watchful and nicer eye" (*WMS* 1:146, 147). The illustration on the title page of the 1831 edition depicts Victor and Elizabeth on the threshold of the Frankenstein family home as he leaves for Ingolstadt. Elizabeth looks lovingly at him, but Victor covers his eyes with his left hand. Although in the caption beneath the engraving Victor says, "I was unwilling to quit the *sight* of those that remained to me; and, above all, I desired to *see* my sweet Elizabeth in some degree consoled," in the illustration he turns his head and willfully covers his eyes (my emphasis). Elsewhere in the text, Victor describes the ways in which he differs from each of these old friends, and neither their gazes nor their questions prompt Victor to tell them the truth. These differences seem to inhibit Victor from telling them his tale, even when his friends' lives depend upon the information. Walton, on the other hand, constantly emphasizes his identification with Victor and hears more of Victor's story than does any other character.

However, Victor cannot completely reciprocate Walton's desire for a deep bond. Walton confesses to Victor the "desire I had always felt of finding a friend who might sympathize with me, and direct me by his counsel" (*WMS* 1:19). Victor, however, deflects Walton's hopes away from himself, telling the sea captain, "You have hope, and the world before you, and have no cause for despair. But I—I have lost every thing, and cannot begin life anew" (*WMS* 1:19). This lack of mutuality is embodied in Victor's inability to return Walton's gaze; during their interactions, Victor's eyes are either dancing with madness or closed in pain. This limit to their sympathetic identification is as crucial as are their similarities for Victor's ability to tell his tale. As Daffron points out, while eighteenth-century theorists highly valued sympathetic connections among people, they regarded an extreme investment in sympathy as a threat to one's identity. In *Enquiry Concerning Political Justice*, William Godwin describes the inevitability of sympathetic connections among people, but warns that "He that resigns himself wholly to sympathy and imitation can possess little of mental strength or accuracy" (300). Walton sees potential for true companionship and he sees Victor's suffering; yet because Victor cannot look back at him in the same way, Walton is protected from over-identification, a form of sympathy that destroys the self. In this version of sympathetic contagion, intimacy, rather than disease, threatens the boundaries of Victor's identity.

In fact, this threat of over-identification prompts Victor to tell his story, even as he is quite explicit about withholding the core element of his narrative—the secret of creating life. Victor begins his story as a cautionary tale:

> I had determined, once, that the memory of these evils should die with me; but you have won me to alter my determination. You seek for knowledge and wisdom, as I once did; and I ardently hope that the gratification of your wishes may not be a serpent to sting you, as mine has been. I do not know if the relation of my misfortunes will be useful to you, yet, if you are inclined, listen to my tale. (*WMS* 1:20)

In the 1831 edition, Mary Shelley writes a stronger, more directive speech for Victor. In this version of the passage, Victor suggests that Walton might "deduce an apt moral" from his narrative: "Do you share my madness? Have you drank also of the intoxicating draught? Hear me,—let me reveal my tale, and you will dash the cup from your lips!" (*WMS* 1:186). When he begins to describe his memory of the creature's animation, Victor says to Walton, "I see by your eagerness, and the wonder and hope which your eyes express, my friend, that you expect to be informed of the secret with which I am acquainted" (*WMS* 1:36). Victor refuses to tell him. At the moment when complete sympathy is possible, Victor withholds a bit of narrative, thus preventing Walton from collapsing his identity into his own. Mary Favret describes the secret Victor withholds as "the myth of paternal power and exclusive, vital authority," and argues that withholding this secret "becomes Victor's weapon against his greatest fear: human intercourse" (*Romantic* 185). His explicit reason for telling his story is to offer a cautionary tale to a friend with similar goals; yet by withholding the secret, Victor protects himself from intimacy.

Although Walton's sympathy makes Victor's narrative possible, Mary Shelley repeatedly emphasizes the instability of spoken narrative, the inability of the narrator to control the response of even a sympathetic audience. When Victor tries to persuade the magistrate to pursue the creature after Elizabeth's death, he is acutely aware of the magistrate's fluctuating reaction to his appeal: "The magistrate appeared at first perfectly incredulous, but as I continued he became more attentive and interested; I saw him sometimes shudder with horror, at others a lively surprise, unmingled with disbelief, was painted on his countenance" (*WMS* 1:152). When Victor then calls upon the magistrate to act, he notices "a considerable change in the physiognomy of the magistrate," who maintains that it is not possible to catch the creature. Victor becomes outraged: "As I spoke, rage sparkled in my eyes; the magistrate was intimidated" (*WMS* 1:153). In spite of Victor's eloquence and his ability to read the magistrate's face, the magistrate recommends that Victor "make up his mind to disappointment" (*WMS* 1:153). Although a willing and absorbed listener, the magistrate does not respond as Victor wishes. An even more poignantly unpredictable response to spoken narrative occurs at Justine's trial. Elizabeth speaks in Justine's defense, with the hope of persuading the jury of her innocence. However, Elizabeth's heartfelt eloquence moves the crowd to identify with Elizabeth, ironically fueling their prejudice against Justine. In this case, their sympathy causes the crowd to misinterpret Elizabeth's words, blinding them to Justine's innocence. The desire for sympathy may drive narrative, but it will not necessarily determine the effects of narrative.

In Mary Shelley's formulation, then, creative expression is admirable, if unsuccessful, when it attempts to bridge difference, as in the creature's eloquent appeal to Victor or Elizabeth's appeal to the prejudiced crowd at Justine's trial. Caldwell suggests, "Shelley may be redefining sympathy as an active reception of difference, rather than a passive transmission necessitating similarity, particularly when she emphasizes listening to language, as she does in every near-sympathetic encounter permitted in the novel" (270–71). However, these transmissions are only "near-sympathetic"—Victor is not compelled to make a companion for the creature, the magistrate is not persuaded to seek the creature, and the crowd's anger toward Justine increases. In each case, Mary Shelley suggests that language may fail when we are in each other's presence. Physical presence threatens the viability of expression because it invites us to apprehend difference, to be falsely persuaded, or to dissolve into the identity-obliterating sympathy against which Godwin warns.

Addressing this problem of physical presence, Mary Shelley's novel suggests that narrative has a different effect when written than when spoken. In his discussion of "the relationship of the nervous body to voice and text in the Romantic period," Nigel Leask argues that both Samuel Taylor Coleridge and Percy Bysshe Shelley regarded the spoken word as more powerful than the written text precisely because of its physiological effects (62). Mary Shelley saw first hand the extreme effect that the physical performance of a text might have when Byron recited Coleridge's "Christabel" at the Villa Diodati, just days before she began writing *Frankenstein*. Byron's rendition of Geraldine's mesmeric power over Christabel caused Shelley to hallucinate eyes in Mary Shelley's breasts and run from the room in the throes of a nervous attack. Perhaps in response to this dramatic example of the physical effect of oral narration, Mary Shelley endorses what Peter de Bolla describes as the move in eighteenth-century elocution texts "from a voice-centered to a text-centered discursivity" (147), in other words, "from a description of the subject in terms of voice to one in terms of the text" (178). Although *Frankenstein* unfolds in a series of embedded in-person conversations between an auditor and a speaker—Victor tells his story to Walton, and within this story recounts the creature's narration to him—these in-person oral narrations are all contained within the written frame narrative of Walton's letters to his sister.

By privileging the written word over the spoken word, Mary Shelley suggests that narration is safest when separated from the body of the speaker. Writing is not more predictable than speaking in its effect, but it attempts to influence the reader very differently—by allowing for reflection and distance. Discussing the effect of physical presence on principled decision-making, Godwin asserts: "Undisciplined feeling would induce me, now to interest myself exclusively for one man, and now for another, to be eagerly solicitous for those who are present to me, and to forget the absent" (212). One's presence can persuade, or as in the case of the creature, dissuade the listener from responding justly. However, while the physical effect of oral narration on others was regarded with caution in the eighteenth century, the move from a voice-centered to a text-centered narrative also created anxiety about interior speech: "If one can speak to oneself and become excited by the interior sound of one's own voice then the possibility of auto-eroticism, and of self-authentication and self-generation becomes manifest" (de Bolla 162). Mary Shelley reflects this fear in her depiction of Walton's and Victor's private reading, both of which lead to destructive forms of self-generation. However, in each case, the scientists are obsessed with solitary reading that is specifically focused on the fulfillment of solitary, individualistic desires. There is much less anxiety in the text about collaboratively written narratives, including Walton's letters (which Victor helps edit), the multinarrator structure of the text, and, of course, Mary Shelley and Percy Bysshe Shelley's limited collaboration on the novel itself.[9] Favret describes the novel's narrative structure as one of "mutual authority" and "correspondence" (*Romantic* 182). The multiple, corresponding narratives that comprise Walton's letters invite rationally based comparisons, inspiring the reader to measure each speaker and to measure her responses to each narrative. Mary Shelley proposes the collaboratively written narrative as a solution both to the dangers of solitary reading and to the dangers of persuasive, in-person narration—that is, to the sympathetic contagion of narrative.[10]

---

9   See E.B. Murray for the details of the Shelleys' collaboration.

10   Steven Goldsmith's chapter on *The Last Man* in his *Unbuilding Jerusalem* brilliantly demonstrates that Mary Shelley was concerned with the contagious effects of certain kinds of narration at least through 1826. Goldsmith argues that *The Last Man* "creates an association between disease and narrative language" (295). Further, he argues that the plague/narrative is communicated by touch, that is, by metonym (a fictional mode) rather than by metaphor (a poetic mode): Narrative can "infect (or represent) only those things that come in contact, that share a border of 'circumstance,' a bond of time or space that defines relationship on the basis of accident, contingency, difference" (306).

The Invisible Author

Written narrative helps overcome the problem of deformity as well as the problem of sympathetic contagion, not because it prevents over-persuasiveness, but because the writer's deformity or "marked" status is invisible behind the printed word. Although characters in the novel are not able to feel sympathy for the creature before them, readers of the novel are moved by his struggle because they cannot see him. Ironically, Mary Shelley recommends physical invisibility as a strategy for those who are culturally invisible. Cultural invisibility is caused not only by deformity, as in the creature's case, but also by any circumstance in which being "marked" as different in some physically evident way makes one's own experience of selfhood difficult to convey to others. Although not marked by hideous difference like the creature, in 1816 Mary Shelley was marked by her parents' fame, making it difficult for others to see her individual creativity. Her sense of being watched by Shelley as she began her writing career led Mary Shelley to explore the benefits of physical invisibility in the novel. She published the first edition of the novel anonymously and, as William St. Clair points out, she hinted that the author was a man with the phrase "his labours" in the preface (359).[11] The dedication of the novel to Godwin and Shelley's efforts on her behalf with publishers led many readers and reviewers to surmise that her husband was the author (St. Clair 360). Mary Shelley shared the desire for anonymity with generations of women writers before and to come. Carolyn Heilbrun explains that before second-wave feminism, it was common for a woman writer "to hide [her] authorial identity from prying eyes" in order to "imagin[e] alternate destinies" for herself and other women (110). Invisibility frees the imagination. In addition to publishing anonymously, Mary Shelley thematized the connection between invisibility and creation. Walton, the most successful storyteller in *Frankenstein*, highlights his invisibility as a writer with his repeated suggestion to his sister that she may not see him again, and the creature is most at peace when he is beyond the judging gaze of humankind. The sense of freedom that invisibility provides—one is not concerned with the audience's immediate reaction, one is not "marked" by difference—allows for the creative expression of suffering. Although she explores the benefits of invisibility for both herself and the creature, Mary Shelley is careful to distinguish this desire for strategic physical invisibility from Victor's desire to look without being seen.

Mary Shelley reveals that even as a child she felt her creativity soar when she was alone and invisible to others. One of her favorite pastimes was to "write stories," yet she had "a dearer pleasure than this, which was the formation of castles in the air—the indulging in waking dreams—the following trains of thought ... . My dreams were at once more fantastic and agreeable than my writings" (*WMS* 1:175). She attributes this difference to her audience: "What I wrote was intended at least for one other eye—my childhood's companion and friend; but my dreams were all my own; I accounted for them to nobody; they were my refuge when annoyed—my dearest pleasure when free" (*WMS* 1:175–76). The absence of audience, and thus of

---

11 The second edition, published after her husband's death, "was advertised as by Mary Wollstonecraft Shelley" (St. Clair 361).

judgment, makes private imagining preferable to writing stories others will read. If the potential criticism of her childhood friend Isabel Baxter's reading "eye" caused anxiety, then certainly she must have felt quite acutely Shelley's watchfulness in the summer of 1816. She describes his expectations for her at length:

> My husband ... was, from the first, very anxious that I should prove myself worthy of my parentage, and enroll myself on the page of fame. He was for ever inciting me to obtain literary reputation ... . At this time he desired that I should write, not so much with the idea that I could produce any thing worthy of notice, but that he might himself judge how far I possessed the promise of better things hereafter. (*WMS* 1:176)

Shelley's concern is with "fame," "literary reputation," and his own power to "judge" Mary Shelley's promise, all externally focused and evaluative rather than sympathetic ways of reading. It is not surprising that her response to this scrutiny, a scrutiny akin to that of scientific experimentation, was "I did nothing" (*WMS* 1:176). Being marked as "the daughter of two persons of distinguished literary celebrity," Mary Shelley becomes a kind of experimental freak show, a living example of the power of inherited literary talent, rather than a person who might claim and develop her own abilities (*WMS* 1:175).[12]

In the introduction to the novel, Mary Shelley goes on to describe the pressure she felt from Byron and Shelley to create an impressive tale: "'*Have you thought of a story?*' I was asked each morning, and each morning I was forced to reply with a mortifying negative" (*WMS* 1:178). During this process of thinking of a story, she is quite focused on audience response. She strives to create a story "which would speak to the mysterious fears of our nature, and awaken thrilling horror—one to make the reader dread to look round, to curdle the blood, and quicken the beatings of the heart" (*WMS* 1:178). Indeed, she felt the story would be unsuccessful if it did not have this effect on the reader: "If I did not accomplish these things, my ghost story would be unworthy of its name" (*WMS* 1:178). And, she implies, Mary Wollstonecraft Godwin would be proven unworthy of hers. Lying down alone in her room after an evening spent as silent auditor to Byron and Shelley's conversation, Mary Shelley is "gifted" with the vision of the scientist and his creature, a vision which she does not at first recognize as material worthy of the writing contest. Later, still despairing of writing a story "which would frighten my reader as I myself had been frightened that night" (*WMS* 1:180), she suddenly realizes that "what terrified me will terrify others" (*WMS* 1:180). Alone and unwatched, she begins to write from her own imagination as an original, rather than "as a close imitator" (*WMS* 1:175). The invisibility of solitude—that is, the lack of a judgmental gaze—frees her imagination to create.

Mary Shelley invites the reader to compare this description of her creative vision with that of her character Victor, who also creates in solitude. He assembles the first creature alone in his lab, keeping his experiment a secret. And, when he retreats

---

12 In an October 1838 journal entry, Mary Shelley regards Shelley's ambition for her more positively: "To be something great and good was the precept given me by my father: Shelley reiterated it ... . but Shelley died & I was alone—my father from age & domestic circumstances & other things could not *me faire valoir*—none else noticed me" (*JMS* 554–55).

to create the bride, he again lives in solitude, "ungazed upon" in a cottage on the Orkney islands (*WMS* 1:127). Both Victor and Mary Shelley emphasize their own vision during these periods of unobserved creation. Victor trains his scientific gaze in charnel houses to prepare himself to make a creature:

> *I saw* how the fine form of man was degraded and wasted; *I beheld* the corruption of death succeed to the blooming cheek of life; *I saw* how the worm inherited the wonders of the eye and brain. (*WMS* 1:35, my emphasis)

Mary Shelley echoes Victor's anaphoric "I saw" in her 1831 account of the inspiration for her novel, the passage with which I began this chapter. Again, Mary Shelley reports:

> *I saw*—with shut eyes, but acute mental vision,—*I saw* the pale student of unhallowed arts kneeling beside the thing he had put together. *I saw* the hideous phantasm of a man stretched out ... (*WMS* 1:179, my emphasis)

Mary Shelley creates these parallel descriptions of creative vision in order to distinguish between the strategic invisibility of the culturally invisible and the disembodied gaze of those with cultural power.

In the midst of creating, Mary Shelley's gaze corresponds with the gazes of the characters she envisions: "[The scientist] sleeps; but he is awakened; *he opens his eyes*; behold the horrid thing stands at his bedside, opening his curtains, and looking on him with yellow, watery, but speculative eyes. *I opened mine* in terror" (*WMS* 1:180). Mary Shelley pictures Victor opening his eyes to see the creature "looking on him with yellow, watery, but speculative eyes" and even invites the reader to "behold" this scene (*WMS* 1:179). Echoing the phrase "he opens his eyes" with "I opened mine," Mary Shelley connects her own eyes with Victor's and with the creature's, which have opened for the first time. The visual field is complex; multiple lines of vision cross and reflect one another. Victor sees the creature; the creature looks at him; Mary Shelley envisions them both and invites the reader to see her creation of this scene. Although invisible herself during the moment of creation, Mary Shelley situates her own vision in relation to those she sees.

Like Mary Shelley, Victor emphasizes the solitude of his creative pursuit and expresses an awareness of his own looking:

> In a solitary chamber, or rather cell, at the top of the house, and separated from all the other apartments by a gallery and staircase, I kept my workshop of filthy creation; my eyeballs were starting from their sockets in attending to the details of my employment. (*WMS* 1:38)

Unlike Mary Shelley, however, Victor does not describe the confluence of his gaze with that of others. In fact, the moment of ultimate horror for Victor is when the creature looks back at him, when their gazes clash: "I beheld the wretch—the miserable monster whom I had created. He held up the curtain of the bed; and his eyes, if eyes they may be called, were fixed on me" (*WMS* 1:61). By returning his gaze, the creature shatters Victor's illusion of objectivity. By creating without being seen, Victor attempts to transcend the material world, including his own body and his own interpretive context. Donna Haraway would characterize his desire to see in this way as the disembodied gaze of the culturally powerful, a gaze that seeks to escape responsibility for what it sees.

In contrast, Mary Shelley's strategic invisibility is both embodied and contextualized. Even as she creates in seclusion from other people, the writer is aware of the natural world. She emerges from her vision and immediately "wish[es] to exchange the ghastly image of my fancy for the realities around" (*WMS* 1:180): "*I see* them still; the very room, the dark parquet, the closed shutters, with the moonlight struggling through, and the sense I had that the glassy lake and white high Alps were beyond" (*WMS* 1:180). While Mary Shelley senses the Alps beyond the room in which she has her vision, Victor is insensible both to the natural world and also to his loved ones as he creates:

> The summer months passed while I was thus engaged, heart and soul, in one pursuit. It was a most beautiful season; never did the fields bestow a more plentiful harvest, or the vines yield a more luxuriant vintage: but my eyes were insensible to the charms of nature. And the same feelings which made me neglect the scenes around me caused me also to forget [my] friends. (*WMS* 1:38)

Dependent on his scientific eye to assemble the creature, Victor is unable to perceive the "charms of nature." As I discuss at length in chapters 3 and 5, the ability to see beauty in the landscape is a sign of health in the Romantic period. In fact, Victor seeks to cure his melancholia on several occasions with trips through the sublime landscape. For example, during the family's excursion to the valley of Chamounix after Justine's trial, Victor credits the landscape with momentarily alleviating his pain: "These sublime and magnificent scenes afforded me the greatest consolation I was capable of receiving. They elevated me from all littleness of feeling; and although they did not remove my grief, they subdued and tranquillized it" (*WMS* 1:70). Moments after her solitary vision, Mary Shelley describes her consciousness of the world beyond her closed shutters—"the glassy lake and white high Alps" (*WMS* 1:35). Her responsiveness to the natural world suggests that the genesis of the novel, though it occurs in solitude, is a healthier activity than is Victor's creation of the creature. Although both creators are invisible to others as they create, Mary Shelley contextualizes her vision among that of her characters and situates her vision within an awareness of the particular landscape. Victor, on the other hand, resists his creature's ability to look and cuts himself off from an awareness of the natural world until much later when he seeks emotional healing in the landscape.

Oblivious to his body's relationship to the world around him, Victor experiences an illusion of disembodied vision, which Haraway describes as "the sensory system that has been used to signify a leap out of the marked body and into a conquering gaze from nowhere" (188). Victor's gaze comes from nowhere and everywhere, and thus creates the illusion of omniscience and objectivity. Although she sees without being seen, Mary Shelley portrays her gaze as, nonetheless, situated in a way that Haraway would regard as consistent with the "politics and epistemologies of location, positioning, and situating, where partiality and not universality is the condition of being heard to make rational knowledge claims" (195). Contextualized vision is much more likely to be responsible vision: "Feminist objectivity is about limited location and situated knowledge, not about transcendence and splitting of subject and object. In this way we might become answerable for what we learn how to see" (Haraway 190). Victor splits subject and object, denying his connection to, and thus his responsibility for, what he has brought to life. In contrast, Mary Shelley emphasizes the ways in which her creative self intertwines with the object of her creation. Although she retreats from view to create, she does not claim transcendence. Instead, she shares with the creature her own problem of being marked. She "bids [her] hideous progeny [that is, her novel] go forth and prosper," and even expresses "an affection for it" (*WMS* 1:180). Situating herself in relation to the objects of her creative vision, Mary Shelley takes responsibility for what she sees and what she creates. This is embodied vision.

Strategic, situated invisibility allows Mary Shelley to create. However, through the parallels she draws between herself and the creature, Mary Shelley makes it clear that she, like Smith, would prefer being held in a sympathetic gaze to being invisible. The creature's period of invisibility—the time he spends living in the hovel outside the De Lacey cottage—marks both the most peaceful period of his life and the time of his greatest longing. Like Mary Shelley, who describes herself as "a devout but nearly silent listener" to the conversations between Byron and Shelley (*WMS* 1:23), the creature listens silently to the De Lacey family's conversation. He secretly helps Felix and Safie with the chores, calling himself "an invisible hand" (*WMS* 1:84). He spends his days observing the family's activities "unseen and unknown" (*WMS* 1:90). In spite of his apparent happiness in this invisibility, his deepest desire is to be held in the family's sympathetic gaze. By observing the De Laceys, he learns about familial love: "I heard of ... the birth and growth of children; how the father doated on the smiles of the infant ... how all the life and cares of the mother were wrapt up in the precious charge; ... of all the various relationships which bound one human being to another in mutual bonds" (*WMS* 1:90). This knowledge painfully highlights his own lack of parental love: "No father had *watched* my infant days, no mother had *blessed me with smiles* and caresses ... . What was I?" (*WMS* 1:90, my emphasis). The creature wishes to be held in the loving gaze of a parent. Diane Long Hoeveler explains that being seen in the eyes of his mother would solidify his positive identity: "He wants to be mirrored in the mother's eyes and to see himself there as a human being ... . It is the mother's eyes that will make him human, but it is a mirror he will never be able to enjoy" ("Fantasy" 19–20). Like her creature, Mary Shelley longs for her mother's sympathetic gaze. She longs, that is, for the impossible: to be reflected and held in her deceased mother's loving, accepting eyes.[13] Because the

_____

13 In a letter to Frances Wright dated two days after the thirtieth anniversary of her mother's death, Mary Shelley expresses her love for her mother and her own memory of the ambitions that Shelley—deceased 5 years—had for her as the daughter of Wollstonecraft: "[I]n addressing me rather on the score of my relations, than myself you touch the right chord to win my (affection) attention, & excite my interest. The memory of my Mother has been always been [sic] the pride & delight of my life; & the admiration of others for her, has been the cause of most of the happiness (of my life) I have enjoyed. Her greatness of soul & my father [sic] high talents have perpetually reminded me that I ought to degenerate as little as I could from those from whom I derived my being. For several years with Mr. Shelley I was blessed with the companionship of one, who fostered this ambition & inspired that of being

person who watches her most avidly, her future husband, sees her not as a mother would, but in comparison to how her mother was, Mary Shelley must escape his gaze in order to create.

Both Smith and Mary Shelley invoke medical categories to explore the cultural conditions that make it possible for women's suffering and women's creativity to be seen. Smith revises her culture's definition of melancholia to allow for the legitimate expression of emotion by women. She intervenes in the cult of sensibility's formulation of the sympathetic gaze to insist on both the authenticity of women's suffering and the authority of women's vision. Although she depicts a range of suffering and seeing bodies for the readers of her sonnets, Smith, like Mary Shelley, expresses the desire to hide from the hostile gaze at times. Mary Shelley utilizes her culture's fear of the Egyptian ophthalmia epidemic as a physical metaphor for the fear of difference that shuts down communication. She suggests that cultures tend to regard those marked by difference or disease as either inferior (in the endemic model) or as threatening (in the epidemic model). Mary Shelley explores the question of how being seen affects one's ability to create narrative, and on this point she is ambivalent—to be held in a sympathetic gaze is to express oneself freely and productively (as Victor does with Walton), but to be marked by the gaze of another is to find one's creative expression shut down (as with the creature). When cultural invisibility is impossible to overcome, real invisibility is a viable strategy.

Both authors distinguish their strategies for creative survival from similar strategies used by men. The male melancholic literary genius and Victor Frankenstein have a great deal in common. Both create alone in their study or lab, cut off from social interaction and emotional engagement. Both deny their bodies, thus seeking to observe without being observed. In contrast to the male melancholic genius, Smith insists on the interrelationship of—rather than the opposition between—emotion and reason, and portrays the sufferer as both seeing and seen in the same moment of sympathetic interaction. Although she chooses to emphasize her invisibility, Mary Shelley situates her creative vision in a physical context that pointedly contrasts with Victor's solipsistic gaze. Neither Smith nor Mary Shelley endorses Romantic solitude. Instead, both authors nourish their creativity with the desire for a sympathetic response to their suffering and their art.

Mary Shelley, however, has less faith in the power of seeing than does Smith—that is, less faith in the power of empirical evidence to change society. Smith emphasizes the female sufferer's ability not just to be seen but to look, thus claiming immersion in sensibility as a position of strength for women while fighting the man of sensibility's tendency to objectify and appropriate women's suffering. She imagines a sympathetic world in which women's genius can flourish. Mary Shelley, in contrast, explores the conditions that limit sympathetic interaction. Most strikingly, she suggests that Victor displaces his potential sympathetic concern for the creature in front of him onto a worried fantasy about the potential worldwide destruction this creature might

---

worthy of him ... yet you must not fancy that I am what I wish I were, and my chief merit must always be derived, first from the glory these wonderful beings have shed [?*around*] me, & then for the enthusiasm I have for excellence & the ardent admiration I feel for those who sacrifice themselves for the public good" (*LMWS* ii.3–4).

cause. In short, Mary Shelley teaches readers that worrying about distant or imagined disasters can blind one to present suffering. Mary Shelley then explores the potential for narrative to redirect attention to the immediate claims of actual subjectivity and suffering. Longing to be held by a sympathetic eye, she instead imagines situated invisibility as a strategy for escaping the judgmental gaze.[14] The contrast between Smith's and Mary Shelley's faith in visual perception surely reflects the difference between Smith's immersion in revolutionary hope while writing the *Elegiac Sonnets* between 1784 and 1797 and Mary Shelley's composition of *Frankenstein* in post-Napoleonic Europe. By 1816, it no longer seemed inevitable that making suffering visible would be enough to inspire the social change necessary to relieve that suffering.

---

14 Mary Shelley's desire to be looked upon by a sympathetic eye did not waver. On New Year's Eve, 1834, she muses: "What can I ask for?—Ah what! for something that is not here—for sympathy! for the eye of affection! for the interchange of thought—the trust & hope in another" (*JMS* 544).

PART 2
Healing

Chapter 3

The Journey to Heal Melancholia: Mary Wollstonecraft's *Letters from Norway*

"[The melancholic] must be removed from his situation and his environment, if possible by a journey to a far distant place, which involves much excitement, much discomfort, and much activity ... . For such patients traveling is a universal medicine."

Johann Christian Heinroth

Mary Wollstonecraft's journey to Scandinavia in 1795 began in the midst of despair. Ostensibly, she sought to help her estranged lover, the American businessman Gilbert Imlay, recover money lost in his effort to profit from breaking the British blockade against France (Kelly *Revolutionary* 174). Although Imlay trusted Wollstonecraft with his business transactions, even giving her power of attorney, he may also have been trying to remove her from London, where he had taken a new lover (Wardle 225). He conceived the idea for the trip after Wollstonecraft, severely distressed about Imlay's infidelity and about the general disintegration of the relationship following the birth of their daughter Fanny, attempted suicide with an overdose of laudanum (Tomalin 224). She was deeply disappointed by Imlay's infidelity and waning affection; his behavior contradicted her hope that they had established a progressive relationship without the legal bond and attendant disadvantages of marriage. Wollstonecraft saw in the trip the potential for producing a travel book (Todd *Mary* 303). Writing the travel narrative to earn money became increasingly important to her over the course of the trip, as she strengthened her resolve to separate her finances from Imlay's. In spite of this emotional turmoil, Wollstonecraft took comfort in her daughter Fanny, who with the nanny Marguerite Fournée, accompanied her on the journey.

The despair underlying these travels resulted from political as well as personal causes. Shortly before her relationship with Imlay began to dissolve, Wollstonecraft's idealism about the French Revolution was destroyed by the violent deaths or imprisonment of many of her friends during the Reign of Terror, which she lived through in Paris (Tomalin 121–43, 162–63). And, as Barbara Taylor explains, "Wollstonecraft was no mere spectator of revolution," but was helping members of the National Convention write policy proposals for their education committee when the Reign of Terror began (148). Wollstonecraft attributes her melancholic mood to betrayals by both "the world" and "friends": "How frequently has melancholy and even misanthropy taken possession of me, when the world has disgusted me and friends have proved unkind" (*WMW* 6:248–49). Her disappointment in love and disillusionment with political ideals intertwined to shake her faith in the potential of "fellow feeling," whether between two people or as the basis of a progressive society (Yousef 544). In addition, her private emotional suffering amplified the sense of dislocation and distress caused by the political turbulence she experienced first hand.[1] This intense personal and public upheaval blurred the boundary between internal and external suffering.

The journey that Wollstonecraft recounts in the twenty-five letters of her 1796 travel narrative *Letters Written During a Short Residence in Sweden, Norway and Denmark* is not only a business trip and new writing project, then, but also an attempt to heal her emotional pain and melancholia while traveling through picturesque, sublime, and beautiful landscapes.[2] The physical motion of travel, I will argue, is a crucial element of this effort to heal herself. In her essay exploring the meanings of movement in *Letters from Norway,* Mary Favret argues that Wollstonecraft "takes the restlessness and dislocation that marked her own life, as well as the society she observed in northern Europe, and tries to shape them into a style, an argument, and a political stance" (*"Letters"* 209). I would add that the discomfort and motion of travel serve to normalize Wollstonecraft's more traumatic experience of dislocation. While traveling, she re-experiences the traumatic feelings of itinerancy and isolation in a more controllable and pleasurable form. More to the point of this study, the salutary effect of travel for Wollstonecraft, I will argue, is dependent on visual perception. Rapturous descriptions of the intense pleasure she feels when looking at natural scenes erupt in the midst of the author's more measured observations about the people, architecture, cultural practices, and economic and political structures she encounters on her journey: "With what ineffable pleasure have I not gazed—and gazed again, losing my breath through my eyes—my very soul diffused itself in the scene" (*WMW* 6:280). Her sight releases her breath and her soul into the external world, her soul eventually "seeming to become all senses" (*WMW* 6:280). As her identity is diffused through her eyes into the "scene," she describes an exchange of sympathy or fellow feeling with nature and an attendant, if temporary, sense of wholeness and health.

Furthermore, in her movement through and description of the Scandinavian scenery, Wollstonecraft responds to medical recommendations for health travel. As I demonstrate below, medical treatises by Romantic-era physicians assert that the motion, exercise, and change of scenery inherent in travel helped to divert the melancholic from unhealthy rumination. These claims for the salutary nature of journeys overlap with the visually based pleasures of picturesque touring described by William Gilpin: especially delight, change of scene, and variety. Critics such as Malcolm Andrews, Ann Bermingham, Elizabeth Bohls, Nigel Everett, Jill Heydt-Stevenson, Alan Liu, and Jeanne Moskal have demonstrated the degree to which the picturesque aesthetic intertwines with political, social, economic, and

---

1   Todd describes the overlap between personal and political distress during the period just before Wollstonecraft's first suicide attempt: "For Wollstonecraft the horrors of the French Revolution now paralleled personal horrors and made them more heroic; public and private coalesced in individual suffering" (*Mary* 282).

2   Following Mary Shelley's example in *History of a Six-Weeks Tour*, I refer to Wollstonecraft's travel narrative as *Letters from Norway*.

gender ideologies. To these studies, I wish to add a consideration of the resonance between the culturally rich practice of picturesque tourism and concurrent health theory.

In treating picturesque journeys as therapeutic pilgrimages, Wollstonecraft portrays the interaction between her mind and the landscape as restorative. Wollstonecraft's discussion of this interchange challenges medical ideology— including gendered definitions of melancholia and essentialist definitions of how women's minds function. As I explain in chapter 1, eighteenth-century medical writers represented women's nervous illnesses as resulting from excessive sensibility and lack of rational capability. In contrast, they defined melancholia as the illness of male intellectuals. In *Letters from Norway*, Wollstonecraft, like Charlotte Smith, repeatedly emphasizes both her intellectual power and emotional depth. For example, she reveals a close relationship between the sublime landscape and her melancholic thoughts and emotions. The comparison she draws between lofty views and the dispirited mind's endless cogitation associates her thinking with what Thomas Trotter and other physicians describe as the extreme rationality characteristic of melancholic "literary men." Yet, while medical writers portray the male melancholic as rational to the exclusion of emotion, Wollstonecraft depicts the extremes of the sublime landscape as a reflection not only of her active mind but also of her tumultuous emotion. Associating both expanse of thought and height of emotion with the sublime landscape, Wollstonecraft revises Edmund Burke's account of the sublime and beautiful in his treatise, *A Philosophical Inquiry into the Origin of our Ideas about the Sublime and the Beautiful* (1757) and challenges gendered notions of nervous illness. Whereas Burke associates the beautiful with a pleasing feminine weakness, and the sublime with awe-inspiring masculine power, Wollstonecraft sees sublime vistas as metaphors for a woman's powerful emotion and melancholic rumination.[3] At the same time, she considers the social risks and medical benefits of cultivating women's sensibility to appreciate the landscape, and she suggests that although sensibility can increase women's vulnerability to illness, it can also heighten their sensitivity to the healing power of the landscape and nurture their ability to imagine social change. Thus, according to Wollstonecraft, the eyes' exploration of picturesque scenes helps to regulate sensibility and to restore order to the suffering mind. In addition, Wollstonecraft's identification with these scenes elucidates the particular nature of her desire for human sympathy and intimacy.

Health Travel

Wollstonecraft's representation of picturesque journeys as therapeutic emerged within the context of the eighteenth- and nineteenth-century practice of health travel

---

3   Wollstonecraft's revision of Burke and Gilpin illustrates geographer Gillian Rose's observation that women have had to challenge masculine visual ideology in order to find "a feminine position from which to perceive the land" (111). Rose characterizes this kind of appreciation of the landscape as "the rearticulation of traditional space so that it ceases to function primarily as the space of sight for a mastering gaze, but becomes the locus of relationships" (112).

in England, when physicians recommended that members of the upper classes take excursions to cure their nervous illnesses. In *A Sentimental Journey Through France and Italy by Mr. Yorick* (1768), Laurence Sterne pokes fun at fellow British travelers, noting that these "idle People ... leave their native country and go abroad" for one of the following reasons: "Infirmity of body, Imbecility of mind, or Inevitable necessity" (33–34). Medical treatises identifying the best climates, guidebooks mapping out the best routes for invalids, travel narratives written by ill persons, and fictional depictions of health travel were common.[4] An expedition abroad for one's health was an extension of the popularity of traveling to spas for treatment. Historian Jeremy Black describes the gradual transition from spa holidays to health tourism in the eighteenth century: "To travel *abroad* for health represented a fusion of two of the more important developments in upper-class activities in this period: tourism and travelling for health" (181, original emphasis). The itinerary for health travel added several important destinations to the basic grand tour's route through Paris and the major cities in Italy. Sites in southern France and Italy—especially Montpellier and Naples—were acclaimed for their climates, and invalids journeyed there for lengthy stays. Consumptive patients' desire to convalesce in "healthy" climates such as Italy and France accounts for much of this tourism. To visit a particular climate for medical treatment was similar to visiting a spa: both focused on the healing potential of a single location and required a stay of several months.

Both medical and invalid authors, however, frequently render the *motion* of travel itself—in the sense that the body both moves itself in exercise and is propelled through scenes—as more therapeutic than the climate or the spa. For example, in his treatise *Change of Air, or the Philosophy of Travelling* (1831), physician James Johnson claims that health travel is more efficient for restoration than is attending a spa: "How many thousand opulent invalids saunter away their time and their wealth, at watering-places in this country ... with little or no improvement of constitution, when a three months' course of constant exercise in the open air would cure all their maladies!" (130). Johnson actually conducted an experiment—taking six men and women on a three-month tour of the continent—to document the value of fast-paced travel for health, particularly for mental health:

> The experiment was tried, whether a constant change of scene and air, combined with almost uninterrupted exercise, active and passive, during the day—principally in the open air, might not ensure a greater stock of health, than slow journeys and long sojourns on the road. (109)

During the tour, he had the opportunity "not only to investigate its physiological effects on [his] own person and those of his party ... but to make constant inquiries among the numerous ... travelers" whom he met (112). Based on this data, he recommends fast-paced travel to melancholic patients as a more effective and affordable therapy than an extended spa visit.

---

4   For an account of health travel through the post-Napoleonic period, see my essay (as Beth Dolan Kautz): "Movement, Melancholia, and Madness: American and British Health Travelers in Post-Napoleonic Europe" in *Revolutions and Watersheds: Transatlantic Dialogues 1775–1815*.

Other physicians praise the virtues of health travel in comparison to talking about problems, resting, and staying near home. They consistently claim that the physical exercise and change of scenery inherent in travel will help to dislodge a patient from the emotional mire of melancholia. The German physician Johann Christian Heinroth notes that if talking with a melancholic patient fails to offer relief, "he must be removed from his situation and his environment, if possible by a journey to a far distant place, which involves much excitement, much discomfort, and much activity" (2:358). "For such patients," he says, "traveling is a universal medicine" (2:358). Similarly, Robert Whytt observes that "when low spirits or melancholy have been owing to long-continued grief, anxious thoughts, or other distress of the mind, nothing has done more service than ... daily exercise, especially travelling" (*Observations* 227). William Buchan recommends long voyages for nervous patients: "[C]hange of place, and the sight of new objects, by diverting the mind, have a great tendency to remove these complaints. For this reason a long journey, or a voyage, is of much more advantage than riding short journeys near home" (*Domestic* 424–25). These physicians prescribe engagement with the outside world and physical movement as cures for melancholia.

Like Johnson, Wollstonecraft compares "taking the waters" with other salutary pleasures of travel. Delayed in Tonsberg for three weeks, Wollstonecraft bathes and takes mineral waters for the melancholia and physical weakness she has experienced over the past months: "Chance ... led me to discover a new pleasure ... beneficial to my health. I wished to avail myself of my vicinity to the sea, and bathe" (*WMW* 6:280–1). She also drinks from a basin of water that tastes of the chalybeate (iron) found in spas. After a few weeks, she finds that her "constitution has been renovated" (*WMW* 6:280). She praises sea bathing and the mineral waters for their healing effect. However, Wollstonecraft, like Johnson, suggests that the recuperation of her health is due as much to by-products of travel as to the healing baths and water: "[T]he good effect of the various waters which invalids are sent to drink, depends, I believe, more on the air, exercise and change of scene, than on their medicinal qualities" (*WMW* 6:281). Although her three weeks in Tonsberg allow her to take a much-abbreviated spa vacation, ultimately she values the motion of travel and viewing the landscape—"exercise and change of scene"—as much as her time spent in the waters. As Bohls argues, Wollstonecraft retains a consistent emphasis on her bodily experience in *Letters from Norway*, in this case connecting the restoration of her physical well-being with aesthetic pleasure (*Women* 168).

Sharing Wollstonecraft's dual focus on health and aesthetics, fictional works of the period describe the landscape health travelers see during their pilgrimages. These texts, like *Letters from Norway*, expand on the medical recommendation for movement and exercise by emphasizing the visual pleasures of travel. Published two years before *Letters from Norway*, for example, Ann Radcliffe's popular *The Mysteries of Udolpho* (1794) depicts a physician's recommendation for travel. After Emily St. Aubert's mother dies, her father's grief begins to impair his physical health: "His physician now ordered him to travel; for it was perceptible that sorrow had seized upon his nerves, weakened as they had been by the preceding illness; and *variety of scene*, it was probable, would, by amusing his mind, restore them to their proper tone" (25, my emphasis). The physician prescribes the air of Languedoc and Provence, but rather than go directly to these locations, St. Aubert chooses a route rich in sublime and picturesque scenes: "St. Aubert, instead of taking the more direct road, that ran along the Pyrenees to Languedoc, chose one that, winding over the heights, afforded much more extensive views and greater variety of Romantic scenery" (27). Radcliffe's extensive descriptions of the landscape allude to the power of picturesque scenes to inspire "delicious melancholy" and "complacency" of mind (45–46). Similarly, twenty-two years after her mother's travel narrative was published, Mary Shelley portrays Victor Frankenstein's insensitivity to the beauties of the landscape as a sign of his ill health, and his travel through the sublime landscape as an attempt to heal his melancholia. In *Frankenstein* and her final travel narrative *Rambles in Germany and Italy*, the subject of chapter 5, Mary Shelley not only reflects her culture's understanding of travel and landscape viewing as salutary practices, but also pays tribute to her own mother's journey, demonstrating that she "sees" her mother's suffering. By reflecting Wollstonecraft's efforts to heal herself in these works, Mary Shelley offers her mother a grown daughter's companionship.

The Salutary Landscape

These literary accounts of the salutary landscape have roots in both medical and aesthetic discourse. In fact, medical theories about the health value of focusing one's attention on the outside world correspond with claims about the psychological and physical effects of learning to see the landscape through three major aesthetic frames—the sublime, the beautiful, and the picturesque. In his *Enquiry*, Burke speculates at length about the effect of the sublime and beautiful on the implicitly male perceiver's state of mind.[5] While the sublime inspires fear and awe, the beautiful engenders feelings of tranquility and love. In the fourth part of his *Enquiry*, Burke describes the ways in which the body registers the psychological effects of the sublime and the beautiful. The fear inspired by the sublime mimics physical pain:

> [A] man in great pain has his teeth set, his eye-brows are violently contracted, his forehead is wrinkled, his eyes are dragged inwards, and rolled with great vehemence, his hair stands on end, the voice is forced out in short shrieks and groans, and the whole fabric totters. Fear or terror ... exhibits exactly the same effects. (131)

In contrast, the "characteristic effect of beauty" on the viewer is relaxation (155). In both cases, the psychological effect registers physically.

Burke's descriptions of the effects of the sublime and beautiful on both mind and body, along with medical theories about the benefits of travel, prepare the way for Romantic-era writers' understanding of the healing effects of viewing various landscapes. As I discuss below, Wollstonecraft modifies aspects of Burke's aesthetic theory but shares his belief in the physiological effects of viewing the landscape. In her essay "On Poetry, and Our Relish for the Beauties of Nature" (1798), Wollstonecraft argues that "the true poets" were "observers of nature" rather than observers of a

---

5   See Bohls (*Women*), Lawrence, and Moskal ("The Picturesque") for discussions of Wollstonecraft's revision of Burke's gendered aesthetic.

literary tradition, and that poetry inspired directly by nature has both aesthetic and therapeutic effects. These poets "charm our cares to sleep," "rouse the passions," and "amend the heart" (7:10). Traveling in Scandinavia shortly after her attempted overdose, and revising this manuscript for publication in the months following her attempted drowning, Wollstonecraft movingly asserts that "the beauties of nature ... force even the sorrowing heart to acknowledge that existence is a blessing" (*WMW* 6:307).[6] Seeing the beauty of nature inspires "the sorrowing heart" to embrace life and health. William Wordsworth echoes this view in the posthumously published essay "The Sublime and the Beautiful": "[I]t is impossible that a mind can be in a *healthy* state that is not frequently and strongly moved both by sublimity and beauty" (*The Prose* 349, my emphasis). More famously, Wordsworth's remembered landscape in "Tintern Abbey" has a physiological effect that leads to psychic healing. These "forms of beauty," even in memory, create "sensations sweet, / Felt in the blood, and felt along the heart, / And passing even into my purer mind / With tranquil restoration" (*Lyrical Ballads* ll. 24, 28–31). The landscape affects the body and then the mind. Although Wollstonecraft and Wordsworth share a general understanding of sublime and beautiful landscapes as salutary, they differ strongly, as I explain below, in their view of the picturesque aesthetic.

For Wollstonecraft and others, the physical motion of perambulating and riding through the fluctuating landscape closely connects the practices of picturesque travel to the medically prescribed journey through changing scenes. The first accounts of scenic tourism in Europe emerged in the mid-eighteenth century, and this practice of traveling in search of landscapes peaked between 1780 and 1820 (Bohls *Women* 89), the same period during which physicians began recommending health travel as an end in itself. Essentially, picturesque travel involved following the directions of a guidebook from one scene, or "prospect," to another. This sense of quick movement through the landscape coincided well with contemporaneous medical recommendations such as Johnson's that melancholic patients seek a change of scenery. The most popular treatise on the picturesque—Gilpin's *Three Essays: On Picturesque Beauty: On Picturesque Travel: And on Sketching Landscape* (1789)—directly addresses the psychological effects of viewing picturesque scenes. Along with his specific instructions for representing a scene in a sketch, Gilpin includes a three-point argument for the psychological pleasures afforded by an interest in the picturesque—the pursuit of novelty and variety, "high delight," and judgment (*Three Essays* 47–50). Gilpin's treatise, which Wollstonecraft reviewed enthusiastically in September 1792, undoubtedly helped to shape understandings of picturesque travel as healthy.[7] Foregrounding the picturesque in the opening paragraph of *Letters from Norway*, Wollstonecraft vows—in spite of her exhaustion and depressed spirits—to offer her observations "as I travel through new scenes, whilst *warmed* with the

---

6 In late May of 1795, Wollstonecraft attempted overdose, leaving directions for Fanny's care and a public letter (Todd *Mary* 286–87). In late October of 1795, she attempted to drown herself in the Thames after finding that Imlay had set up house in London with another woman (Todd *Mary* 352–58).

7 Wollstonecraft wrote positive reviews of several of Gilpin's travel guides for the *Analytical Review* (*WMW* 7:161, 196–98, 386–88, 455–57).

impression they have made on me" (*WMW* 6:243, my emphasis). Gilpin notes in *Observations on the River Wye* (1782) that his descriptions of the landscape will "have the better chance of being founded in truth; as they are taken ... *warm* from the scenes of nature" (2, my emphasis). Like Gilpin, Wollstonecraft wishes to experience the landscape with physical immediacy; while he uses the word "warm" to highlight the freshness of the scene, however, she uses the word to draw attention to the landscape's effect on her body.

Wollstonecraft's depiction of picturesque views as physically and mentally nurturing parallels medical discourse about the relationships among the mind, the body, and the outside world. In the 1786 treatise *The Elements of Medicine*, John Brown outlines his theory of excitability, which is grounded in the common assumption that disease originates in and health is sustained by the interaction between the individual person and the external world. In Brown's system, each human has a base state of excitability that is affected by both external and internal agents. A related theory that informs the medical writings of Trotter, Whytt, and others outlines an active "sympathy" among the parts of the body. Trotter suggests that some parts of the body, such as the digestive system, are more sensitive to mental stimulation than are others (86). Diverting the mind's attention to the external world was thought to improve problems with the mind itself and, as a consequence, alleviate problems with sympathetic organs like the intestines. Although Gilpin does not make specific health claims for the effect of the landscape on the body, he does suggest that "tranquil" scenes might inspire "complacency of mind" (*Three Essays* 47). Wollstonecraft's representation of the picturesque intensifies and literalizes the therapeutic qualities only hinted at in Gilpin's version of the aesthetic. She looks both to the variety and also to the order of the picturesque landscape to help her manage the despair that threatens to engulf her.

In contrast to Wollstonecraft, Wordsworth depicts the picturesque as unhealthy, an indication of the pervasiveness of the aesthetic's association with health, which he wishes to counter. He describes his own interest in picturesque travel as a susceptibility to that "strong *infection* of the age" in *The Prelude* (XI.156, my emphasis). Elizabeth Fay explains "[I]n passing through the crucible of the French Revolution and [Wordsworth's] desertions of Annette and Caroline, melancholy became translated into the very detrimental psychodynamic of dejection" (160). Wordsworth suggests that his desire for moral certitude following these events fueled his interest in the systematic thinking of William Godwin's philosophy, which asserted that the application of reason to all aspects of social life would result in the discernment of truth (Wordsworth X.889, 893–901, Gill 85). In the 1850 version of *The Prelude*, Wordsworth refers to this period of his life as "the crisis of that strong disease," during which he finds "our blessed reason of least use / Where wanted most" (XI.306, 308–9). He connects his initial enthusiasm for Godwin's ideas to his concurrent interest in Gilpin's systematic aesthetic, describing himself during this period as "Giving way / To a comparison of scene with scene, / Bent overmuch on superficial things, / Pampering myself with meager novelties / Of colour and proportion" (XI.157–61). Wordsworth asserts that his exclusive reliance on reason in his effort to sort out the truth of a distressing political situation altered his aesthetic and moral vision:

What wonder, then, if, to a mind so far
Perverted, even the visible Universe
Fell under the dominion of a taste
Less spiritual, with microscopic view
Was scanned, as I had scanned the moral world? (1850, XII.88–92)

As many scholars have noted, Wordsworth eventually became disillusioned by the power of both philosophical reason and the picturesque aesthetic, establishing an alternative landscape aesthetic based in intuitive sense.[8] However, while Wordsworth rejects the picturesque for its systematic approach to vision, Wollstonecraft values the rational elements of the aesthetic because of their tempering effect on sensibility.

Sensibility

Echoing in a more personal way the concerns she expresses about cultivating women's sensibility in *A Vindication of the Rights of Woman* (1792), Wollstonecraft refers to her state of mind during the journey in Scandinavia as "a sensibility wounded almost to madness" (*WMW* 6:303). Great feeling leads to great pain. In her representation of both the despair she feels and also the healing she experiences from the landscape, Wollstonecraft stages both the negative impact and also the paradoxical and dynamic influence of sensibility on health and the psyche. Sensibility—exhibited in this case by the aesthetically trained eye—becomes the greatest point of connection between mental health and the landscape. The sensitivity that enables Wollstonecraft to appreciate the landscape's visual beauty and sublimity also exposes her to painful emotions: "Why has nature so many charms for me—calling forth and cherishing refined sentiments, only to wound the breast that fosters them?" (*WMW* 6:298). Nature refines Wollstonecraft's sensibility, but that refinement makes her as vulnerable to heartbreak and melancholy as it makes her receptive to "rapture": "Nature is the nurse of sentiment,—the true source of taste;—yet what misery, as well as rapture, is produced by a quick perception of the beautiful and sublime ... when every beauteous feeling and emotion excites responsive sympathy, and the harmonized soul sinks into melancholy, or rises to extasy" (*WMW* 6:271). Because she sees the potential for pain in nature's education of her own fervent responses, she worries about nurturing her daughter Fanny's sensibility: "With trembling hand I shall cultivate sensibility, and cherish delicacy of sentiment, lest, whilst I lend fresh blushes to the rose, I sharpen the thorns that will wound the breast I would fain guard—I dread to unfold her mind, lest it should render her unfit for the world she is to inhabit" (*WMW* 6:269). Acting in this moment as a mother who wishes to protect her daughter from the pain she has experienced herself, Wollstonecraft sees the problem of sensibility in quite concrete terms. This awareness of the social risks and health benefits of educating her daughter's sensibility is central to Wollstonecraft's representation of landscape

---

8   Scholars such as Alan Liu, Theresa M. Kelley (*Wordsworth's*), and Matthew Brennan examine Wordsworth's rejection of the picturesque as a means of establishing an alternative vision of the Romantic landscape, but they do not take literally his invocation of health and disease.

aesthetics in her travel narrative. Just as her role as mother intensifies her concerns about educating women's emotions, the experience of loving her child, discussed below, shapes her solution to this challenge.

Medical theories about melancholia lend even more poignancy to Wollstonecraft's concerns about cultivating Fanny's sensibility. The eighteenth-century medical writers discussed in chapter 1 portray women as "naturally" inclined to exhibit sensibility, men as innately capable of rational thought. Because Wollstonecraft attributes her state of mind to "wounded" sensibility and great disappointment, she is vulnerable to essentializing medical ideology that would categorize her as irrational. Medical writers such as Buchan would, no doubt, identify Wollstonecraft as a hysteric despite her lucid intelligence. However, by celebrating her ability to observe and to reason and by calling herself melancholic, Wollstonecraft complicates the gendered distinctions applied to nervous illnesses. Even as she expresses despair in *Letters from Norway*, she, like Smith, portrays herself as capable of analytical as well as emotional responses to the scenes, people, and cultures she encounters in her travels. Reflecting on both personal disappointment and the more general oppression of women, Wollstonecraft, again like Smith, portrays qualities of mind and heart as interdependent: "[W]e reason deeply, when we forcibly feel" (*WMW* 6:325). Demonstrating her sensibility, Wollstonecraft describes her compassionate identification with the deceased Queen Matilda of Denmark, persecuted for both her choice of lover and her attempted political reforms: "Poor Matilda! Thou hast haunted me ever since my arrival" (*WMW* 6:321).[9] She also reveals pride in her rational capability when she shares with the reader one Scandinavian host's comment that she is "a woman of observation" because she asks him "*men's questions*" (*WMW* 6:248, original emphasis). These accounts of Wollstonecraft's compassionate and intellectual interactions with the people she encounters highlight for the reader the combination of great emotive and rational capabilities that she possessed.

Wollstonecraft relies not only on words, but also on images to make these capabilities and her suffering visible to readers. Medical anthropologist Byron J. Good explains the "role of symbolization" in communicating to others the suffering caused by an invisible illness such as melancholia: "Given the close link between the visible and the real in ... medicine, resistance to imaging yields challenges to the ... disaffirmation of the sufferer. Absolute certainty to the sufferer, pain remains ambiguous and unverifiable to others; it remains interior, resisting social validation" (125). Wollstonecraft externalizes her melancholic pain, making it visible in her descriptions of the Scandinavian landscape. Most notable is her response to the waterfall at Sarpsfossen, which would have appeared to Wollstonecraft as it does in the scene depicted in Christian August Lorentzen's painting completed the same year Wollstonecraft visited the site (Figure 4).[10] Viewing this magnificent cascade

---

9   For a discussion of Wollstonecraft's identification with Queen Matilda and echoes of Wollstonecraft's description in Wordsworth and Percy Bysshe Shelley, see Swaab (25–26).

10   Later in the trip, Wollstonecraft also views the Trollhättan Falls. The waterfall near Fredrikstad to which she refers in this passage is the Sarpsfossen Falls. The falls were associated with Sarpsborg until 1567, when the town of Sarpsborg was destroyed in the war between Sweden, Norway, and Denmark. This disaster forced the people to move their town

near Fredrikstad, her mind follows the movement of the water from the dark recesses into the light: "The impetuous dashing of the rebounding torrent from the dark cavities which mocked the exploring eye, produced an equal activity in the mind: my thoughts darted from earth to heaven, and I asked myself why I was chained to life and its misery?" (*WMW* 6:311). Her thoughts imitate the sublime torrent as they dash in and out of dark mental cavities that elude understanding. Wollstonecraft, like her daughter Mary Shelley and like Smith, expresses the difficulty in making one's suffering—"the dark cavities"—visible to "the exploring eye." While Mary Shelley recommends strategic invisibility for those whose suffering is difficult to apprehend, and Smith makes her suffering visible by foregrounding the body, Wollstonecraft expresses and finds relief for suffering in the correspondence between external world and internal emotion.

Discovering the resonance between her emotional state and the waterfall is ultimately a pleasurable experience for Wollstonecraft:

> Still the tumultuous emotions this sublime object excited, were pleasurable; and, viewing it, my soul rose, with renewed dignity, above its cares—grasping at immortality—it seemed as impossible to stop the current of my thoughts, as of the always varying, still the same, torrent before me—I stretched out my hand to eternity, bounding over the dark speck of life to come. (*WMW* 6:311)

Providing a metaphor for her experience of melancholia—grounded in excesses of feeling and thinking—the cataract excites "tumultuous emotions," yet it also inspires an overflowing of the unstoppable "current of [her] thoughts." The identification of her thought process and emotion with the waterfall seems to offer relief. She begins to think of happiness in the afterlife, which she describes on a sublime scale as "eternity." In this example, the landscape, rather than Wollstonecraft's own body, gives her despair a sublime, corporeal presence. Anthropologist Godfrey Lienhardt explains that finding a visual image that represents the cause or experience of suffering allows the sufferer to "grasp its nature intellectually" and "to some extent transcend and dominate it in this act of knowledge" (170). By externalizing her tumultuous emotion and overflowing thought in the vision of the waterfall, Wollstonecraft simultaneously helps readers see her experience and helps herself gain some power over her suffering.

Wollstonecraft's description of the waterfall also enacts her practice of using visual perception to divert her attention from melancholic rumination. In these instances, she portrays sensibility as a tool that ameliorates rather than causes depressive feelings. Before visiting the waterfall discussed above, she reports that she suffers from "fatigue and melancholy": "How I am altered by disappointment!—When going to Lisbon, the elasticity of my mind was sufficient to ward off weariness, and my imagination still could dip her brush in the rainbow of fancy, and sketch futurity in glowing colours" (*WMW* 6:310). Just as she begins to regret not only the grief she

---

and its lumber industry to Fredrikstad. In 1702, the rebuilt Sarpsborg was again destroyed, this time in a landslide. Sarpsborg was not granted town status again until 1839. Thus, when Wollstonecraft visited the falls that are now associated with Sarpsborg, the closest town would have been Fredrikstad.

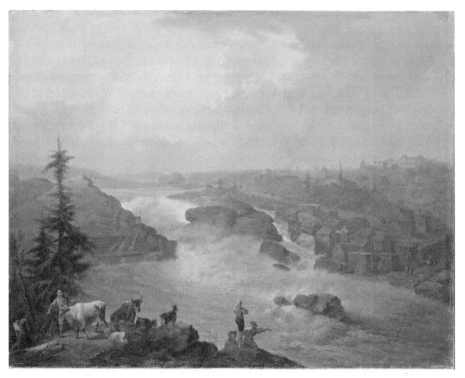

Fig. 4.   **C. A. Lorentzen.** *The Waterfall at Sarpsfossen.* **1795**

has experienced, but also its effect on her ability to create a positive vision of the future, Wollstonecraft deliberately focuses her attention on the landscape: "Now—but let me talk of something else—will you go with me to the cascade?" (*WMW* 6:310). She signals this transition from regret about the past to present hope with the word "now," interrupting her train of melancholic thought with an invitation to the reader to view the thunderous torrent. Looking at the waterfall, she finds release from circular, melancholic rumination: "Reaching the cascade, or rather cataract, the roaring of which had a long time announced its vicinity, my soul was hurried by the falls into a new train of reflections" (*WMW* 6:311). The velocity and reverberation of the turbulent waterfall immediately shifts her thoughts. Although it does not eliminate her despair, looking at the cascade helps Wollstonecraft move from obsession with the past to immersion in the present moment of the sublime landscape.

Healing in the Landscape

Wollstonecraft's practice of taking walks and viewing the landscape when melancholic thoughts and feelings become overwhelming upholds medical writers' enthusiasm for exercise and attention to new scenes. Listening to the distressing story of a wet nurse who has been abandoned by the father of her child, Wollstonecraft is reminded of her estrangement from Imlay and of her status as a single parent: "There was something in this most painful state of widowhood which excited my compassion, and led me to reflections on the instability of the most flattering plans of happiness, that were painful in the extreme" (*WMW* 6:283). Wollstonecraft attempts to soothe her "heart wringing in anguish" by taking a walk: "It was too early for thee to be abandoned, thought I, and I hastened out of the house, to take my solitary evening's walk" (*WMW* 6:283). Noting Wollstonecraft's reference to Rousseau's *Rêveries du promeneur solitaire* in this passage, Eleanor Ty suggests that Wollstonecraft's shift from sympathizing to walking is "an effort not to identify too closely with the young woman who is represented by Wollstonecraft as a helpless victim and widow. Instead, she wishes to be the independent nature lover, at peace with herself" ("History" 80). Moving from the young woman's presence into a walk, Wollstonecraft shifts out of melancholic rumination into a more active and powerful sense of herself.

Like the healthful shift created by walking, shifts between awe-inspiring vistas and tranquil views rouse Wollstonecraft's mind from the grief in which it is mired. Exploring the environs of her first landing point in Scandinavia, the bay of Möllosund, she observes: "I walked on, still delighted with the rude beauties of the scene; for the sublime often gave place imperceptibly to the beautiful, dilating the emotions which were painfully concentrated" (*WMW* 6:247). While exercising her body to recover from the eleven-day voyage from England, Wollstonecraft also exercises her mind by focusing her eyes on the aesthetic changes in the landscape. Like Burke, she is interested in the shift between these opposite states of arousal and repose. However, the shift from sublime to beautiful does not create as striking a difference in Wollstonecraft's response as Burke's influential account of the categories suggests. In her descriptions of the landscape, Wollstonecraft seeks to "toughen" Burke's portrayal of beauty as weakness by aligning the beautiful with rationality, an association that Burke disavows (Lawrence 92). Rather than abruptly plunging her from painful to pleasurable sensations and back again, the variation between sublime and beautiful—that is, between great feeling and rationality—has a holistic, soothing effect. Crossing the often "bare and sublime" mountains between Sweden and Norway, she experiences a transition that is more dramatic than (but just as healing as) the fluctuating landscape in the bay of Möllosund: "[A]fter mounting the most terrific precipice, we had to pass through a tremendous defile, where the closing chasm seemed to threaten us with instant destruction, when turning quickly, verdant meadows and a beautiful lake relieved and charmed my eyes" (*WMW* 6:265). Her eyes' apprehension of this migration between the sublime rocks on the one hand, and the beautiful meadows and lake on the other, serves to "dilate" painful feelings about the past by immersing the mind in the ever-changing present. In addition, the visual transition between these scenes externalizes her emotion. She sees the oscillation between extreme feeling and organized thought embodied in the contrast between sublime and beautiful scenes; seeing her mood externalized, she feels her painful internal fluctuations relieved.

In such moments of dilation, one savors Wollstonecraft's passage between sublime and beautiful settings, recognizing with her how essential this mobility is to her sense of well-being. Wollstonecraft's emphasis on movement in these therapeutic shifts between sublime and beautiful landscapes invokes the picturesque aesthetic.

Moskal argues that in Wollstonecraft's portrayal of the picturesque landscape in *Letters from Norway*, "the sublime merges, in a most un-Burkean way, with the beautiful" ("The Picturesque" 276). Heydt-Stevenson discusses the ways in which theorists such as Uvedale Price promoted the picturesque as a mediating aesthetic, commingling the sublime and the beautiful. Specifically, she states that Price's version of the picturesque "is feminine but founded on energy and vitality" (269). Writing during the same years, Wollstonecraft and Price agree that the picturesque landscape is lively and dynamic, though Wollstonecraft expands the potential of such vigor when she finds that viewing picturesque landscapes provides an antidote to her emotional suffering.[11]

In her enthusiasm for what Gilpin terms "delight" and in her modification of Gilpin's descriptions of "the pursuit of novelty," "framing," and "variety," Wollstonecraft creates a salutary picturesque. Invoking the language of picturesque delight, Wollstonecraft describes the healing effect of viewing the landscape at Möllosund Bay: "I felt its picturesque beauty ... . How silent and peaceful was the scene. I gazed around with rapture, and felt more of that spontaneous pleasure which gives credibility to our expectation of happiness, than I had for a long, long time before" (*WMW* 6:247). This picturesque scene, inviting her rapturous gaze and inspiring immediate felicity, gives her hope for future happiness. In his *Three Essays,* Gilpin notes that "We are most delighted, when some grand scene, rising before the eye, strikes us beyond the power of thought ... and every mental operation is suspended. In this pause of intellect ... an enthusiastic sensation of pleasure overspreads it" (49–50). The "pause of intellect" that accompanies picturesque delight proves therapeutic for Wollstonecraft. For a moment at least, the picturesque scene at Möllosund suspends remembered terrors and grief: "I forgot the horrors I had witnessed in France, which had cast a gloom over all nature, and [were] ... damped by the tears of disappointed affection to be lighted up afresh ... . [C]are took wing while simple fellow feeling expanded my heart" (*WMW* 6:247). Viewing the picturesque landscape opens her heart and encourages "fellow feeling," or a sympathetic connection with others. Although the picturesque aesthetic is often associated with nostalgia, here it helps release her mind from its vexing focus on loss, allowing her to concentrate for a moment on the possibility of fellow feeling.

The hope for fellow feeling informs Wollstonecraft's interaction with many of the natural objects she observes. In an ebullient mood, she says of herself: "Let me catch pleasure on the wing—I may be melancholy to-morrow. Now all my nerves keep time with the melody of nature" (*WMW* 6:294). The musical metaphor, "nerves keep time with the melody of nature," suggests that her emotions accord with both the rhythm and the song of the landscape. In other words, she experiences harmony with both the structure of the landscape and also with the relationships between its elements, or notes. Healing for Wollstonecraft depends on a harmonious and sympathetic connection between self and world. Wollstonecraft envisions wellness as a sociable rather than an individualistic state. Accordingly, Wollstonecraft contrasts the separateness one feels in despair with the promise of belonging offered by sympathy: "I have then considered myself as a particle broken off from the grand mass of mankind;—I was alone, till some involuntary sympathetic emotion, like the attraction of adhesion, made

---

11 Price's *Essays on the Picturesque* were published in 1794, 1795, and 1810.

me feel that I was still part of a mighty whole, from which I could not sever myself" (*WMW* 6:249). Giving the landscape human characteristics and human agency, Wollstonecraft elaborates further on this sense of reciprocal, sympathetic communication between nature and the beholder. The picturesque scenery on the way to Tonsberg displays a human expression: "The country still wore a *face of joy*—and my soul was alive to its charms" (*WMW* 6:298, my emphasis). The phrase "face of joy" gives the landscape an independent presence and emotional life and suggests the possibility that the countryside looks back at Wollstonecraft. The motion of travel normalizes her sense of isolation and dislocation. However, in the course of that travel, spontaneous flashes of sympathetic feeling join her again to "the mighty whole."

This sense of belonging results both from her sensitivity to the landscape's vitality and also from the projection of herself, or perhaps the sympathetic recognition of herself, in the landscape. On the seashore in Sweden, she notices that "[t]he scattered huts ... stand shivering on the naked rocks, braving the pitiless elements" (*WMW* 6:253). Burdened with grief, yet also exhibiting a great deal of courage as a 1790s Englishwoman traveling alone in Scandinavia, Wollstonecraft identifies with the "shivering" yet brave rocks. Similarly, on the boat to Stromstad, sailing among the rocks, which form "very picturesque combinations" (*WMW* 6:292), she sympathetically observes the trees that stand exposed on almost every ridge of the rocks and islands: "Few of the high ridges were entirely bare; the seeds of some pines or firs had been wafted by the winds or waves, and they stood to brave the elements" (*WMW* 6:292). Feeling isolated, she identifies with those seedlings who "brave the elements": "Sitting then in a little boat on the ocean, amidst strangers, with sorrow and care pressing hard on me,—buffeting me about from clime to clime,—I felt 'Like the lone shrub at random cast, / That sighs and trembles at each blast!'" (*WMW* 6:292).[12] Wollstonecraft moves from anthropomorphizing the seedlings as braving the weather to characterizing herself as a lonesome plant, cast onto the rocks at random and trembling at adverse conditions. Looking at the landscape, Wollstonecraft transforms the scene into a metaphor for her emotional situation, finding comfort in what she perceives as the sympathetic melancholy of nature—a companionship that she lacks with Imlay. The delight she feels in looking emerges not just from the momentary suspension of thought that Gilpin describes, but also from the visual representation in the landscape of her difficult emotions and of her intense desire for intimacy.

As this identification with the landscape suggests, Wollstonecraft's sense of movement through the Scandinavian outdoors differs most significantly from Gilpin's much parodied description of the pursuit of fresh views as a hunt. He comments: "[S]hall we suppose it a greater pleasure to the sportsman to pursue a trivial animal, than it is to the man of taste to pursue the beauties of nature?" (*Three Essays* 48). In contrast, Wollstonecraft uses the word "pursuit" to disparage the activity of commerce, which she partially blames for Imlay's lack of feeling. Favret observes that

---

12 Wollstonecraft alters two lines from Oliver Goldsmith's "The Traveller, or A Prospect of Society." The original lines are "Here let me sit in sorrow for mankind, / Like yon neglected shrub at random cast, / That shades the steep and sighs at every blast" (ll. 102–4). Changing "neglected" to "lone" and "shades the steep" to "trembles," Wollstonecraft emphasizes the subjective emotion of the shrub.

Wollstonecraft's most negative portrayal of movement erupts in her "charges against the ubiquitous movements of trade" ("*Letters*" 221). Wollstonecraft explains the effect of the "chase after wealth" on social relationships: "A man ceases to love humanity, and then individuals, as he advances in the chase after wealth ... . [T]o business, as it is termed, every thing must give way; nay, is sacrificed; and all the endearing charities of citizen, husband, father, brother, become empty names" (*WMW* 6:342). Just as the pursuit of wealth destroys sympathetic relationships, so it also damages the eyes of the pursuer. She observes that the commercial people of Hamburg are "ever on the watch, till their eyes lose all expression, excepting the prying glance of suspicion" (*WMW* 6:340). Wollstonecraft suggests that the rigidly hierarchical subject-object relationship inherent in commerce damages both one's fellow feeling and also one's ability to see beauty and to convey sympathy through the eyes.

In contrast, Wollstonecraft's engagement with new scenes in the mode of picturesque travel soothes rather than hardens the eyes. Rather than pursue scenes to consume them, Wollstonecraft finds that the tableaux themselves captivate her attention. She does not hunt them so much as they call out to her. As evening falls on Gothenburg, Wollstonecraft "calms her agitated breast" by listening to the "waters murmur, and fall with more than mortal music" (*WMW* 6:252). Nature offers its soothing sounds to her and beckons her to come outside: "A crescent hangs out in the vault before, which woos me to stray abroad:—it is not a silvery reflection of the sun, but glows with all its golden splendour" (*WMW* 6:252–53). The moon calls to her and offers a physical metaphor for a sympathetic relationship in which two bodies are equal: in Wollstonecraft's description, the moon recreates rather than just reflects the sun. Similarly, on the way to Frederikstad, the landscape has the power "to attract my attention, and beguile, if not banish, the sorrow that had taken up its abode in my heart" (*WMW* 6:315). Embracing rather than hunting picturesque scenery allows for a restorative reciprocity between landscape and viewer. While she rejects the pursuit of scenes, however, Wollstonecraft extols the healing effects of looking purposefully at the landscape as one travels. In her review of Gilpin's *Observations on the River Wye*, Wollstonecraft differentiates between rambling and scenic travel, between desultory observations and those informed by an aesthetically trained eye:

> If all travelers had ... some decided point in view ... to concentrate their thoughts, and connect their reflections, readers, who look for more than barren amusement, would be assisted to arrange [what they see] instead of rambling with an unfixed eye through a variety of desultory matter and detached observations, which no running interest, or prevailing bent in the mind of the writer rounds into a whole. (*WMW* 7:161)

Looking at the landscape with aesthetic purpose rather than with "an unfixed eye" and, at the same time, remaining open to the landscape's influence together help viewers like Wollstonecraft "concentrate their thoughts" and "connect their reflections."

Wollstonecraft further develops her sense of the aesthetic object as dynamic and active by supplementing Gilpin's notion of picturesque "variety" in terms of health travel.[13] According to Gilpin, the "great foundation of picturesque beauty"

---

13 See Bohls for a detailed discussion of Wollstonecraft's politically resonant revision of the picturesque aesthetic object (148–58).

is "the happy union of simplicity and variety" (*Three Essays* 28). Wollstonecraft's desire to find visual diversity not only within a scene, as Gilpin instructs, but also among scenes conveys a visceral sense of the body passing through the landscape. She recreates a moving panorama of "new scenes" in her narrative, thus offering a more visually textured and aesthetically sophisticated account of health travel than do the physicians recommending the motion of travel. Approaching Helgerac, Wollstonecraft emphasizes her movement through a changing landscape: "We passed ... through several beech groves, which still delighted me by the freshness of their light green foliage, and the elegance of their assemblage, forming retreats to veil, without obscuring the sun. I was surprised, at approaching the water, to find a little cluster of houses pleasantly situated, and an excellent inn" (*WMW* 6:291–92). We traverse with the author through these quickly shifting scenes: several beech groves, the water, the village. Wollstonecraft associates mental health and physical freedom with her body's vital, active passage through natural settings.

This passage through the landscape is not exclusively, but rather primarily, a visual experience. On the way to Stromstad, Wollstonecraft rhapsodizes about the visual pleasure of travel, again anthropomorphizing natural objects:

> The rocks which tossed their fantastic heads so high were often covered with pines and firs, varied in the most picturesque manner. Little woods filled up the recesses, when forests did not darken the scene; and vallies and glens, cleared of the trees, displayed a dazzling verdure which contrasted with the gloom of the shading pines. The eye stole into many a covert where tranquillity seemed to have taken up her abode, and the number of little lakes that continually presented themselves added to the peaceful composure of the scenery. (*WMW* 6:263)

The phrase, "rocks ... *were often* covered," communicates a sense of temporality (contrast, for example, "*many* rocks were covered"), and thus the feeling that she moves through, rather than pauses to look at, this landscape. Mentioning "[t]he *number* of little lakes that continually *presented themselves*," Wollstonecraft again calls attention to her transit through a series of scenes, highlighting the landscape's ability to "present" itself. Although no Claude glass frames these views, vision is crucial: as Wollstonecraft travels her "eye st[eals] into many a covert," searching the recesses of the landscape. Wollstonecraft is not merely a melancholic body being transported through scenes in a carriage, but a viewer whose eyes both receive the "dazzling verdure" of the trees and also actively explore the landscape's coverts and dark spaces in search of "tranquillity."

Wollstonecraft highlights both the receptive and creative aspects of visual perception not only when she passes through scenes, but also when she stops to describe scenes from a fixed point of view. In so doing, she modifies Gilpin's instructions to create a foreground in one's picturesque sketch by adding a branch or similar overhang to frame a prospect. On the way back to Sweden after a day trip to Halden, Norway, she notes: "The huge shadows of the rocks, fringed with firs, concentrating the views, without darkening them, excited that tender melancholy, which, sublimating the imagination, exalts, rather than depresses the mind" (*WMW* 6:267). The "huge shadows of rocks, fringed with firs" provide the frame, a necessary element in the picturesque aesthetic. By focusing her view on a structured scene, the frame transforms her painful melancholy into a tender melancholy. This sensitivity to the landscape exalts her spirits, allowing Wollstonecraft to consider "the play between the frame and chaos" (Heydt-Stevenson 270).

This example of framing suggests a modification of Bohls's argument that Wollstonecraft "destroy[s] the distance between a perceiver and a statically framed scene" (*Women* 151). I agree with Bohls that unlike Burke, whose aesthetic theory depended on distancing himself from the aesthetic object through hierarchical class and gender distinctions, Wollstonecraft depicts herself in much closer relation to the landscape (Bohls *Women* 158). And, unlike Gilpin, who recommends the erasure of crops and all but a few picturesque workers in one's sketch of a scene, Wollstonecraft closes, as Bohls so eloquently explains, the hierarchical distance between viewer and scene by allowing the landscape's energy, motion, and political resonance to exceed the viewer's frame. Yet, I argue, rather than do away altogether with the picturesque convention of framing, Wollstonecraft modifies it in some instances to help her revise the relationship between viewer and object. There is still distance in this framing, but it unfolds across horizontal rather than vertical space. It is the distance between the mirror and the body, between child and mother, between an intimate and oneself—a distance through which we see ourselves in the other and feel comforted rather than repelled by the resonance.

Many of the individual scenes that Wollstonecraft pauses to describe, then, are framed by a protective natural presence. This is not an aesthetic frame that excludes social relationships and material conditions, but rather a sheltering frame that intimately involves the viewer with the scene, the scene with the viewer. For example, arriving late in Tonsberg, she finds comfort in the view from her room: "The inn was quiet, and my room so pleasant, commanding a view of the sea, confined by an amphitheatre of hanging woods, that I wished to remain there" (*WMW* 6:270–71). In the shelter of the room, she overlooks the sea—which is protectively framed by the amphitheatre of woods—and feels the desire to stay. This vision of "confinement" feels secure rather than limiting. As Ty has argued, Wollstonecraft literalizes the metaphor of confinement in *The Wrongs of Woman* to illustrate women's social imprisonment (*Unsex'd* 31–45). In the inn at Tonsberg, however, Wollstonecraft experiences confinement not as maternal imprisonment, but as the woods' embrace of the sea, a comforting encirclement that reflects her own feelings of security provided by the pleasant inn. Looking out the window of her cozy room, she envisions a lateral correspondence with the sheltered sea. Having just discovered that she would be delayed for three weeks in Tonsberg, Wollstonecraft laments not bringing Fanny with her in the sentence preceding her description of the scene. Missing her child, she feels more poignantly the sense of happy enclosure sometimes associated with maternal love. There is protection in the distance of this "amphitheatrical view," as Ingrid Kuczynski terms it (35). However, because the distance helps Wollstonecraft see the reflection of her comforting room in the sheltering landscape, she feels protected by, rather than protected from, the view.

This womblike framing is one way in which Wollstonecraft imagines what Moskal so aptly describes as a picturesque landscape shaped by maternal affection. Moskal invokes Nancy Chodorow's object-relations theory and Melanie Klein's concept of maternal regression to explain Wollstonecraft's concurrent and sometimes overlapping representation of both herself and the landscape as maternal ("The Picturesque" 267). In short, feelings of love for one's own child intensify the mother's desire also to be mothered, and thus evoke a double identity as mother and child. As Moskal notes, this "multiplicity" is "more intense, Chodorow has shown, when the child is a daughter, as in Wollstonecraft's situation with Fanny Imlay in tow on most of her journey" ("The Picturesque" 267–68). Wollstonecraft's maternal feelings for Fanny unlock a desire to be mothered herself, and accordingly, she sees the protection she wishes both to give and to feel in the scenes she observes. On an estate in Norway, she admires the "aged pines" more than the house itself: "Time had given a grayish cast to their ever-green foliage; and they stood, like fires in the forest, sheltered on all sides by a rising progeny" (*WMW* 6:285). Portraying the trees as sheltered by their "progeny," Wollstonecraft creates a visible metaphor to help readers see her hope for the sheltering love she might share with her daughter Fanny.

A similar multiplicity of maternal identification pervades her description of walks near the ruins in Tonsberg: "Here I have frequently strayed, sovereign of the waste, I seldom met any human creature; and sometimes, reclining on the mossy down, under the shelter of a rock, the prattling of the sea has lulled me to sleep" (*WMW* 6:279). The rock offers Wollstonecraft a womblike shelter in which she is lulled to sleep by the lullaby of the maternal sea, which at the same time "prattles" like a child. Wollstonecraft wanders into a quintessentially picturesque scene, the ruins of a fort. Falling asleep within this scene—under the shelter of a picturesque rock—she then awakes, her "eye" following the sailboats as they seem to find shelter in the scene framed by pines:

> Balmy were the slumbers, and soft the gales, that refreshed me, when I awoke to follow, with an eye vaguely curious, the white sails, as they turned the cliffs, or seemed to take *shelter* under the pines which covered the little islands that so gracefully rose to render the terrific ocean beautiful ... . Everything seemed to harmonize into tranquility. (*WMW* 6:279–80, my emphasis)

She sees in the distant landscape the maternal shelter that she feels in her immediate contact with nature. Both the shelter she feels and its corresponding reflection in the external world offer her a deep sense of security and well-being. The disarray of external and internal worlds she experienced following the Reign of Terror is, for a moment at least, alleviated. The ordered and peaceful correspondence between the external landscape she sees and the emotion she feels seems to offer hope for change in the political realm as well.

Individual and Social Improvement

Wollstonecraft's hope for health and social change is grounded in what she sees as the close relationship between imagination and sensibility. Ty notes that "Wollstonecraft's idea of the imagination is closer to the late-eighteenth-century conception of sensibility" than to the "flash of imagination" described by Wordsworth ("History" 77). Wollstonecraft's aesthetic sensibility inspires her imagination; that is, her sensitivity to the external world helps her reconfigure, or re-imagine what she sees. Of pine and fir groves at night, she says: "nothing can be more picturesque, or, more properly speaking, better calculated to produce poetical images" (*WMW* 6:286). The picturesque landscape inspires "poetical images," restoring Wollstonecraft's productive creativity. The landscape also fuels the associative power of her imagination. In Risor she says, "Wandering there alone ... my mind was stored with ideas, which this new scene associated with astonishing rapidity" (*WMW* 6:295). She notes that "growing intimate with nature, a thousand little circumstances, unseen by vulgar eyes, give birth to sentiments dear to the imagination, and inquiries which expand the soul" (*WMW* 6:256). For these scenes to nurture the imagination, the eye must be refined rather than "vulgar" in its aesthetic sensitivity. The activity of the trained eye "gives birth" to both "sentiment" and rational "inquiries." Inspiring both thought and feeling, the landscape leads her to imagine social improvement: "The view of this wild coast, as we sailed along it, afforded me a continual subject for meditation. I anticipated the future improvement of the world, and observed how much man still had to do, to obtain of the earth all it could yield" (*WMW* 6:294). Wollstonecraft's sensibility, or sensitivity to the landscape, unlocks the imaginative thinking needed to conceive "the future improvement of the world."

By using the word "improvement" in connection with the aesthetic imagination, Wollstonecraft endorses Gilpin's enthusiasm for changing the world one is given. In *Observations, on Several Parts of England* (1792), Gilpin asserts: "He who works from imagination ... will in all probability, make a much better landscape, than he who takes all as it comes" (1). To create a pleasing sketch, the picturesque tourist's imagination must complement what the eye encounters in nature. Bohls argues that Gilpin's emphasis on the viewer's imagination "substitutes imaginary for real ownership and manipulation of the land" (*Women* 91). Gilpin advises, for example, that when painting a simple field, one should "break the surface of it ... [by] add[ing] trees, rocks, and declivities" (*Three Essays* 28), just as a propertied man would physically modify the landscape on his estate. Imaginatively remaking scenes afforded middle-class travelers a sense of visual "ownership" of the land. This visual remodeling of the scene, I argue, also gave melancholic travelers such as Wollstonecraft a greater sense of their own power to alter the external world. The ability to improve the external world would be a powerful sign of health for a person suffering from depressive feelings. Good cites examples of patients who first recognize their clinical depression when the world outside seems different: "It was the world that first seemed to change [because] the body as physical object and as agent of experience did not belong to separate worlds. The illness was present in the living body. It was experienced as a change in the lifeworld" (116–17). For Wollstonecraft, the disorder of the world was only partially the creation of her "jaundiced eye of melancholy" (*WMW* 6:331). In France, she witnessed a series of violent political actions that resonated deeply with the betrayal and interruption of future hope that she experienced in her personal life. Experiencing a positive correspondence between internal emotions and the external natural world, then, offers Wollstonecraft hope that the recovering self might also be projected into a healed social body.

Elaine Scarry's explanation of the relationships among suffering, vision, and the imagination in *The Body in Pain* offers a context for understanding Wollstonecraft's pleasure in replacing personal distress and political disappointment with aesthetic beauty. Scarry explains the equation of vision and imagination in literature: "It is because vision and hearing are, under ordinary conditions, so exclusively bound up with their object rather than their bodily location that they are the senses most frequently invoked by poets as the sensory analogues for the imagination" (165). The viewer's temptation to forget her own body is disrupted, however, when the eye itself becomes damaged and feels pain (by looking at the sun, for example), or when "the objects in the external field" begin "to appear distorted or blurred to her (that is, if the objects begin to become lost to her)" (165). In this moment, the viewer "will cease to experience vision only as objectified interior content and will begin to become more self-conscious of the event of 'seeing' itself: she no longer experiences the images ... without also experiencing her own body in the mode of aversiveness and deprivation" (165). Wollstonecraft's awareness of her own body in the act of looking results from the loss of the desired object. She illustrates the correspondence between desire for the aesthetic object and desire for the beloved in terms of this loss. At the end of her journey, she compares the actual unpleasantness of Hamburg, which looked much better "at a distance," with the loss of Imlay's love: "After a long journey, with our eyes directed to some particular spot, to arrive and find nothing as it should be, is vexatious, and sinks the agitated spirits. But I, who received the cruelest of disappointments, last spring, in returning to my home, term such as these emphatically passing cares" (*WMW* 6:339). Longing for Imlay to return her feelings, she looks with expectation at the beautiful vision of Hamburg in the distance, creating a substitute object for this longing. When Hamburg disappoints her "agitated spirits," she sinks back into painful thoughts about the loss of Imlay. Significantly, she uses vision to express these disappointments in aesthetic pleasure and in love.

This loss of the object of desire can be healed, Scarry explains, either by shifting one's desire to a new object or by imagining a new object if an actual object is not available: "Desire ... will, if deprived of its object, begin to approach the neighborhood of pain, as in ... prolonged objectless longing; conversely, when such a state is given an object, it is itself experienced as a pleasurable ... because self-eliminating physical occurrence" (166). There is nothing painful about desire itself "if the person experiencing [it] inhabits a world where ... a companion is near" (166). But, if, as in the case of Wollstonecraft, the lost objects of desire—Imlay and the French Republic—cannot be replaced with a "naturally-occurring" object of desire, then "imagining is ... the ground of last resort" (166). Thus, the imagination of a future, mutually protective relationship with her daughter Fanny begins to replace her desire for Imlay, and the hope for slow political change begins to replace her former hope for the success of the French Revolution.[14] This transition from loss to

---

14 Wollstonecraft articulates her hope for reform rather than revolution in the Appendix to *Letters from Norway*: "[H]urry the benevolent reformer into a labyrinth of errour, who aims at destroying prejudices quickly which only time can root out, as the public opinion becomes subject to reason. An ardent affection for the human race makes enthusiastic characters eager to produce alteration in laws and governments prematurely. To render them useful and permanent, they must be the growth of each particular soil, and the gradual fruit of the ripening understanding of the nation, matured by time, not forced by an unnatural fermentation" (*WMW* 6:346).

imagination is catalyzed by the landscape, because Wollstonecraft realizes the extent of her loss when she sees it projected onto the natural world.

Wollstonecraft's portrayal of her body moving through a living landscape reconfigures medical discourse and articulates the therapeutic possibilities inherent in the picturesque aesthetic. This aesthetic allows her to resist both the essentialized body-as-object promoted by medical writers who attribute women's nervous illness to their uteruses, and the Burkean disembodied aesthetic eye surveying scenes from a distance. Rather than separate the observed, feminized landscape (body) from the observing masculine eye (mind), Wollstonecraft imagines both viewer and landscape as maternal, vulnerable, and mutually sympathetic. The aesthetic object and the spectator both contain mind and body; the object thinks and the subject moves. Like Smith, Wollstonecraft challenges the conception of women's nervous illnesses as body-based and nonrational, even as she invokes the practice of health travel to reframe the picturesque journey and to offer us the image of a whole person interacting on an equal level with a sympathetic landscape.[15] In this demonstration of the sympathetic relationship or fellow feeling between the landscape and the viewer, Wollstonecraft exhibits hope for individual healing and social change, which she regards as interdependent. Whereas Smith longs for a sympathetic world to recognize her suffering, Wollstonecraft imagines the world and the self undergoing positive change together.

Thus, Wollstonecraft looks at the therapeutic landscape and imagines the "future improvement of the world." Although she acknowledges that there are ill-made picturesque scenes, just as she acknowledges the dangers of sensibility, she never relinquishes her faith in the possibility that humans can change the conditions we inherit, that we can build a more mutually sheltering and maternally sympathetic world. Her enthusiasm for the "improved" land on an estate in Sweden expresses the value she places on maternal sympathy: "I visited, near Gothenburg, a house with improved land about it, with which I was particularly delighted. It was close to a lake embosomed in pine clad rocks ... . One recess, particularly grand and solemn, amongst the towering cliffs, had a rude stone table, and seat, placed in it, that might have served for a druid's haunt" (*WMW* 6:256–57). The lake is "embosomed" in the rocks, and the simple stone table is nestled under the towering cliffs. All of the elements of the scene work to protect and complement one another. In addition, as Bohls points out, the type of improved land that Wollstonecraft endorses is "localized and ultilitarian" (*Women* 150). At the same estate, she appreciates the gentle way in which the landscape leads the eye: "In one part of the meadows, your eye was directed to the broad expanse; in another, you were led into a shade, to see a part of it, in the form of a river, rush amongst the fragments of rocks and roots of trees; nothing seemed forced" (*WMW* 6:257). Wollstonecraft's pleasure comes not from the human power to hunt and pursue, as Gilpin frames it, but from the power both to appreciate and to create harmonious beauty. She imagines a version of social "improvement" that, like these aesthetic improvements, is based in a maternal

---

15 In addition to the medical works on melancholia by Buchan, Trotter, and Whytt that I discuss in chapter 1, see Evelyne Ender and Elaine Showalter on the history of associating women's emotional suffering with their bodies and irrationality, rather than with their minds.

ethic of care. Not imposed artificially on a landscape, this kind of improvement is responsive to the given scene.

In the tight connection she draws between personal healing and social improvement, Wollstonecraft clearly differs from Wordsworth, who retreats from painful social interaction into remembered landscapes. In Hamburg, feeling the strain of "man and wretchedness," she seeks refuge in a scene recreated in her imagination: "In fancy I return to a favorite spot ... . Rocks aspiring towards the heavens, and ... shutting out sorrow, surrounded me, whilst peace appeared to steal along the lake to calm my bosom, modulating the wind that agitated the neighbouring poplars" (*WMW* 6:343). She remembers how the scene surrounded her with protection, "shutting out sorrow," calming both the wind and her bosom. Two years later Wordsworth expresses in "Tintern Abbey" a very similar hope for the consoling effect of a remembered landscape: "These forms of beauty have not been to me, / As is a landscape to a blind man's eye: / But oft, in lonely rooms, and mid the din / Of towns and cities, I have owed to them, / In hours of weariness sensations sweet" (*Lyrical Ballads* ll. 23–27). Retreating from the "din" of the city, Wordsworth immerses himself in the visual recreation of the scene at Tintern Abbey and feels restored. In the course of her journey and in her remembrance of it, Wollstonecraft seeks the comfort that Wordsworth expresses so assuredly. For Wollstonecraft, though, the consolation offered by these remembered scenes is transitory: "[T]he din of trade drags me back to all the care I left behind, when lost in sublime emotions" (*WMW* 6:343). Wordsworth retreats from the "din" of urban life into a remembered landscape. In contrast, Wollstonecraft is dragged from her sublime reverie by the "din of trade," which, as I note above, she regards as a hierarchical and dehumanizing rather than a lateral and loving way to structure social relationships. Wollstonecraft does not hope to heal herself in retreat from the world, but rather hopes to be healed by a sympathetic exchange between external and internal worlds, an exchange between the viewer and the scene. Bohls argues that Wollstonecraft "situate[s] aesthetic pleasure in a practical, material matrix extending from the body and its sensations to political engagement" (*Women* 141). Wollstonecraft imagines health as harmony between solitude and sociability, as a productive reverberation between individual growth and social improvement.

Chapter 4

Scientific Botany as Therapy in Charlotte Smith's Literature

"I took a liking to this recreation of the eyes [botany], which in misfortune
rests, amuses, distracts the spirit and suspends the feelings of pain."

Jean-Jacques Rousseau

Charlotte Smith infused the literature she wrote during the last twelve years of
her life with references to scientific botany. She portrayed this life-long interest as
pleasurable, as intellectually engaging, and increasingly as therapeutic. As a child,
she studied painting with the landscape artist George Smith and discovered that her
nearsightedness better equipped her to draw "close studies of flowers and leaves"
than to paint grand landscapes (Fletcher 13). Although she employed it in novel
ways, Smith's interest in botany was common among women of her class and era.
Between 1760 and 1830, women "read botany books, attended public lectures about
plants, corresponded with naturalists, collected native ferns, mosses, and marine
plants, drew plants, developed herbaria for further study, used microscopes," "studied
Latin," and "wrote about botany" (Shteir 3–4). Fully participating in this tradition,
Smith and her sister Catherine Dorset proposed in 1797 to write a botanical textbook
in order to improve upon the badly done plates in other elementary guides. In a
letter to her publisher, Smith describes a book designed for students and botanical
artists that would juxtapose her sister's drawings of plants—"*one* to illustrate *each*
of Linneas's orders"—with her own explanation of the science for beginners (*CLCS*
283, original emphasis).[1] This project never came to fruition; however, Smith
displays her knowledge of botany copiously in her published works, particularly in
the poetry, novels, and children's literature she wrote after 1795.

    The effect of Smith's literary botanizing on our understanding of Romanticism
has been the topic of much scholarly conversation following the republication
of her work in *The Poems of Charlotte Smith* (1993). Stuart Curran argues in his
introduction to this edition that the "multitudious, uncanny particularity" of her
natural descriptions in *Beachy Head* (1807) "testifies to an alternate Romanticism

---

1   The letter from Charlotte Smith to Thomas Cadell Jr. and William Davies, written
from Oxford and dated 1 August 1797, proposes the following: "Mrs. Dorset, whose skill in
botanical drawings is greater than that of almost any person I know, has a plan of our doing
together a set of drawings, *one* to illustrate *each* of Linneas's orders—to be etched with a page
of Letter press to each & the characters done with precision for the use of botanical students &
those who cultivate this branch of drawing" (*CLCS* 283). She promised that Dr. James Edward
Smith, president of the Linnaean society, would correct it for her. See Fletcher's biography
for more on the deterioration of Smith's relationship with her publisher during this period,
probably the reason the book was never published.

that seeks not to transcend or to absorb nature but to contemplate and honor its irreducible alterity" (xxvii–xxviii). In her invaluable article on Smith's merging of botany and poetry, Judith Pascoe similarly contends that Smith's late works "set forth a poetic manifesto which, in its insistence on close observation and faithfully rendered detail, challenges the prevailing strictures of the artistic establishment of her day" (193). Jacqueline Labbe offers an important caveat to these views in her study of the contingencies of gender and visuality, arguing that in spite of Smith's dedication to the "detailed point of view" inherent in botany, she never relinquishes her claim to the more masculine and powerful "prospect view" (*Romantic Visualities* 31). Implicitly and explicitly, these scholars invoke vision to explain the influence of Smith's natural history poetry on what we call "Romanticism." Smith's detailed and scientific view of nature contributes to a nontranscendent version of Romantic subjectivity, that is, a subjectivity inseparable from material circumstances.

Scholars have also taken notice of references to botany in the generically hybrid works Smith published for children, especially *Rural Walks* (1795), *Rambles Farther* (1796), *Minor Morals* (1798), and *Conversations Introducing Poetry, Chiefly on Subjects of Natural History, for the Use of Young Persons* (1804).[2] As both Pascoe and Ann B. Shteir point out, the poems in these volumes shaped a tradition of verse designed to educate children about natural history.[3] Pascoe observes that in the dialogues that accompany the poetry in each work, the teacher figure demonstrates to the children "how to look at the world" and portrays "the distancing vantage of the painter" as "inferior to the amplifying awareness of the botanical poet" (203). Donelle Ruwe argues that the children's works herald Smith's deepening engagement with scientific botany. She contrasts Smith's more fanciful references to flowers in the first edition of the *Elegiac Sonnets* (1784) with her attention to botanical detail in the later children's works and finally in *Beachy Head*. Ruwe provocatively asks, "What happened between *Elegiac Sonnets* in 1784 and *Beachy Head* in 1807 to inspire this lush concreteness in floral imagery?" ("Charlotte" 124). While Ruwe attributes the change to Smith's mastery of "a botanic poetic" ("Charlotte" 124), I would argue that the origin of this shift lies in the material circumstances of Smith's life in the mid 1790s—the details of which Judith Phillips Stanton's edition of Smith's letters makes accessible. The letters and literature Smith wrote during this period reveal that her involvement in therapeutic regimens for a variety of illnesses inspired her to deploy her already substantial botanical knowledge to a new end. She began to consider the therapeutic value of the botanical gaze.

2　The other two of her six books for children do not focus on botany. Smith wrote the first two of three volumes of the work *History of England, from the Earliest Records, to the Peace of Amiens, in a Series of Letters to a Young Lady at School*, published in 1806. *The Natural History of Birds, Intended Chiefly for Young Persons* (1807) was published posthumously.

3　In 1777, John Aiken, brother of Anna Letitia Barbauld, wrote "An Essay on the Application of Natural History to Poetry," encouraging poets to represent nature with scientific accuracy in order to realize poetry's instructive power. Similarly, the anonymous editor of the volume *Descriptive Poetry: Being a Selection from the Best Modern Authors: Principally Having Reference to Subjects in Natural History* (1807)—which includes poems by Smith, William Hayley, Robert Southey, Robert Burns, Amelia Opie, Samuel Taylor Coleridge, and William Wordsworth—expresses his hope that the poems will serve as "an incitement to a more extended research for detailed information" by young readers (iv).

Although she eventually identifies botanizing as the only activity that alleviates her emotional suffering, Smith addresses more common health therapies—spa going and viewing the salutary landscape—in the *Elegiac Sonnet*, "Written at Bristol in the summer of 1794." Like Mary Wollstonecraft and Mary Shelley, Smith engaged in both healing practices, in her case to treat the crippling rheumatoid arthritis and enormous psychological stress she experienced during most of her adult life. In fact, in March of 1794, the year she wrote this sonnet, she went to Bath for what she thought would be a "month or six weeks" to treat both rheumatism and the ill effects of anxiety (*CLCS* 103). She explains the decision to a friend:

> I have been a martyr to the Rheumatism, the gout, or something ... & now am entirely crippled, so as not to be able to walk across the room; I have reason to fear it is an ill form'd gout ... which, brought on by anxiety, my constitution has not the strength to throw out. And as my life is so necessary to my family, tho Heaven knows how little desirable to myself, I have at length determined to follow the advice of my Physicians and go to Bath. (*CLCS* 103)

Although Smith's physical suffering was somewhat alleviated by the spa treatments she underwent in this period, she was still plagued by symptoms of melancholia, including insomnia. In addition, her best-loved daughter Anna Augusta began to experience health problems related to her pregnancy and to the subsequent loss of her newborn son in July 1794. By August, after staying in Bath not just for six weeks but for over four months to treat her own and her daughter's conditions, Smith informs her publisher William Davies that Anna Augusta "is now order'd to Bristol hot wells, having all the symptoms of a decline" (*CLCS* 147). Smith moved her daughter to Clifton, near the Bristol hot wells, for what became eight months of treatment for consumption.

Reflecting Smith's experience with spa therapy, the first quatrain of Sonnet 64, "Written at Bristol in the summer of 1794," portrays a chronically ill person who seeks healing in the warm baths:

> Here from the restless bed of lingering pain
> The languid sufferer seeks the tepid wave,
> And feels returning health and hope again
> Disperse 'the gathering shadows of the grave!' (ll. 1–4)

Like many spa-goers, the speaker undertakes this therapy to treat more than one complaint; she looks for both "health and hope," a recovery from both physical and mental debility. In the first quatrain, she expresses confidence in the healing power of the waters. Sitting in the soothing hot wells at Bristol, she looks up at the landscape:

> And here romantic rocks that boldly swell,
> Fringed with green woods, or stain'd with veins of ore,
> Call'd native Genius forth, whose Heav'n-taught skill
> Charm'd the deep echos of the rifted shore. (ll. 5–8)

This attention to the landscape reflects the advice of eighteenth-century medical writers who, as I explain in chapter 3, regard the fresh air and new scenery inherent in the trip to the spa to be as crucial to healing as bathing or taking the waters. Before leaving for Bath in 1794, Smith notes that she has "been advised to try change of air & scene & should leave home for a few weeks" (*CLCS* 99). Smith describes the scenery that the ailing speaker seeks not only as different from his or her normal environment, but also as quite obviously picturesque. The rocky cliffs that surround the spa at Bristol are "romantic," picturesque in their varied texture and in their framing by the "green woods" (l. 5, 6).

Although she draws attention to the picturesque setting of the Bristol hot wells, Smith's speaker does not feel the same sense of comfort in the picturesque scenery that Wollstonecraft describes during her journey in Scandinavia. In fact, the speaker in Smith's sonnet concludes in the sestet that none of these healing alternatives—neither the warm baths of Bristol, nor the picturesque hills that surround it, nor the warm air—has the power to alleviate her depressed spirit:

> But tepid waves, wild scenes, or summer air,
> Restore they palsied Fancy, woe-deprest?
> Check they the torpid influence of Despair,
> Or bid warm Health reanimate the breast;
> Where Hope's soft visions have no longer part,
> And whose sad inmate is—a broken heart? (ll. 9–14)

Smith emphasizes the deep feeling of the British artist whose "broken heart" cannot possibly respond to these conventional therapies. In the speaker's imagination, "Health" would "reanimate the breast," restoring "Hope's soft visions." The Bristol hot wells do not offer the speaker relief from "the torpid influence of Despair," and they do not heal Anna Augusta, who after months of treatment dies in Bristol in April 1795.

Following Anna Augusta's death, Smith begins to intermingle references to botany and health in her literature, beginning with two *Elegaic Sonnets* that discuss botanical sketching in relation to the loss of her daughter. She writes Sonnet 65, "To Dr. Parry of Bath, with some botanic drawings which had been made some years," to the physician who attended her daughter during her final illness. She explains in a footnote that she is obliged to him "for the kindest attention, and for the recovery from one dangerous illness of that beloved child whom a few months afterwards his skill and most unremitted and disinterested exertions could not save!" (57). In the first quatrain she notes that she completed the drawings she sends "in happier hours, ere yet so keenly blew / Adversity's cold blight" (ll. 1–2). She refers to the illness as a "blight," thus implicitly portraying Anna Augusta as a flower, or one of "Luxuriant Summer's evanescent forms" (l. 3). This association continues as she observes that, under siege like her own family during this crisis, "the lovely family of flowers / Shrink from the bleakness of the Northern blast" (ll. 5–6). Although "present care and sorrow past" disrupt the "botanic pencil's mimic powers" (ll. 7, 8), "one flower of deathless blossom" survives: "the unfading Amaranth of Gratitude" (ll. 12, 14). She associates the living Anna Augusta with a flower, thus evoking her beauty and fragility, and then offers her thanks to Dr. Parry also in the form of a flower. She locates botanical sketching in a happier time, asserting that the "botanic pencil's" power to imitate life has been lost.

Smith discusses botanical sketching in terms of loss again in Sonnet 91, "Reflections on Some Drawings of Plants," explaining that although she can draw flowers with skill, she has no sketch of her deceased daughter Anna Augusta, except in her heart:

> I can in groups these mimic flowers compose,
> These bells and *golden eyes*, embathed in dew;
> Catch the *soft blush* that warms the early Rose,
> Or the pale Iris cloud with *veins of blue*;
> Copy the scallop'd leaves, and downy stems,
> And bid the pencil's varied shades arrest
> Spring's humid buds, and Summer's musky gems:
> But, save the portrait on my bleeding breast,
> I have no semblance of that form adored. (ll. 1–9, my emphasis)

The beautiful irony is that, in spite of her lament that she has no portrait of Anna Augusta, Smith draws her daughter into her botanical sketch, bestowing upon the plant "golden" teary eyes, a "soft blush," and "veins of blue." One can imagine Smith meditating on the memory of her daughter's beautiful face as she concentrates on the details of drawing. She recreates the botanical specimen in terms of what is lost, and yet she is aware that she cannot bring Anna Augusta back to life with her pencil. What is reflected, then, into "some drawings of plants" is Smith's grief. Although the concentrated vision required by botanical sketching does not heal this pain, drawing does provide a way to make her sense of loss visible.[4]

By the mid 1790s, Smith claims botany as the only reliable therapy for her melancholia and begins her excursion into literary botany in earnest. In the midst of her fifteen-month struggle with her daughter's and her own health in Bath and Bristol, Smith writes her first children's book, *Rural Walks* (1795), which includes among moral lessons and social criticism an informal curriculum in natural history. She also works on volume 2 of the *Elegiac Sonnets* (1797), the volume that includes for the first time the sonnets I discuss above, as well as Sonnet 79, "To the goddess of botany," discussed below. She continues to focus on botany in her proposal for the botanical handbook in 1797, as well as in three of her other children's narratives, especially *Conversations Introducing Poetry*, which I also discuss at length below. Shteir points out that with one of the novels she wrote in this period—*The Young Philosopher* (1798)—Smith responds to James Edward Smith's suggestion that "she turn her botanical knowledge to literary and financial advantage" (70). In her correspondence with Dr. Smith, the president of the Linnaean Society, she writes: "I have not forgotten ... your hint of introducing botany into a novel" (*CLCS* 314). As in her poetry and children's literature, Smith includes in this novel footnotes that identify the scientific names of the plants mentioned in the narrative. In addition, the character Laura Glenmorris teaches her daughter Medora scientific botany, and turns to the scientific study of nature to comfort herself during challenging times. Loraine

---

4   Even in something as straightforward as the letter proposing that she and her sister write a botanical textbook, Smith refers to botanical drawing as consoling: "I sometimes go to drawing by way of relaxation when other's [sic] would walk, or converse, or play at cards" (*CLCS* 284).

Fletcher points to a passage in which Laura, separated from her daughter and hiding in a cave from malicious pursuers, begins to catalogue the plant life on the walls of the cave (268–70). Laura asserts: "Amidst the many sad hours I have passed, I have never failed to feel my spirits soothed by the contemplation of vegetable nature ... I hoped I might find security, and endure life till I could reach England, though still my heart's deep wounds unceasingly bled, and still the image of my lost happiness haunted me" (*WCS* 13:157–58). Botany might not heal the "heart's deep wounds," but it does offer Laura a sense of security and visual consolation while the "image of her lost happiness"—her daughter and her home country—haunts her. Two years later, in *The Letters of a Solitary Wanderer* (1800–02), which I discuss in the final section of this chapter, Smith draws a portrait of a peripatetic melancholic, who explores the healing power of both collecting and looking through the scientific lens of Linnaean botany.

For Smith, the practice of botany served as visual therapy, and the Linnaean system of classification offered a model for a language that might make one's suffering intelligible to others. In "To the goddess of botany," Smith emphasizes the visual pleasure of botanizing, quoting Jean-Jacques Rousseau's *Rêveries du promeneur solitaire* (1778) in a footnote: "I took a liking to this recreation of the eyes [botany], which in misfortune rests, amuses, distracts the spirit and suspends the feelings of pain" (68). Rousseau's use of the word "recreation" reflects William Buchan's assertion that for melancholics "[t]he best kinds of exercise are those connected with amusement" (*Domestic* 18). The exercise and amusement provided by botanizing were for Rousseau and for Smith specifically a "recreation of the eyes." Re-creating, or looking according to the rules of Linnaean botany, "rests, amuses, distracts the spirit and suspends the feelings of pain," even if it does not cure them. In this chapter, I address the metaphorical and practical aspects of botanizing that Smith portrays as helpful for treating melancholia in works from three genres: the poem "To the goddess of botany," the children's book *Conversations Introducing Poetry*, and the collection of novellas *Letters of a Solitary Wanderer*. With her focus on scientific botany's systematic nomenclature and description of a plant's location in these works, Smith calls for an accurate language to describe suffering in all its complexity, including its roots in social circumstances.

Botanical Handbooks and the Discourse of Health

While Smith's portrayal of botanizing as a therapeutic practice reflects the general medical advice to melancholics that they amuse themselves, her emphasis on Linnaean botany invokes a more specific discourse of health used to "sell" the study of natural history at the end of the eighteenth century. "[Botany is] as healthful as it is innocent," proclaims William Withering, author of the first comprehensive and most popular English publication based on the Linnaean system, *A Botanical Arrangement of All the Vegetables Naturally Growing in Great Britain.*[5] In the first of fourteen editions of the handbook produced between 1776 and 1877, Withering, a protégé of

---

 5 The translation into English of Swedish botanist Carl Linnaeus's *Philosophia Botanica* (1751) popularized the practice of botanical classification in England, which was widespread by 1760 (Kelley "Romantic" 231).

Linnaeus, argues for the health value of botanizing: "[It] beguiles the tediousness of the road ... and furnishes amusement at every footstep of the solitary walk" (iii).[6] Withering emphasizes both the mental engagement and physical exercise that botany offers. Although the title of Withering's botanical text changes by the third edition of 1796 to emphasize Linnaean nomenclature (*An Arrangement of British Plants, According to the Latest Improvements of the Linnaean System*), his promotion of the salutary qualities of botanizing persists. Similarly, William Mavor's handbook, *The Lady and Gentleman's Botanical Pocket Book: Adapted to Withering's Arrangements of British Plants* (1800), written as the title indicates to be a portable companion to Withering's more comprehensive text, also notes the healthful benefits of botanizing: "Whether we consider the effect of Botany as enlarging the sphere of knowledge, or as conducive to health and innocent amusement, it ought to rank very high in the scale of elegant acquirements" (vi). Mavor, like Withering, promotes botany to both women and men of the leisured classes as "conducive to health." In the introduction to the 1830 edition of *An Arrangement of British Plants*, William Withering Jr., who took over the editing of the handbook when his father died in 1799, asserts that botanizing will aid both the average person and the "convalescent" by "dissipat[ing] the gloom from which the most meritorious are not uniformly exempt," and by "induc[ing] the convalescent to wander forth in quest of renovated vigour" (liv–lv). Part of the attraction of botanizing, then, was simply that it encouraged moderate exercise.

The physical movement and outdoor activity of botanizing fulfill recommendations by physicians such as Buchan, James Johnson, Thomas Trotter, and Robert Whytt that melancholics exercise or travel for their health, a topic I discuss at length in chapter 3. Botanical enthusiasts themselves portray botanizing as an affordable opportunity to heal in the outdoors. An epigraph to Withering Jr.'s 1830 edition of *An Arrangement of British Plants* relays the broad claims made for botany in an earlier botanical guide, *Johns's Practical Botany* (1826): "No science can be prosecuted with so little expense, and with so much advantage, as to the means of acquiring it, as botany; none certainly is at once so subservient to the improvement of both the mental and corporeal powers." Similarly, in the introduction to her botanical catalogue *The British Garden* (1799), Lady Charlotte Murray alludes to the healthful exercise and relatively low expense of botanizing: "[T]he study of Botany, that science by means of which we discriminate and distinguish one plant from another, is open to almost every curious mind; the Garden and the Field offer a constant source of unwearying amusement, easily obtained, and conducing to health, by affording a continual and engaging motive for air and exercise" (vi). Murray suggests that botanizing is "conducing [sic] to health" because it motivates people to exercise in the fresh air. In addition, Murray's description of botany as "that science by means of which we discriminate and distinguish one plant from another" highlights the visual and mental activity required by the practice of botany, a characteristic that avid amateur botanists Smith and Rousseau associate with healing.

Several botanical guides recommend these benefits of botanizing to women in particular. In a quotation included in Withering Jr.'s introduction, Elizabeth Kent,

---

6   This publication information is found in T. Whitmore Peck and K. Douglas Wilkinson's *William Withering of Birmingham* (Baltimore: Williams and Wilkins, 1950).

another "eulogist" of systematic taxonomies, describes the effect of scientific botanizing on the female mind[7]:

> The study of the vegetable world has something of that soothing power which we experience from its actual presence. There is, undoubtedly, an influence in the pure air, the stillness, the calm freshness of the country, that tends to quell all unkindly feelings and to foster the gentler affections. Such scenes are favourable to reflection; and *dispassionate reflection* will turn anger into pity, and lend to sorrow itself a patience from which it may extract some portion of sweetness. (xxxviii-xxxix, my emphasis)

Kent is particularly concerned with botany as an antidote to the dangers of passion for women. Botany not only exposes women to the fresh air, but also helps to regulate their emotions with rational reflection. Likewise, Trotter specifically recommends botanizing to prevent nervous illness in young girls. He suggests that if girls are sent to boarding school, the school should be in the country so that they might botanize:

> An adjoining flower garden will be a motive for recreation for some, while the taste may be improved by the study of Botany; a task peculiarly adapted to young ladies. Such avocations will train the female mind to the love of simplicity, and store it with that species of information, which affords food for reflection at a future day; and will fill up much of the leisure to be met with in the domestic scene ... . And while her nervous aunts are moping their evenings over the card table, she will gather health by her cheerful excursions; and preserve her bloom of countenance by the only means that can give it an additional charm. (275–76)

Trotter recommends botanizing as a remedy for what he perceives as the health risks of domestic leisure. By storing "the female mind" with "food for reflection at a future day," botanical study strengthens the young woman's mind to resist the disorders that plague "her nervous aunts." "Young ladies," he suggests, can make the best of domestic restriction by exercising their bodies and minds in the garden.

The discourse of health employed to promote botany is not purely a response to concerns about nervous illness, but also a strategy for defending the practice of botany against claims that it was morally inappropriate for women. On the one hand, the relative simplicity of Linnaean botany made the science accessible to lay people, including women. Many botanical handbooks, such as Mavor's *The Lady's and Gentleman's Botanical Pocketbook,* were directed toward a female audience; however, as Pascoe points out, these handbooks assume widely different levels of scientific engagement among their readers (198). On the other hand, Linnaean botany's focus on the sexual organs of plants inspired Richard Polwhele and other conservative male writers to object to women's study of scientific botany, equating their passion for the amateur science with an impure interest in sexuality. In *The Unsex'd Females* (1798), Polwhele frames his attack on literary women of the 1790s—including Smith and Wollstonecraft—as an attack on female botanizing (Shteir 27–28). Partially in response to widespread enthusiasm for Erasmus Darwin's erotic versification of Linnaeus's system in *The Loves of the Plants* (1789),

---

7   Author of *Domestica* (1823) and *Sylvan Sketches* (1825), Elizabeth Kent was the sister-in-law of Leigh Hunt and a friend of the Shelleys. For more on her life and work, see Shteir (135–45).

Polwhele accuses women who study plants of deliberately immersing themselves in sexual activity (Shteir 28). He warns that "if botanizing girls ... do not take heed ... they will soon exchange the blush of modesty for the bronze of impudence" (Polwhele 9). Even Withering, a great proponent of Linnaean botanizing for women, modestly chose "to drop the sexual distinctions in the titles to the Classes and Orders" in later editions of his handbook (Withering 1776 v). Most botanical guides stop short of Withering's censorship, choosing instead to emphasize the health value of the science in order to defend female botanists against charges of immorality.

Floral, Medicinal, and Scientific Botany

Smith draws on the botanical handbooks' discourse of health in order to further her ideas about mental illness and healing. In her literature for children, Smith reflects the two major elements of the botanical handbooks' defense of botanizing: the exercise and fresh air that accompany botanical excursions and the appropriateness of the study for girls as well as boys. As the titles of her first two children's books *Rural Walks* and *Rambles Farther* suggest, Smith portrays women and children undertaking the study of botany as they exercise. The conversations about natural history between the mother-teacher and children in these works take place on walks during which the teacher figure helps the children learn to see nature scientifically. The children ask questions about the plants, animals, and insects that they encounter, and their mother rewards their curiosity about these topics with detailed facts about the natural world. In these works and in *Minor Morals* and *Conversations Introducing Poetry*, Smith teaches her child and adult readers that natural history is not only an essential component of education, but also an effective therapy for emotional suffering.[8]

In a passage from *Minor Morals* that resonates with Trotter's recommendation that young women botanize, the teacher, Mrs. Belmour, proclaims:

> The young person, who, tired of her work, and without any book that may be amusing or instructive at hand, can go into the garden and shrubbery, or among the meadows and hedges, and bring back a bouquet of flowers; who can either describe them singly with their various parts (of stalks, leaves, calyx, corolla, stamen, pistil, anther and stigma, with the pollen or duit), or who can arrange them in a pleasing form together, and give her composition correctness and relief, need never give way to that mawkish indolence, that inanity of the mind, which, if indulged, will render her burthensome to herself and uninteresting to others. But a taste for the culture of flowers ... is particularly adapted to women; is soothing to their mind, and refines their taste, while it prevents them from suffering from that want of motive to go into the air, and from yielding to that torpid ignorance which hurts alike the body and the mind. (*WCS* 12:222–23)

---

8   Alan Bewell observes that teaching botany and other forms of natural history was an important element of a woman's role as educator of her children. As examples, he cites Francis Arabella Rowden's *Poetical Introduction to the Study of Botany* (1801) and Mrs. Montolieu's *The Enchanted Plants* (1803), both of which are much more moralistic and stylized than Smith's work. See "Keats's 'Realm of Flora,'" *Studies in Romanticism* 31 (1992): 71–98. For a discussion of the political resonance of botanizing, see Bewell's "'Jacobin Plants': Botany as Social Theory in the 1790s," *Wordsworth Circle* 20 (1989): 132–39.

Refining Trotter's recommendation that young women botanize, Mrs. Belmour instructs the young person to see the bouquet of flowers she picks in two ways. Looking through the lens of scientific botany—"she can ... describe them singly with their various parts"—or seeing in terms of the aesthetic conventions of floral botany—she can "arrange them in a pleasing form together." Either way, she will soothe her mind, refine her taste, and stave off "mawkish indolence," "inanity of the mind," and "torpid ignorance."

In addition to Linnaean botany and floral botany, the long-standing practice of medicinal botany (also called herbal medicine, or simply herbalizing) continued into the eighteenth century.[9] Writers of scientific handbooks sought to establish firm boundaries between the three branches of botany, but it was more crucial to distinguish Linnaean botany from mere herbalizing than it was to differentiate floral botany from either.[10] Introductions to botanical handbooks promote botany as scientifically superior and more professional than the feminine field of herbal medicine. Linnaeus comments that gardeners and physicians practice a version of botany that does not belong to botanical science (Morton 262). Rousseau spurns the "habit of considering plants only as a source of drugs and medicines," suggesting if the botanist lingers "in some meadow studying one by one all the flowers that adorn it ... people will take you for an herbalist and ask you for something to cure the itch in children, scab in men, or glanders in horses" (*Rêveries* 109). He fears his interest in botany will be associated with the more feminine practice of herbalizing and wishes to emphasize his rational rather than compassionate capacities.

Botany's origin in herbal medicine, a practice focused on the care of others, at first made it an acceptable science for women (Schiebinger 241). That is to say, women's botanizing was construed as an outgrowth of their "natural" desire to nurse their loved ones with herbal medicine. As it became clear that many eighteenth-century women were interested in botany as an intellectual and professional rather than domestic endeavor, several botanical writers sought to revive herbal medicine as the proper outlet for women's botanical interests. John Chambers dedicates his handbook *A Pocket Herbal; Containing the Medicinal Virtues and Uses of the Most Esteemed Native Plants* (1800) to ladies, gently encouraging them to return to their "natural" area of study, herbal medicine:

> Botany is now become a very general study with the Ladies, and may I hope that the fair Votaresses of Flora may acquire an additional interest in those plants which they now admire for the beauty of their colours, and the wisdom of their structure, from the idea that they may be made subservient to the relief of the afflictions of their fellow creatures ... . To such I present my work, sincerely wishing them the continual enjoyment of those heartfelt gratifications which never fail to flow from the virtues of the female mind exerting themselves in their natural sphere—to the care of their families, and the relief of the distressed. (iv–v)

---

9   The Society of Apothecaries began formalizing the study of herbal medicine with the establishment of the Chelsea Physic Garden in 1673. The garden offered monthly classes for apprentices (Landry 50).

10   Floral botany was not without its critics. Smith, for example, disdains the florist's practice of "forcing" growth out of season, and Withering suggests that by altering the structure of blossoms, florists create monstrosities (Pascoe 195–96).

Chambers alludes to the three major ways one might study plants—the florist's admiration for "the beauty of their colours," the scientist's respect for "the wisdom of their structure," and the herbalist's hope that they will bring "relief of ... afflictions"— but suggests that women's interest in plants would be best directed to support their "natural sphere," the home. In contrast to scientific botanizing, floral arrangement and herbal medicine were less intellectual, uninterested in the sexual organs of plants, and aligned with domestic duties; in other words, they were the domain of respectable women.

In her poetry, Smith combines her knowledge of scientific botany with the appropriately feminine activity of floral arrangement. While she also demonstrates her knowledge of medicinal botany, Smith suggests that the practice of Linnaean botany is more effective than herbal medicine for healing the mind. Smith refers to herbal remedies for melancholia only to comment on their ineffectiveness. The two plants that she includes in Sonnet 8, "To Spring," are both used to treat nervous disorders: "[T]he primrose pale, / And lavish cowslip, wildly scatter'd round, / Give their sweet spirits to the sighing gale" (ll. 5–7). In his pocket herbal, Chambers notes that cowslip and primrose roots "dried and powdered" "are good in Nervous disorders" (161–62, 212–13). In the sonnet, Smith first expresses hope that with these flowers the season will bring relief from melancholia:

> Ah! season of delight!—could aught be found
> To soothe awhile the tortured bosom's pain,
> Of Sorrow's rankling shaft to cure the wound,
> And bring life's first delusions once again,
> 'Twere surely met in thee! (ll. 8–12)

But then her hope that the products of spring will restore her mental health is disappointed. Spring and its flowers "[h]ave power to cure all sadness—but despair" (l. 14). Smith thus rejects the medicinal branch of botany as a therapy for melancholia.[11] She contrasts scientific botany with medicinal botany in order to outline the particular kind of visual and mental activity needed to heal the wounded mind.

However, she does see value in medicinal botany for physical ailments. Fletcher notes that in 1799, Smith's "rheumatism was worsening and she complained of dropsy, for which she tried foxglove as a remedy to avoid medical bills" (287). Mrs. Talbot, the teacher in *Conversations Introducing Poetry*, praises a scientific collection of plants for its ability to inspire viewers to reflect on both the beauty and utility of flora:

---

11 The botanical allusions in Smith's poetry rarely have such a clear medicinal meaning. Of the approximately forty flowers she alludes to in "Flora," for example, six are listed as medicinal herbs in *A Pocket Herbal*; however, they reveal no pattern in terms of illnesses treated, and none has any connection to nervous illness. The six herbs to which both Smith and Chambers refer are "convulvulas" (Smith l. 41; Chambers 136–37); "foxglove" (Smith l. 65, Chambers 175); "cistus" (Smith l. 83, Chambers 151–52); "gentian" (Smith l. 115, Chambers 178); "thyme" (Smith l. 138, Chambers 232); and "chamomile" (Smith l. 138, Chambers 150–51).

[A] collection of plants offers only pleasing ideas: even the most common, that spring up under our feet, and are thrown from our gardens as weeds, are many of them very elegant, and others are of medical utility. I cannot say that I think the pleasure of botanizing destroyed, by considering plants as convertible into drugs; on the contrary, I reflect with satisfaction, that objects so beautiful in themselves, are also endowed with the power of alleviating pain, or diminishing fever. And when I am sick, much of the disgust which the taste of medicine excites, is conquered, when I know, that what is proper for me to take is only the roots, bark, flowers, leaves, or seeds of a plant. (*WCS* 13:179–80)

Although Smith, unlike Rousseau, respects the acquisition of knowledge about herbal remedies, she asserts that the practice of medicinal botany does not have the same effect on the mind as does the practice of Linnaean botany.

And, indeed, the types of cognitive engagement required by Linnaean botany and medicinal botany differ significantly. Linnaean botany is a rubric that, while artificial and imperfect, allows for newly discovered plants to be described or understood in terms of their own structure's relation to that of other plants. Linnaeus's system classifies and names plants based on "fructification." Classification involves identifying the number, form, proportion, and situation of the seven reproductive parts of the plant: the calyx, corolla, stamen, pistil, ovary, receptacle, and seed (Morton 263). Linnaeus developed a relatively simple nomenclature that divides plants into 24 classes and orders based on the number of male stamens and female pistils (Shteir 15). The first twelve classes refer to the number of stamens, classes 13–19 to the "length or groupings of stamens," and classes 20–23 to the "more complicated sexual arrangements, including those hermaphroditic flowers ... and the one class that puzzled Linnaeus's taxonomic itinerary, the Cryptogamia, so called because members of this class lacked proper flowers and so reproduced themselves by rather cryptic (as opposed to sexually explicit) means" (Kelley "Romantic" 231). A flower with one stamen is classed as monandria, a flower with two, diandria, and so on. These classes are further divided into orders based on the characteristics of each plant's pistils; orders are designated by the terms monogynia, digynia, and so forth (Shteir 15). Below class and order in the Linnaean hierarchy are the categories genus and species. The scientific name for a plant, an italicized binomial extracted from the plant's entire description, includes the genus (always capitalized) and then the species (e.g., *Digitalis purpurea* for foxglove). Smith's avid interest in Linnaean botany celebrates the human mind's power to organize and name the external world—specifically, the ability to analyze the details of an individual plant in order to place it in a relational framework.

In contrast, medicinal botany requires the gestalt recognition of a plant based on one's experience with the plant's healing properties. The illustration entitled "Plants of medicinal value to particular human body parts" from Michael Valentini's 1713 work demonstrates that medicinal botany is organized in relation to the human body (Figure 5). Each plant is identified with the part of the body that it is thought to help; for example, the Portulaca depicted in the second row is paired with the kidney because it was used to help dissolve kidney stones.[12] Medicinal botany does not require one to classify plants based on their structure, and, in fact, does not absolutely

---

12 See Lev and Dolev for the history of the medicinal use of this herb (177).

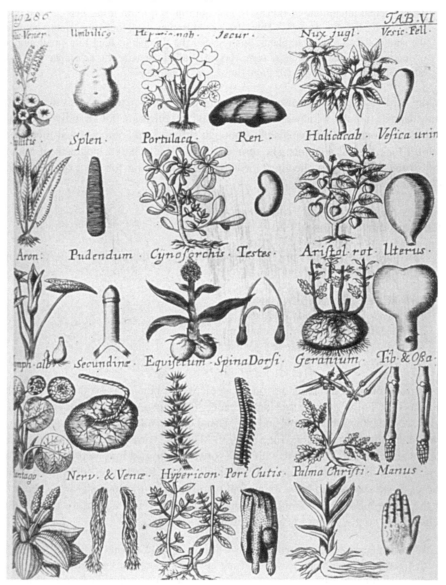

Fig. 5.   Michael Bernhard Valentini. *Plants of Medicinal Value to Particular Human Body Parts*, 1713

require the herbalist to know plant names. In contrast, the essence of Linnaean botany is naming, and the system for naming is based in a system for seeing that can be applied to plants the botanist encounters for the first time. Rousseau's introductory remarks to his *Letters on the Elements of Botany* (trans. 1785) distinguish between the modes of perception required by these two types of botany:

The principal misfortune of Botany is, that from its very birth it has been looked upon merely as a part of medicine ... . This false idea of Botany, for a long time, almost confined the study of it to medicinal plants, and reduced the vegetable chain to a small number of interrupted links. Even these were very ill studied, because the *substance* only was attended to, and not the *organization*. (Intro., my emphasis)

While medicinal botany focuses on the "substance" of a plant and its effect on the body, Linnaean botany focuses on the physical "organization" of an individual plant and its relationship to other plants. Although Smith found some herbal medicines helpful for physical ailments, she turned to the visually based language of botany and to the practice of collecting, identifying, and naming for the expression and alleviation of emotional suffering.

"To the goddess of botany"

In "To the goddess of botany," Smith addresses the therapeutic value of seeing scientifically in her appeal to Flora:

Of Folly weary, shrinking from the view
Of Violence and Fraud, allow'd to take
All peace from humble life; I would forsake
Their haunts for ever, and, sweet Nymph! with you
Find shelter ... (ll. 1–5)

In the footnote, Smith elaborates on her depiction of botany as a "shelter" from the "haunts" of "Folly," "Violence," and "Fraud," thus suggesting that botany soothes a mind wounded by other people and by external circumstances: "'Rightly to spell, Of every herb that sips the dew,' [or botany in Milton's words] seems to be a resource for the sick at heart—for those who from sorrow or disgust may without affectation say 'Society is nothing to one not sociable!'" (68). In addition to Milton, Smith quotes Shakespeare and most extensively Rousseau in the longest single footnote in the *Elegiac Sonnets*.[13] Smith compares herself to Rousseau, drawing a parallel between the conflicts they each encountered in society:

Without any pretensions to those talents which were in [Rousseau] so heavily taxed with that excessive irritability, too often if not always the attendant on genius, it has been my misfortune to have endured real calamities that have disqualified me from finding any enjoyment in the pleasures and pursuits which occupy the generality of the world. I have been engaged in contending with persons whose cruelty has left so painful an

---

13 Smith felt that the four-paragraph footnote was essential to the poem. While correcting proofs of volume 2 of the *Elegiac Sonnets* (1797), Smith finds that the footnote to this sonnet has been omitted. She writes to her publisher to insist on its reinstatement: "I observe, in returning the within proof, that the additions I wish'd to have made to the Notes on the Sonnet to the Goddess of Botany seem to have been left out. I wish they had been inserted as they had a direct & particular reference to the subject" (*CLCS* 277). The "direct & particular reference" she wishes to make in the notes is to the healing power of botanizing.

impression on my mind, that I may well say, "Brilliant flowers, adornment of meadows, cool shades, streams, arbors, foliage, come purify my imagination sullied by all these hideous objects." (68)

Smith ventriloquizes Rousseau at the end of this passage, calling on botany to "purify [her] imagination" from negative influences. It is not Smith's imagination itself that causes her suffering, but "real calamities," including the cruelty of the courts and the trustees of her father-in-law's estate that leave "so painful an impression on [her] mind."

Smith refers to her embodied vision to express both her awareness of this oppression and her strategy for healing. The speaker shrinks "from the *view* / Of Violence and Fraud" (ll. 1–2, my emphasis) and rests her "tired and tear-swoln *eyes*, / Among [botany's] silent shades of soothing hue" (ll. 5–6, my emphasis). The speaker's eyes do not rest passively, but rather engage in active scientific perception to learn "the bright varieties" of plants (l. 8). Instead of "calamities," the viewer hopes to see "every veined leaf" in "mead or woodland; or in wilds remote," as well as in caves, on cliffs, in rivers, and in the ocean (ll. 10, 11–14). The eyes travel through the landscape, collecting visual memories of botanical specimens. In the footnote attached to this poem, Smith describes the restfulness she finds in looking scientifically: "The *wearied eyes* and languid spirits find relief and repose amid the shades of vegetable nature.—I cannot now turn to any other pursuit that for a moment soothes my wounded mind" (68, my emphasis). As the "wearied eyes" find relief in looking at botanical specimens, so the "wounded mind" is soothed. Smith gauges pain and healing through the eyes and regards looking rationally as the first step toward healing melancholia.

Smith's focus on the visual in "To the goddess of botany" reflects Rousseau's account of the salutary value of botany in the seventh walk of *Rêveries du promeneur solitaire*. Rousseau explains how looking at the details of botanical specimens in order to classify them alleviates his emotional suffering. He fears "that [his] imagination, alarmed by [his] misfortunes, might fill [his] reveries with them" (107). However, in the midst of "the continual consciousness of [his] sufferings," Rousseau finds that:

> an instinct that is natural to me *averted my eyes from every depressing thought, silenced my imagination* and, fixing my attention on the objects surrounding me, made me look closely for the first time at the details of the great pageant of nature, which until then I had hardly ever contemplated otherwise than as a total and undivided spectacle. (107–8, my emphasis)

The botanizer's focus on details "silences" Rousseau's imagination, averting his eyes "from every depressing thought." His use of the word "eyes" in place of "mind" emphasizes that the rational engagement required by Linnaean botany begins with seeing. Rousseau's claim that botanizing regulated his imagination would have been significant to Smith. As I explain in chapter 1, she actively resisted the categorization of women as overly emotional and fanciful, commonly cited causes of culturally disempowering nervous illnesses. By identifying the social circumstances of her depressed spirits, and by demonstrating her engagement with Linnaean botany's rational classification system, Smith aligns herself with the figure of the rational, melancholic genius rather than the emotional, hysterical woman.

Conversations Introducing Poetry

Smith's children's book *Conversations Introducing Poetry* mobilizes into instruction her assertion that botany offers a restorative recreation for the eyes. Although Smith does not posit botany as a therapeutic endeavor until the triumphant final poem in this volume, the ten conversations leading up to "Flora" demonstrate what it means to Smith to see scientifically. This way of seeing is not only therapeutic to the botanizer, but also provides a model of perception and expression that might make suffering more visible to others. Smith posits a language of suffering that is based on three major aspects of botanical practice—collecting specimens, identifying their specific context, and naming them in a relational framework. Thus, just as individual botanical specimens are named or become visible based both on their particularity and also on the characteristics they share with other plants, so individual experiences of suffering might be better understood when seen in a relational framework. Although she develops the language of suffering most fully in *The Letters of a Solitary Wanderer*, discussed below, Smith prepares readers to understand this language by training them to see botanically in *Conversations Introducing Poetry.*

Smith announces her commitment to visual observation with the first word of the narrative: "Look." With this word, George directs his younger sister Emily to observe both the details of a specific natural object and the way that object compares to more familiar examples: "Look, Emily, look at this beautiful shining insect ... it is shaped very like those brownish chafers ... but this is not so big, and is much prettier.—See what little tassels it has on its horns; the wings shine like some part of the peacock's feathers" (*WCS* 13:65). Their mother, Mrs. Talbot, repeatedly directs the children to "look," "observe," or "shew" her what they have seen. When George reports that he has seen "coffee, cocoa, and the bread fruit tree; the sugar cane, indigo, and ginger" in a greenhouse they visit, Mrs. Talbot notes "I am very glad you have seen these plants, as they give you a much clearer idea of those productions thus growing, than can be conveyed by any description" (*WCS* 13:92). Mrs. Talbot encourages the children's desire to see the details of the natural world first hand. And when Mrs. Talbot does not mention the scientific names of the plants, animals, and insects in the narrative, Smith supplies them for her child readers in the footnotes, in this case: "Cocoa, *Theobroma cacao*. Bread fruit, *Artocarpus incise*. Sugar cane, *Saccharum officinarum* ... ." (*WCS* 13:92).

The interplay between text and notes in this example demonstrates the mutually constitutive nature of naming and seeing in the practice of natural history. George explains to a friend that his mother "walks with us, and tells us the names of different trees and flowers" (*WCS* 13:73). After returning from a walk on her own, Emily reports: "I was going to gather the blossoms of a tall pink, and white bell-shaped flower in the lower shrubbery, the name of which I do not know; but I found that in many of the flowers there were dead flies" (*WCS* 13:139). Mrs. Talbot immediately teaches her daughter the scientific and common names of the plant: "It is the *Apocynum*, or tutsan leaved dog's bane" (*WCS* 13:139). Emphasizing the importance of looking at specimens oneself, George asks his sister, "Shew it to me, Emily, when we go for our walk" (*WCS* 13:139). When George suggests that they have seen this type of plant before, Mrs. Talbot helps to train his eye to distinguish between the two plants he has seen and thus to name them correctly: "[The plant you remember] is a very different plant; it comes from the swamps of North America, and has received the name of *Dionæa muscipula*, or Venus's fly-trap; it is white, and without any great share of beauty" (*WCS* 13:139). She also encourages the children to compare the plant at hand to botanical sketches they know and even corrects one of these sources:

> The author of "Les Etudes de la Nature," who saw this plant in the royal botanic garden at Paris, where it has long been cultivated, speaks of it as another Dione; but except in its quality of catching insects, it has no resemblance to the plant so called, and is quite of a different species. The one receiving the flies on a foliole, or part of the leaf armed with spines; while this, the *Apocynum*, takes them in its cup, or flower; partly by the construction of anthers in which the insects get entangled, and partly by the viscid quality of the honey-like substance that attracts them. (*WCS* 13:140)

This lesson teaches children to name plants by looking closely at the details of individual specimens in order to distinguish their features from those of other plants. Mrs. Talbot's correction of Bernardin de Saint-Pierre, author of *Études de la Nature* (1784), encourages the botanizer to believe her own eyes and to trust her own knowledge rather than to rely on someone else's judgment. Smith posits educated, confident seeing as an assertion of one's subjectivity.

Following Linnaeus's practice, Mrs. Talbot also tells her children where plants originate, thus asserting that the well-trained botanical eye must also learn to see specimens in their native context. Her attention to origins reflects a trend in botanical practice in late-eighteenth-century England. In response to reader requests, Withering began to emphasize the geographical context of plants in the second edition of his work (1787/1792): "The particular places of growth of the rarer plants are carefully enumerated, and many new ones are added at the request of several friends" (1787/1792 iv–v). The subtitle of Murray's *The British Garden* emphasizes the importance of both context and naming in botanizing: *A Descriptive Catalogue of Hardy Plants, Indigenous, or Cultivated in the Climate of Great-Britain, with Their Generic and Specific Characteristics, Latin and English Names, Native Country, and Time of Flowering*. When George asks his mother the name of "that beautiful tree which seems to bear white lilies," she answers not just with the name, but with the geographical origin of the tree and with some sense of its relation to other trees: "The *Datura arborea*, or tree thorn-apple ... is a native of Mexico and Peru, and is of the same genus as the common thorn-apple, a plant frequently found in lanes, and among rubbish by the sides of roads" (*WCS* 13:91). Mrs. Talbot identifies both the plant's native country and also the locations in which it thrives. In another exchange, Mrs. Talbot remembers encountering some favorite spring flowers: "[T]he yellow hellebore and the snow-drop were the most remarkable. The latter of these, you know, is indigenous in this country, and often grows spontaneously on the edges of fields and in extensive orchards, whitening the ground with its elegant drooping blossom" (*WCS* 13:103). While Mrs. Talbot notes the location in which these plants are usually found, Smith provides the scientific names for the hellebore and the snow-drop in a footnote: "Yellow hellebore, *Helleborus hyemalis*. Snow-drop, *Gulanthus nivalis*" (*WCS* 13:103).

The notes to the two volumes of *Conversations* enact the study of natural history as a progression from memorizing nomenclature to acquiring a more sophisticated understanding of a plant's geographical context and cultural relevance. The notes I quote above, all from the first volume of *Conversations*, are collected at the end of the volume in what adds up to a four-page catalogue of scientific names for animals, insects, and plants. The only note to this volume that offers more than the common and scientific names for plants promotes the value of eyewitness accounts in the construction of natural history: "Nasursium, *Tropæolum majus*.—This is one of the flowers which is said to have a sort of glory, or light halo of fire apparently surrounding it, of an evening in dry weather—a phenomenon first observed by one of the daughters of Linnaeus. I once thought I saw it in the Summer of 1802" (*WCS* 13:87). Seeing presumably leads to questions, and then to a more complete understanding of the plant. Accordingly, the notes to the second volume, depicted in Figure 6, are more extensive than those in the first volume.[14] In them, Smith continues to offer scientific names and to focus on the act of seeing, but she adds descriptions of the use, social and cultural context, and geographical location of natural objects. The notes inform readers that *Satice*, or sea lavender, grows on sterile cliffs and serves as a border plant in English flower beds. And, *Salsola kali*, or saltwort, a Mediterranean plant also found on the Sussex coast, is used in the production of glass. In additional notes not depicted in Figure 6, Smith quotes several natural history sources, including Gilbert White's *Natural History of Selbourne* and William Woodville's *Medicinal Botany*, thus situating her knowledge in a learned discussion about natural history.[15] The notes to "Flora," organized in a third list, also combine names with more elaborate notes on context.

The increasing complexity of the notes parallels the increasing technical difficulty of the poetic forms included in the two volumes. Labbe observes: "The child-reader ... advances from the simple iambic quatrameter, *abab* pattern of the first few poems through to rhyming iambic pentameter and the internal structural and rhyme variety of the later poems" (*Charlotte Smith* 169). Not only a natural history handbook but also a poetry primer, *Conversations* posits an analogy between the structure of poems and the structure of plants. Just as she teaches the children to distinguish between species of plants and animals, Mrs. Talbot teaches them to distinguish among various poetic forms. Describing blank verse, Mrs. Talbot contrasts it with "heroic verse of ten syllables, where the lines rhyme to each other, or rhyme alternately" (*WCS* 13:162). As with botany, one learns poetic form by placing poems in a relational framework. The visual organization of *Conversations* highlights the natural and poetic specimens that the children collect to further their education in each area. In the back of each volume, the notes seem to catalogue a collection of natural objects:

---

14 Labbe argues that in *Beachy Head* Smith's progression from providing the scientific names of plants to correcting Linnaeus and Gilbert White helps to establish her intellectual authority ('Transplanted' 82–84).

15 For example, she relies on Woodville's work to supply the following note: "*Morus nigra*, the common Mulberry—The mulberry tree, a native of Italy, is cultivated not only for its grateful fruit, but for the more lucrative purpose of supplying food to silk-worms. The leaves of the white mulberry are preferred for this purpose in Europe; but in China, where the best silk is made, the silk-worms are fed with the leaves of the *Morus tartaricus*. From the bark of another species, *Morus papyrifera*, the Japanese make paper, and the inhabitants of the South Sea Islands, the cloth which serves them for apparel. Woodvilles *Med. Bot.*" (*WCS* 13:208).

206   N O T E S.

Line 174. *Statice*, Sea Pink, Sea Lavender, commonly called Thrift, is frequently used for borders of
flower beds.   It covers some of the most sterile cliffs.

177. *Salsola kali*, Saltwort, this plant when burnt
affords a fossile alkali, and is used in the manufacture
of glass.   The best is brought from the Mediterranean,
and forms a considerable article of commerce.   It is
very frequent on the cliffs on the Sussex coast.

181. *Algæ*, Sea weeds of many sorts.   Sea Lace,
line 183, is one of them.   *Algæ*, *Fuci* and *Conferva*,
include, I believe, all sea plants.

182. *Polyp*, the Polypus, or Sea Annemone.

184. *Coralline* is, if I do not misunderstand the
only book I have to consult, a shelly substance, the
work of sea insects, adhering to stones and to sea
weeds.

189. *Flos aquæ*, Green Byssus, Paper Byssus, a
semi-transparent substance floating on the waves.

Panier'd is not perhaps a word correctly English,
but it must here be forgiven me.

191. *Pinna*.   The *Pinna*, or Sea Wing, is contained in a two-valved shell.   It consists of fine long
silk-like fibres—The *Pinna* on the coast of Provence
and Italy, is called the silk-worm of the sea.   Stock-
ings and gloves of exquisite fineness have been made of
it—See note 27th to the Œconomy of Vegetation.

The subsequent lines attempt a defcription of sea
plants, without any correct classification.

END OF THE SECOND VOLUME.

Fig. 6.   **Notes from Charlotte Smith's** *Conversations Introducing Poetry*,
          1804, vol. 2

Wasp, *Vespa vulgaris.*
Hornet, *Vespa crabro.*
Hare-bell, *Hyacinthus non scriptus.*
Broom, *Sparium scoparium.*
Clover, *Trifolium pretense.* (I.193)[16]

Likewise, on the page preceding each of the ten conversations, a list of titles catalogues the poetic collection that complements the collection of natural objects. The page introducing "Conversation the Ninth," for example, includes the following poems:

The Geranium.
The Mulberry-tree.
The blighted Rose.
Studies by the Sea. (*WCS* 13:199)

This list of titles signifies both a collection of verse and a collection of natural specimens. As Pascoe observes, "*Conversations* presents itself as a collection and takes up collecting as a topic of interest throughout" (*WCS* 13:xv). In the introduction to the work, Smith describes the various ways in which she found the poetry for this volume, noting "my collection insensibly increased" (*WCS* 13:61). Mrs. Talbot refers to the poems as "our collection of animals" and "our Museum of animals" (*WCS* 13:83, 13:142). In addition, she describes the final poem in the collection as itself a collection: "[O]ur little cabinet picture of Flora" (*WCS* 13:227).

This collector's cabinet in verse—the 228-line poetic fairy tale "Flora"—concludes *Conversations* by mingling scientific and therapeutic aspects of botanizing. In the fairy tale itself, Smith dramatizes the activities that are essential to botanical study: collecting, naming, and contextualizing. She frames this fanciful narrative with initial and concluding lines that argue for botany's healing effect on the wounded mind. In the first few lines of this frame, the speaker restates the desire Smith describes in "To the goddess of botany" to escape from oppressive social structures into the refuge of botanizing:

Remote from scenes, where the o'erwearied mind
Shrinks from the crimes and follies of mankind,
From hostile menace, and offensive boast,
Peace and her train of home-born pleasures lost;
To Fancy's reign, who would not gladly turn,
And lose awhile the miseries they mourn
In sweet oblivion? (ll. 1–7)

The mind wearied by the "crimes and follies of mankind" escapes into a remote garden. The speaker refers to Flora as "the enchanting Goddess of the flowery tribe, / Whose first prerogative it is to chase / The clouds which land on languid beauty's face" (ll. 14–16). She is to "Bid the wan maid [spring] the hues of *health*

---

16 These pages numbers refer to the original edition rather than the Pickering & Chatto edition, which does not reproduce the visual effect of a catalogue.

assume" (ll. 19, my emphasis). Flora's first duty is to chase the clouds away, or improve mood, the result of which Smith describes as "health." As the blooming of botanical gardens brings spring to life, so they bring the botanizer to life.[17]

Immediately following this twenty-line introductory frame, the speaker declares, "The vision comes!" (l. 21). In the next 180 lines, Flora marshals the plants to defend themselves against attacking insects.[18] The vegetation is armed and dressed for battle:

> For conquest arm'd the pygmy warriors wield
> The thorny lance, and spread the hollow shield
> Of Lichen tough; or bear, as silver bright,
> Lunaria's pearly circlet, firm and light.
> On the helm'd head the crimson Foxglove glows,
> Or Scutellaria guards the martial brows,
> While the Leontodon its plumage rears,
> And o'er the casque in waving grace appears; (ll. 61–68)

Portrayed as both beautiful and fierce, the fighting flowers in this poem are meant to inspire Emily to take an interest in fanciful topics, with the ultimate goal of developing her taste for mythological references in poetry. Yet the poem also continues to train the children's scientific eye. Seeming to answer the speaker's wish in "To the goddess of botany" to botanize in a variety of locations, Flora directs the reader's eye to plants in "the deep woodland" (l. 127), "along the mountain stream," (l. 140), within the stream itself, "[t]hro' richer pastures," (l. 164), down to the seashore, and into the "depths" of the sea (l. 179). The scientific names, collected in the notes along with comments on geographical context, march parallel to the plants in the verse. Thus, the botanical lessons that Mrs. Talbot teaches in the prose—how to visually identify, name, and geographically contextualize plants—are brought to life in this botanical fantasy.

Smith closes the frame with the speaker's 28-line concluding plea to Flora— who pleases children, young people, and brides—to give special attention to those suffering from melancholia and loss: "But most for those, by Sorrow's hand oppress'd, / May thy beds blossom, and thy wilds be drest" (ll. 215–16). She also urges Flora to help "the Mourner," who "droops in some sequestered spot" "O'er blighted happiness, for ever gone" (ll. 218, 220). She implores Flora to teach the mourner to shift his focus from "the dear image" of the one he has lost to the flowers in the vision (l. 221):

---

17 Smith footnotes this passage with lines from William Cowper's *The Task* that support her portrayal of botanizing as therapeutic. Smith quotes these lines also in *Minor Morals*:

> The spleen is seldom felt where Flora reigns;
> The lowering eye, the petulance, the frown,
> And sullen sadness, that do shade, distort,
> And mar the face of beauty, when no cause
> For such immeasurable grief appears:
> These Flora banishes. (*WCS* 12:223)

18 See Ruwe's "Benevolent Brothers" for a discussion of the gender crossing that occurs in this war between plants and insects (107–9).

Thou visionary Power, may'st bid him view
Forms not less lovely—and as transient too,
And, while they soothe the wearied Pilgrim's eyes,
Afford an antepast of Paradise. (ll. 225–28)

The framing lines assert that botanizing heals; the internal verse narrative demonstrates how this healing works. In her vision, the speaker collects plants from multiple locations, identifies them using Linnaean nomenclature, and considers their geographical context. Collecting, naming, and contextualizing—all visual-based activities—are the three major aspects of botanical practice that Smith portrays as therapeutic. The analogy Smith draws between the physical structure of plants and the formal structure of poems in *Conversations* calls for the invention of a literary language analogous to the scientific language of Linnaean botany, but designed to describe suffering rather than plants.

The Solitary Wanderer

Smith presents botanizing as a healing practice also in *The Letters of a Solitary Wanderer*, which she completed two years before *Conversations*. More radically, she proposes the collecting, contextualizing, and naming essential to botanical practice as a template for a language that will illuminate the experience of suffering so that others might apprehend it. The Solitary Wanderer describes himself as suffering from a "deep depression" (*WCS* 11:5). The frame narrative tells the story of the Solitary Wanderer's attempt to alleviate his melancholic pain through travel and botanizing. The internal narratives, five intricate tales that the Solitary Wanderer gathers in the course of his journey, tell the stories of other people's suffering, both in the primary storyline and in the many secondary narratives embedded in each of the five tales.[19] Smith intended to write a sixth volume, "the story of the Solitary Wanderer himself," but did not complete it due to ill health and a change in publisher between the appearance of the first three volumes in 1800 and the final two volumes in 1802 (*WCS* 11:309). However, Smith seems to offer a plot summary of this intended volume two years later in *Conversations*. Mrs. Talbot gives her children a poem written by "a young man, with whom I was once acquainted," and then describes his circumstances:

> A peculiar and disastrous chain of events, seemed to pursue him through life; but after his fortune apparently changed for the better, other circumstances arose, which deprived him of the happiness, independence, and affluence promised him ... . [T]he loss of a mother and a sister, to whom he was most affectionately attached, added to a disappointment in the character and conduct of a young woman ... were circumstances so affecting his mind, that he never could determine to pursue any of those objects, either of ambition or amusement, which usually attract young men of his rank and situation—but relinquishing his establishment, he passed the greatest part of his time in wandering into different countries. (*WCS* 13:196–97)

---

19 For a compelling analysis of the formal structure of this work, see D. L. Macdonald's introduction to vol. 11 of the *Works of Charlotte Smith*.

"Wandering into different countries," the Solitary Wanderer collects narratives of suffering, just as the children in *Conversations* collect poems about the plants, animals, and insects they find. The five tales in five volumes describe the circumstances of individuals oppressed by slavery, forced marriage, tyrannous religious structures, or despotic governments, and detail the grief of people who have lost children, parents, siblings, or cherished friends. Smith emphasizes the status of these tales as found objects by reproducing much of the narrative in the form of letters that the Solitary Wanderer discovers or is given, or by having the Solitary Wanderer relay tales in the voices of the original sufferers. Traveling to collect plants and tales, the Solitary Wanderer seeks healing for his melancholia.

These collecting activities offer a model for a new language of suffering that the Solitary Wanderer suggests will go further to heal him than will conventional therapies for melancholia. He refers to the two therapies Smith rejects in the sonnet "Written in Bristol"—going to the spa and viewing the landscape. He writes to his friend who suggests that he undergo a spa regimen for his melancholia: "So, you really think I should do better to resort to some of those public places, of which the North of England boasts a considerable variety?" (*WCS* 11:8). The Solitary Wanderer chooses to avoid the spa, expressing skepticism that he will find consolation in such company: "Believe me, such an assemblage as these places usually produce, may irritate and render incurable the misanthropy (which you say is a great fault in my character), but cannot afford one moment's alleviation to the sufferings of a wounded heart" (*WCS* 11:8). Instead, the Solitary Wanderer, like the health travelers I discuss in the previous chapter, seeks to divert his mind from despair by immersing himself in travel: "When I undertake to give you a regular account of my wanderings, or at least as regular as my rambling life will admit of, you will own that I have done right in determining to try if *continual change of scene* will not relieve me from the deep depression I have now for some months vainly endeavored to conquer" (*WCS* 11:5, my emphasis). And indeed, the Solitary Wanderer does find some physical benefit in health travel: "I feel the advantage of changing the air and of new scenes on my outward man, though my mind is still inert and torpid" (*WCS* 11:6). The change of air and scene revives his body, but not his "inert and torpid" mind.

Health travel does not alleviate his "deep depression" because the Solitary Wanderer's pain results in part from the difficulty of describing his suffering to others. He comments on this problem in a letter to his friend:

> Already I feel myself better able than I was to converse upon paper, though I still would fly from the well-meant importunity of those who will not let me be sick or miserable in my own way, but continually distress me with inquiries and remonstrances, and say: "What aileth thee? and wherefore is thy countenance overcast, and thine heart disquieted?" when, if they cannot understand, I cannot explain why I am unhappy.—Ah! how difficult it is to communicate to others what one feels! After all, how little impression does it make! (*WCS* 11:5)

The Solitary Wanderer resents the difficulty inherent in identifying his condition ("what") and explaining its etiology ("wherefore") to others. The claim that one's suffering is beyond words signifies the intensity of pain the condition causes. Yet the Solitary Wanderer's lament—"how difficult it is to communicate to others what one feels"—also resonates with medical writers' struggle to redraw the boundaries among nervous illnesses in the late eighteenth century. Buchan describes the challenge of identifying any nervous illness as a discrete disease process:

> Of all diseases incident to mankind, those of the nervous kind are the most complicated and difficult to cure. A volume would not be sufficient to point out their various appearances. They imitate almost every disease; and are seldom alike in two different persons, or even the same person at different times. (*Domestic* 420)

The Solitary Wanderer wishes for a language that will help him communicate to others the difference between his suffering and, for instance, garden variety hypochondria, or common melancholia, just as Mrs. Talbot is able to convey to her children the difference between the *Dionæa muscipula* (Venus flytrap) and the *Apocynum*, two fly-catching plants that look alike to the untrained eye. He longs for a grammar of suffering as clear and accessible as the grammar of botany.

Rejecting conventional therapies, the Solitary Wanderer turns to collecting narratives, a practice he implicitly compares to collecting plants. At the beginning of his journey, the Solitary Wanderer notes that botany "used to interest and soothe my mind beyond any other study; but now I am in a state of spirits when it would rather depress than charm them" (*WCS* 11:7). Yet he pursues the amateur science anyway, defending his interest in botany to his friend and correspondent: "Without books, and with no other companions but my servant and my two horses, you will think my lingering in such places as I have described a very strange plan: and you despise, I know, the pursuits of the botanist ... which I have occasionally taken up with some degree of interest" (*WCS* 11:7). The Solitary Wanderer "lingers" in ditches and bogs to collect botanical specimens. Just as he "lingers" in unusual places to collect plants, so the Wanderer "lingers" around a haunted house in order to construct a narrative about the history of suffering that took place inside: "I have *collected* a number of circumstances which I am persuaded are authentic, and which I think ... will make a history not uninteresting or without its moral. I shall *linger* about this melancholy abode, and make my picture amid the very scenery where the incidents happened" (*WCS* 11:11, my emphasis). The Solitary Wanderer uses the words "collect" and "linger" to describe both the gathering of plants and the collecting of narratives of suffering, thus linking the two activities. In a reference to his narrative project and to botanical sketching, he promises to "make [his] picture" from the "circumstances" he collects. In the introduction to *Letters of a Solitary Wanderer*, Smith explains that she intends each volume to contain "a single Narrative, which the Solitary Wanderer is supposed to *collect* in the countries he visits" (*WCS* 11:3, my emphasis).

Although *The Letters of a Solitary Wanderer* is essentially a fictional travel narrative, the stories the Wanderer collects are much fuller than his account of his own travels. This focus on the suffering of others temporarily alleviates his melancholic pain. In the fourth volume, "The Hungarian," the Solitary Wanderer tells the story of two lovers separated by a tyrannous older brother and by the wars following the French Revolution. After he helps the lovers reunite, the Solitary Wanderer looks for a new tale of suffering to distract him from his own pain: "[W]here shall I find persons who can excite in my heart an interest so lively as to suspend, for some months at least, that sense of dreary vacuity which has for many years rendered my life rather a burthen I was to exert myself to bear, than an existence I was to enjoy?" (*WCS*

11:402). Both clergymen and physicians recommended that depressed patients visit others less fortunate than themselves to cure despair and prevent suicide. Quoting a Dr. Baxter, Benjamin Fawcett recommends that caretakers of depressed patients "Engage them in comforting others, that are in deeper distress than themselves" (19). As he interacts with the subjects of the tales he gathers, the Solitary Wanderer gains a sense of purpose: "My life, whatever it may be to myself, is not however always useless to others; I have more than once met in my wanderings with those whose sorrows I had the power at least to suspend" (*WCS* 11:100). Collecting the stories of others, the Solitary Wanderer "remark[s] the various miseries of life" and thus better "learn[s] to endure [his] own" (*WCS* 11:100). As he retells these stories, the Solitary Wanderer gains insight into his own pain. Smith planned for the Solitary Wanderer to tell his own story in the final volume—that is, after he had established and practiced a language of suffering.

Much as naturalists sent botanical reports and specimens from expeditions abroad to the Linnaean Society, the Solitary Wanderer mails his collection of narratives in letters to his friend in England. Each narrative is taken from a different geographical context, including Yorkshire ("The Story of Eduoarda"), Liverpool and Jamaica ("The Story of Henrietta"), sixteenth-century France ("The Story of Corisande"), Germany ("The Hungarian"), and Ireland ("The Story of Leonora"). For the Solitary Wanderer, as for botanists who collected specimens from around the world, recording the context in which he finds a specimen is crucial to the classification process. *The Annals of Natural History; or Magazine of Zoology, Botany and Geology* published botanists' letters under the section heading: "Information respecting Botanical Travellers." Writing from Brazil, for example, George Gardner reports, "During my first walks I collected specimens of the following plants: *Turnera trioniflora*, which grows profusely in waste and cultivated spots and by road sides .... In marshy places, which were beginning to dry up, I found fine specimens of *Pontederia paniculata*, *Hydrolea spinosa*, and a small purple-flowered *Ammannia*" (*Annals* 464). The editor reports that Gardner's collection of about 200 species of plants has arrived and "will be distributed to the different subscribers with as little delay as possible" (*Annals* 62). Likewise, the Solitary Wanderer says to his friend, "You opine, that it is of no manner of importance to the world whether some plant of no known use, or evident beauty, is found in a ditch in Yorkshire, or in a bog in Lincolnshire" (*WCS* 11:7). He corrects his friend's opinion, arguing that recording a plant's specific location is crucial for identifying and naming that plant.

As with the botanical specimens he collects, the Solitary Wanderer identifies the geographical origin of each story he gathers and seeks to preserve its individual integrity as he adds it to his narrative collection. He consistently identifies his own location, writing at the top of his fourth letter, for example, "May 9, From a Cottage made out of one of the most distant Offices of Palsgrave Priory" (*WCS* 11:13). Likewise, the authors of the letters he collects note the locations from which they write. Henrietta, the heroine of the second tale, composes a letter, "On board the Argonaut, at Sea, quitting the Madeira Islands" (*WCS* 11:109). Although identifying the place from which one writes a letter was a common practice in the eighteenth century, in this text it serves as an example of how a language that expresses suffering might begin—with attention to the social context of that suffering. The Solitary Wanderer preserves the original structure of each story by reprinting letters and other documents when he can; when he does not have access to these documents, he carefully identifies the source of his narrative. The Solitary Wanderer translates "The Story of Corisande" from the Old French in which Corisande's relative De Vezelai has written it in order to "preserve a great part of the narrative" that he takes from "a great number of manuscript memoirs, letters and papers that belonged to my family" (*WCS* 11:203). The fifth volume, which tells "The Story of Leonora," is comprised mostly of letters Leonora wrote to her friend Sophia, who then passed them on to the Solitary Wanderer. The Solitary Wanderer's collection of narratives replicates scientific botany's attention to context, type, and individual structure. He seeks to establish a common language of suffering, but also to preserve the "irreducible alterity" of each individual's suffering in the process.

By putting the stories in a collection, the Solitary Wanderer allows the reader to consider one person's suffering in a relational framework. For example, several tales resonate with Smith's own life story, particularly her disastrous forced marriage to Benjamin Smith. Although the circumstances differ wildly, the basic problem—forced marriage—is the same. When Henrietta, the subject of the second volume, finds that her father plans to marry her to the nephew of a widow he likes, she characterizes his intention as "selling his daughter to the most dreadful of all slavery," a powerful statement to make about marriage in a letter written from a slave plantation in Jamaica (*WCS* 11:121). Hours before Henrietta's compulsory wedding, a slave named Amponah helps her escape her father's house during the confusion of a slave uprising. As the maroons escape the bonds of slavery, she escapes the bonds of marriage. Eventually, her paternal uncle, who is living as a hermit in a cave, finds her and unwittingly reunites her with Denbigh, the Jacobin reformer she regards as her soul mate. Corisande, the heroine of the third volume, is held hostage by relatives who wish her to marry the Marquis de Champignac, whom she does not love. Disguised as a peasant boy, she attempts to escape. The narrator describes her understanding of the impact such a marriage might have on her life: "Though yet a child in years, she very properly considered, that, if she was old enough to make an indissoluble engagement, and to pronounce vows the most solemn and binding that can be imposed by social laws, she was certainly old enough to have a will of her own, and to act as that will directed" (*WCS* 11:212–13). Her initial escape is not entirely successful; she requires rescue by Montgomeri, a friend of her father whom she encounters at a propitious moment. Eventually, the Marquis's long illness releases her from the threat of unwelcome marriage, and she weds Montgomeri instead. Unlike Smith, both of these young women ultimately escape arranged engagements designed to enhance familial power and marry instead for love. Nonetheless, the similarities among Smith's story and her two character's tales establish that, whether in eighteenth-century England, eighteenth-century Jamaica, or sixteenth-century France, marriage can be threatening to a woman's well-being. The young women from these diverse settings struggle mightily against family desires and paternal power to escape the potential disaster of bad marriages. The commonalities among the stories in these novellas expose the social origins of suffering—women's oppression in marriage—while the differences honor each woman's individual experience of suffering.

Apparently the resonance between these stories and Smith's forced marriage was subtle enough, or followed gothic and sentimental narrative conventions closely enough, that it did not inspire the criticism of reviewers. *The Critical Review* begins its assessment of the first three volumes of *The Letters of a Solitary Wanderer* with an expression of gratitude. Although the work does not rank among Smith's best fiction, the reviewer notes, it does not, like the prefaces to her poetry and novels, voice personal complaints about the chancery case, or make "declamations on the injustices of attorneys and trustees" (36). The critic also praises her for resisting the impulse to depict herself as a character, presumably an objection to the teacher-figures in her children's works, whom the reviewer sarcastically describes as the "peculiarly prudent ladies of a middle age whose prototypes are not hard to find" (36). In her introduction to volumes four and five, Smith fires back at this snide praise:

> [A]s to the resemblance they thus pretend to find between certain characters in different books, as all alluding to one person, what right have they to say it? Surely no impartial reader will judge in the manner, or imagine I could be guilty of such foolish egotism as to represent myself under these different characters, and under circumstances which, in no single instance, bear any relation to my private life. (*WCS* 11:310)

In spite of this claim, or perhaps to spite the critics, Smith writes a fifth volume that resonates more overtly with the circumstances of her own childhood marriage than do the narrowly averted forced marriages in the first three volumes. When the mother of the main character Leonora dies, her father remarries. Like Smith at age 15, Leonora does not get along with her stepmother, and her father pressures her to marry the dissolute young man Mr. Wardenell in order to get her out of the house: "To this marriage Leonora was the first sacrifice, tho' she had not yet completed her fifteenth year; for the new Mrs. Leicester could not bear a daughter-in-law as tall as herself, and of such eminent beauty, that she was every where an object of admiration" (*WCS* 11:409). Because she loves her father, Leonora goes along with his plan. She laments, "My mother's death was the first real evil that befell me, and from that period a series of calamities incessantly pursued me" (*WCS* 11:430). After Leonora marries Wardenell, she suffers from his infidelity and his involvement in a series of money-losing schemes. When Wardenell's father dies, his behavior deteriorates even further. Though the details differ, these circumstances reflect Smith's relationship with Benjamin Smith. Unlike Henrietta and Corisande in the previous volumes, Leonora does not stand up to her family to escape the forced marriage. The story of Leonora's life illustrates how a woman suffers when her father chooses his own immediate desires over his daughter's future well-being. Smith also explores the consequences of Leonora's decision, like that of Smith herself, to obey her father's wishes rather than to follow her own feelings.

In addition to this autobiographically resonant set of stories, Smith places many other apparently less personal narratives of suffering in a relational framework. For example, although we have only Smith's brief summary of the Solitary Wanderer's own story, what little we know resonates with the embedded story of the Hermit in the second volume. Like the Solitary Wanderer, the Hermit chooses a life of solitude to recover from his pain, asserting that "wounded as I have been ... it is only in perfect solitude I find life supportable" (*WCS* 11:183). In both cases, the Hermit's and the Solitary Wanderer's suffering results from familial losses and from "disappointment in the character and conduct of a young woman" (*WCS* 13:196–97). Born into a very wealthy plantation-owning family, the Hermit, originally named Mr.

Maynard, marries young. His wife Fanny proves immature and overly influenced by her socially ambitious mother. After consumption claims their daughter's life, the marriage falls apart. Fanny runs away with her sister's brother-in-law, leaving Maynard behind with a son to raise. After divorcing Fanny, Maynard unhappily remarries and discovers years later that his first wife has become a prostitute. He provides her with a separate residence and an income, only to find that his second wife, jealous of this arrangement, has murdered his son. Fanny and Maynard mourn their son, and then Fanny dies of grief. Although we do not know the comparable details of the Solitary Wanderer's suffering, his loss of a sister and mother parallels Maynard's loss of his children, and his disappointment in a young woman parallels Maynard's response to Fanny's desertion. Like the Solitary Wanderer, Maynard rejects suggestions that he go to a spa, and instead attempts to recover from his first wife's betrayal by traveling and interacting with a close friend. When his friend dies unexpectedly, Maynard is inspired by the abolitionist treatises he discovers among his friend's papers to return to Jamaica to help in the fight against slavery. Maynard observes that before reading these treatises, he was blind to the suffering of slaves: "I was amazed at the indifference with which I had *looked on* and been a party in oppression" (*WCS* 11:182, my emphasis). With this plot turn, Smith posits that a person's extreme suffering can open his eyes to the suffering of others. Suffering can, in Maynard's case, turn a plantation-owner's son into an abolitionist, and in the Solitary Wanderer's case, turn a wealthy young man into a collector of narratives illustrating social oppression.

Collected together, these accounts of suffering encourage the reader to compare the social circumstances of different lives. The suffering presented in the three narratives that address forced marriage reveals the dangers of patriarchal society for women as a group. And the various manifestations of these dangers present the experience of individual women's suffering under patriarchy—Henrietta's father tries to marry her off to facilitate his financially auspicious match; Corisande's relatives bestow upon her a fiancé who will help them gain control over the family property; and Leonora's father pushes her out of the house into a marriage in order to please his competitive second wife. The differences among these stories are as important as the similarities. Unlike Henrietta, who escapes the threat of unwelcome marriage with the help of a slave and her uncle, and unlike Corisande, who left her family home under her own power but was rescued by her future husband, Leonora has no help. By putting these stories in a relational framework, Smith argues that it is not possible for a woman to resist paternal and familial authority—which is fully supported by the law—without help from sympathetic men. In the parallel stories of the Hermit Maynard and the Solitary Wanderer, Smith presents us with men who each suffer from a woman's "character and conduct." The physician and friend who attends Maynard after Fanny leaves him attributes her failures to lack of education and to unproductive societal expectations for women:

> I believe, my friend ... that what is called their education gives [women no character] ... . If any of them venture even to look as if they had any will of their own, or supposed themselves capable of reasoning, how immediately are they marked as something monstrous, absurd, and out of the course of nature! while the most insipid moppet that ever looked in a glass is preferred to one of those reasoning damsels, especially by empty and superficial young men. (*WCS* 11:161–62)

He explains that when women are taught to base their self-worth on their appearance rather than on their minds, they respond to aging by finding a new man to reassure them that they are attractive. When told in a relational framework, stories of men suffering at the hand of women's bad character and conduct become a collective critique of women's education rather than individual portraits of evil women.

The language of suffering as Smith conceives it requires that individual suffering be understood in the context of oppressive social structures. Like a botanical specimen in a collection, a story placed among other stories allows the reader to see not just an individual complaint, but a social problem with a range of resultant suffering. And, in return, the discernment of this social problem, this "class" or "order" of suffering, makes individual suffering more visible because it can, finally, be given a name. The goal of Linnaean botany was to name and classify flora according to principles that would apply to any plant one encountered. As Theresa Kelley explains, "Linnaeus's systematics explicitly addressed the discovery of new and strange species from around the globe that had already begun to put extraordinary pressure on the task of classifying its flora and fauna" ("Romantic" 226). Likewise, with her language of suffering, Smith seeks to make unfamiliar suffering visible to those who have not experienced it themselves. With both suffering and natural history, to name is to know. Linnaeus himself claims, in an echo of John Locke, that "without names there can be no permanent knowledge" (Morton 273). Likewise, medical historian Charles Rosenberg asserts: "In some ways disease does not exist until we have agreed that it does, by perceiving, naming, and responding to it" (xiii). Who creates these names, of course, is no small matter.

Indeed, the European project of naming and classifying plants based on their anatomical relation to other plants from around the world effectively erased national boundaries and local origins.[20] Mary Louise Pratt describes the "transformative,

---

20 Smith, however, describes viewing botanical collections as an internationally rich experience, one that signifies origins even as the plants are removed from these origins. In *Conversations*, for example, Mrs. Talbot takes her children into a botanical garden and conservatory and expresses enthusiasm for the international array of specimens: "There are few sights, my children, that afford me so much pleasure as a collection of plants, where the produce of every quarter of the world is assembled. In the stove the natives of the torrid zone; in the conservatory the inhabitants of milder regions, which are yet too tender to bear the winter in this country. There, planted in a swampy soil, brought from heaths and moors, are the beautiful productions of North America; in another spot of compost earth are Alpine plants; and on that artificial rock those that flourish on dry and stony places, where little else will vegetate" (*WCS* 13:91). Though surely identified by a Linnaean binomial that erases the details of local context, the plants in this collection are organized according to climate, thus reflecting their original context. As with her celebration of specimens from around the globe, the great number of international settings Smith chooses for her novels reflects a more cosmopolitan than imperialist agenda. Curran asserts, "No novelist of her time has so broad a range of setting. It is not only that she transports her novels to Europe, to North America, and to the Caribbean, but even within Great Britain, she will move Ethelinde, say, between Grasmere in the Lake District, to London, then Dorset .... Cosmopolitanism for Smith is, from the first, a major personal virtue and a determining ethical element for the cultures explored in her fictions" (gen. intro. *WCS* 1:xxi–xxii).

appropriative dimensions" of Linnaean classification: "One by one the planet's life forms were to be drawn out of the tangled threads of their life surroundings and rewoven into European-based patterns of global unity and order" (31). It is a breathtaking display of dominance and entitlement to name all the plants on the earth according to a European system of classification. This ordering, Pratt convincingly argues, was an assertion of European hegemony: "The eighteenth-century classificatory systems created the task of locating every species on the planet, extracting it from its particular arbitrary surroundings (the chaos), and placing it in its appropriate spot in the system (the order—book, collection, or garden) with its new written, secular European name" (31). Placing one's suffering within a relational context—naming it to communicate it to others—also involves an assertion of power, yet the stakes are quite different. To name one's own illness is to name the other within oneself and thus to create distance between the "self" and "the illness." Medical anthropologist Byron Good explains the importance of "naming the source of suffering, particularly for those in chronic pain": "To name the origin of the pain is to seize power to alleviate it, and the intensity of the pain demands urgency. To name the origin of pain is also a critical step in the remaking of the world, in the authoring of an integrated self" (129). Although Smith based her language of suffering on botanical classification, the relationship between specimen and name is much more dynamic for suffering than for botany. While Linnaean orders and classes offer a stable structure into which each new specimen can be placed, in Smith's language of suffering, each new specimen reconstitutes or shifts the "order" of suffering through which it is first seen. The details of each tale of suffering have an irreducible, individual texture in which Smith places a great deal of faith. Although Corisande, Henrietta, Leonora, and Smith all experience the threat of forced marriage, the details of each individual story reshape our understanding of women's autonomy in patriarchal culture. To create a relational framework of suffering is to see individual suffering; to see examples of individual suffering is to restructure that framework repeatedly and recursively.

On a practical level, botanizing alleviates Smith's melancholic pain. For Smith, as for Rousseau, discerning the structure of plants, placing them in a relational framework, sketching their details, and identifying them by name are all therapeutic activities. Botanical study offers the satisfaction of ordering and describing the outside world when one's own mental state feels disordered. If drawing botanical sketches makes Smith's grief visible, creating a grammar of suffering based on the principles of Linnaean botany might establish a common language for people to express and apprehend one another's suffering. Natural history, as Michel Foucault argues, does not make apparent natural phenomena that people have simply overlooked, but rather "constitute[s] ... a new field of visibility ... in all its density" (132). A language of suffering, like a language of natural history, can create a new field of vision in which not only individual suffering, but also the social patterns that underlie this suffering become visible and are named. Donna Haraway observes that "Linnaeus referred to himself as a second Adam, the 'eye' of God, who could give true representations, true names, thus reforming or restoring a purity of names lost by the first Adam's sin" (9). While I do not think Smith would make such a claim for herself, her interest in Linnaean botany inspired her to create a narrative form that makes suffering intelligible to a wide range of people. Seeing with a botanical eye—that is to say, collecting, naming, contextualizing—offers a template for this new genre. When narrative form creates "a new field of visibility," there is hope that the sufferer's pain might be acknowledged and alleviated.

While in the *Elegiac Sonnets* Smith heralds the creative benefit of being held in a sympathetic gaze, in *Conversations* and *The Letters of a Solitary Wanderer*, Smith details how that gaze might be trained. Smith's relational framework of suffering exposes the complexity behind the suffering bodies that she presents in her poetry. The Hermit in the second volume of *The Letters of a Solitary Wanderer*, for example, prepares us to sympathize with and ask questions of the enigmatic cliff-dwelling hermit at the end of *Beachy Head*. In addition, knowing the details of the Hermit's story from *Letters of a Solitary Wanderer* gives new depth to our questions about the suffering bodies—including the maniac, the shipwrecked mariner, the pilgrim, the Laplander, and the exile—who populate the *Elegiac Sonnets*. Just as seeing plants first hand leads the children in *Conversations* to ask questions about the context of plants, seeing the bodies of sufferers after hearing other detailed narratives of suffering inspires comparisons and questions about the social causes of their suffering. Smith argues that individual suffering is best understood in a collection that allows for comparison and exploration of the causal context. For Smith, however, there is no philosophical category or general name for suffering that will ever be completely separable from the individual's material experience of that suffering.

As we shall see in chapter 6, Smith creates a variation on this language of suffering in her children's work *Rural Walks*. Rather than collecting first-person narratives of individual suffering that the reader might compare in order to draw conclusions about social context, Smith positions the teacher figure in *Rural Walks* as an ethnographer of the impoverished ill, collecting and commenting on stories so that others might apprehend the relationship between illness and poverty.

Chapter 5

Invisibility and the History of Trauma: Mary Shelley's *Rambles in Germany and Italy*

"If traumatic experience, as Freud indicates suggestively, is an experience that is not fully assimilated as it occurs, then ... what [does] it mean to transmit and to theorize around a crisis that is marked, not by a simple knowledge, but by the ways it simultaneously defies and demands our witness [?]"

Cathy Caruth

In her final published work, the epistolary travel narrative *Rambles in Germany and Italy, in 1840, 1842, and 1843* (1844), Mary Shelley details her search for health and her hopes for Italy's political well-being. In addition, she describes her visits to several locations associated with life-changing losses, traumatic experiences that simultaneously defy and demand witness. This narrative, an account of two trips that Mary Shelley took to the Continent with her son Percy Florence Shelley and his friends, moves between describing the visible world such travel narratives customarily depict and invoking invisible presences. It alternates between disclosing and withholding, showing and concealing. Although she produced an impressive body of literature in her authorial life following the publication of *Frankenstein*, Mary Shelley simultaneously sought shelter from public exposure after the death of Percy Bysshe Shelley.[1] Answering Edward John Trelawny's 1829 request that she provide documents and stories about Shelley for Trelawny's own autobiography, she notes that "there is nothing I shrink from more fearfully than publicity" (*LMWS* ii.72). She expresses a desire "to wrap night and obscurity of insignificance around me" and a strong resistance to being "the subject of *men's* observations" (*LMWS* ii.72, original emphasis). With *Rambles*, however, she emerges from the public invisibility she sought, including a three-year hiatus from writing. For both political and personal reasons, she fought the desire to "run away & shut myself up yet more entirely" in order to write a travel narrative for public consumption (*LMWS* iii.101).

Mary Poovey argues that Mary Shelley's tendency in her later novels "to express and efface herself at the same time" emerges from the tension between, on the one hand, her radical upbringing and marriage, and on the other, her father's, and indeed patriarchal Britain's, increasingly conservative attitudes towards women's roles (*Proper* 131). While this tension is also apparent in *Rambles*, I regard the narrative's fluctuation between expression and effacement, visibility and invisibility, also as a

---

1   Mary Shelley published six novels after *Frankenstein*, as well as numerous short stories and essays.

trauma response—or more precisely, as the narrative embodiment of the unsettling tension between what is known and unknown in trauma. The formal properties of these fluctuations in Mary Shelley's travel narrative are also the formal properties of traumatic utterance—ambivalence, circumlocution, and temporal delay. Mary Shelley's written account of her return to the site of youthful trauma intentionally or unintentionally "traces the rhythms" of how one experiences trauma, to use Patricia Clare Ingham's formulation, even as it cannot or does not present those past traumatic events directly (10).[2]

Previous trauma makes itself known in Mary Shelley's responses to the places that surrounded the loss of her children and her husband. It surfaces also in her striking fear that her only surviving child will die like his father while sailing in Italy, a loss that would seem to repeat the loss of her other children and her partner. She looks at Percy Florence's boat on Lake Como and "shudders": "I can bring no help, except constant watchfulness ... . A tragedy has darkened my life: I endeavor, in vain, to cast aside the fears which are its offspring; they haunt me perpetually" (*WMS* 8:113).[3] These traumatic losses haunt her again as, upon re-entering Italy, she feels that "the days of my youth hover near" (*WMS* 8:261). Her identification with the "inanimate objects that had surrounded me, which *survived*, the same in aspect as then" make her feel that her life "since was but an unreal phantasmagoria" (*WMS* 8:148, my emphasis). The displacement of her own survival onto the objects she revisits in Italy, as well as the unreality of the present moment, together signal the survivor's sense of inexpressible experience, which Cathy Caruth describes as "the oscillation between a *crisis of death* and the correlative *crisis of life*: between the story of the unbearable nature of an event and the story of the unbearable nature of its survival" (7). Embodied first in Victor Frankenstein's creature, the sense of suspense between life and death that is inherent in trauma is even more powerfully present in *Rambles* as Mary Shelley moves fluidly, yet painfully, between the living and the dead. Mary Shelley's assertion that she wrote the narrative "in a state of pain that makes me look at its pages now as if written in a dream" evokes the painful process of working through trauma, which requires an emotional awareness of the unknown at the heart of traumatic experience (*LMWS* iii.146).

In her introduction to *Rambles*, Mary Shelley does not reference her own losses, but focuses her attention instead on supporting the Risorgimento, the movement for Italian nationalism. However, the way this political discussion both reveals and conceals desire reflects the structure of a trauma response. She explicitly demands that her readers witness Italy's struggles and potential as a nation, qualities she makes visible through discussions of Italy's literature, art, music, history, and politics. She aspires to "induce some among my countrymen to regard with greater attention, and to sympathize in the struggles of a country, the most illustrious and the most unfortunate in the world" (*WMS* 8:69–70). Yet, she defies witness of her

---

2   I am indebted to Ingham for sharing this formulation with me, for lively conversations about the signs and implications of traumatic experience, and for directing me to Caruth's book.

3   Jeanne Moskal describes Mary Shelley's trip as part pilgrimage to relieve "survivor's guilt." She eventually overcame her anxiety about her son's death by joining him for a sail, an experience that Moskal argues helps expiate this guilt ("Travel Writing" 252–54).

more private motivation for writing this partially political work—to raise funds for Ferdinando Gatteschi, an Italian revolutionary exile whom she met in Paris after the 1843 journey, and for whom she had a great deal of sympathy, perhaps even strong feeling.[4] Although she includes Gatteschi's account of the Carbonari in *Rambles*, she mentions neither him nor their relationship in the text. In spite of this tension between her openly stated political goal and her private motivation for writing, Mary Shelley proposes the work to her publisher not as a political document nor as an objective travel guide, but rather as "personal to myself" (*LMWS* iii.96). While this phrase suggests that the personal nature of the text might offer readers insight into the author and her infamous circle, I argue that the reflexive structure of this phrase—"personal to myself"—is exactly what she produces in *Rambles*. Although the narrative refers to both past and present suffering as well as to historical trauma, these traumatic events seem unconsciously coded to be partially seen but not fully understood from the outside. The phrase "personal to myself," then, indicates a willingness to explore previous trauma as privately as one can in a published narrative, yet it does not promise that Mary Shelley will herself be able to access fully the trauma she veils.

This fluctuation between demanding and defying witness informs not only her motivation for writing, but also her account of suffering during the two trips. Mary Shelley undertook the journeys to expand Percy Florence's education as well as to restore her health in Germany's spas and in Italy's salubrious climate. In *Rambles* she includes accounts of the two types of treatment that she explored on these trips—the institutional medicine she encountered in her visits to Germany's spas and the salutary landscape she enjoyed both at the spas and while traveling. Ultimately, Mary Shelley champions the balm derived from viewing the landscape over the prescriptive spa regimen. Like her mother, Mary Shelley describes the landscape—particularly when picturesque—as healing. However, while Mary Wollstonecraft seeks novelty and therapeutically sheltering scenes in the Scandinavian landscape, her daughter looks at the Italian landscape through the lens of memory and through the eyes of those she has lost, including her mother. Mary Shelley's trips to Italy in the 1840s were her first since she departed that country in 1823, leaving behind the graves of Shelley and of their children Clare and William. Writing about her visit to Rome in 1843, she answers an implied question from her correspondent: "'What are the pleasures I enjoy at Rome?' you ask" (*WMS* 8:347). She replies that while the experience offers therapeutic visual beauty, it also triggers traumatic memories. The pleasures are "so many, that my mind is brimful of a sort of glowing satisfaction, mingled with tearful associations. Besides all that Rome itself affords of delightful [sic] to the eye and imagination, I revisit it as the bourne of a pious pilgrimage. The treasures of my youth lie buried here" (*WMS* 8:347–48). Looking in order to heal on this pilgrimage, Mary Shelley must gaze through past suffering to alleviate present pain.

The 1840 and 1842 trips both began in the midst of emotional strain and illness. Prior to her 1840 trip, Mary Shelley suffered from depression, her condition exacerbated by editing Shelley's complete works. On 12 February 1839, while editing volume 2 of the *Works*, and while also receiving criticism for her revisions of *Queen*

---

4   In her introduction to the Pickering & Chatto edition of *Rambles*, Jeanne Moskal suggests that Mary Shelley was more willing to enter the public eye again because of her relationship with Gatteschi (*WMS* 8:54n1).

Mab in volume 1, she speculates: "I almost think that my present occupation will end in a fit of illness ... . I am torn to pieces by Memory—Would that all were mute in the grave!" (*JMS* 559). Editing her dead husband's works, she hovers between the living and the dead, acutely aware of her status as a survivor. With her wish that "all were mute in the grave," Mary Shelley hopes to silence the memories around these losses that haunt her, simultaneously acknowledging the muteness at the center of trauma. As she predicted, illness followed editing. Later in the spring of 1839, a particularly bad bout of recurring nervous illness characterized by "weakness and languour" prevented her from writing at all (*JMS* 563). Less than two weeks before leaving on the 1840 trip, Mary Shelley observes in her journal that during the preceding sixteen months she has been "oppressed by care, disappointment & ill health—which all have combined to depress and irritate me" (*JMS* 564). She continues: "[I]t is my strange fate that all my friends are sufferers—ill health or adversity bears heavy on them—& I can do little good—& lately ill health—& extreme depression have even marred the little I could do ... . My health impaired by a thousand mental sufferings has cast chains on my soul" (*JMS* 564). The 1842 journey followed a similar period of depression, caused in part by the disappointing news she received about her much-needed inheritance from Shelley (Sunstein 356). In addition to having ample cause for a depressive mood during these years, Mary Shelley was generally subject to extended bouts of what she describes as "darkest Melancholy" (*JMS* 546). Prior to and during the trips recounted in *Rambles*, she also suffered from chronic headaches, symptoms which were finally diagnosed in 1850 as the brain tumor that would cause her death (Sunstein 383).

In the first letter of *Rambles*, she encapsulates her feelings of ill health in a sentence, confiding to the reader (and to her ostensible correspondent Claire Clairmont), "You know ... how grievously my health has been shaken: a nervous illness interrupts my usual occupations, and disturbs the tenor of my life" (*WMS* 8:76). Mary Shelley goes on to express hope that "traveling will cure all," and more specifically that her "mind will ... renew the outworn and tattered garments in which it has long been clothed" (*WMS* 8:2). After the 1840 journey, she describes traveling as "the [thing] I like best in the world" (*LMWS* iii.5). In a letter written to her aunt from Florence in 1842, Mary Shelley credits travel for her improved health: "My health is a good deal improved—my long journey, though fatigueing [sic] at the time, has strengthened me ... a great deal of fresh air & exercise are quite necessary to me" (*LMWS* iii.46). Planning for the 1842 trip, she imagines herself happy in Italy: "by Lago Maggiore—in Venice—at Rome & Naples—what days might pass—what hours flow on, radiant with good spirits—teeming with glowing images—exalted above dull cares & gossip in the region of the beautiful" (*JMS* 572). She hopes to find in travel both a life "teeming with glowing images" in the "region of the beautiful"—that is to say a life of pleasurable looking—and also an escape from "gossip" and unwelcome scrutiny.[5]

---

5   During the trip her health fluctuated. For example, she refers to her fatigue in several locations (*WMS* 8:85, 90), complains of depression and "solitude and perplexity" in Milan (*WMS* 8:134–35, 139), and reports that she is "very much fatigued, and not well" on the way to Dresden (*WMS* 8:195).

As this passage illustrates, Mary Shelley, like Wollstonecraft and Charlotte Smith, depicts herself actively looking. However, while both Wollstonecraft and Smith present their suffering bodies and minds to readers, Mary Shelley adamantly resists the penetrating gaze of others. In contrast, Wollstonecraft includes in *Letters from Norway* moving expressions of heartbreak and appeals to an unnamed lover which, however restrained in comparison to her actual letters to Gilbert Imlay, are still much more personally forthcoming than Mary Shelley's narrative. Mary Shelley, as Jeanne Moskal points out, presents herself in *Rambles* as a loyal widow, keeping hidden from view the more recent pain of two love relationships—a broken engagement to Aubrey Beauclerk, and romantic feelings for Gatteschi ("Travel" 251). Smith, as I have argued, invents generic strategies to help others see her suffering body. Because Smith understood the origins of her suffering to lie in social structures, she felt compelled to make that suffering visible so that its social causes might be addressed. In contrast, Mary Shelley invites readers to see the outlines of her suffering, but not its interior detail. In a profoundly physical way, she regarded herself as the origin of her own suffering.

In a journal entry written shortly before the trips recounted in *Rambles*, Mary Shelley expresses guilt for eloping with Shelley many years earlier, an action that contributed to Harriet Shelley's suicide: "Poor Harriet to whose sad fate I attribute so many of my own heavy sorrows as the atonement claimed by fate for her death" (*JMS* 560).[6] Among the heaviest of these sorrows were the deaths of three children and the loss of an additional pregnancy.[7] And, as Moskal argues, she may also have felt "guilt for 'causing' her own mother's death from puerperal fever" ("Speaking" 207). All these events place the center of the trauma within Mary Shelley's body. If, as Caruth argues, we cannot witness the moment of our own trauma, but rather repeatedly circle the place of its absence—the blank screen of repression—it makes sense that Mary Shelley, unlike Smith, is not interested, and in fact is perhaps quite uncomfortable, in having others see her suffering body. She herself contains the trauma she must evade. As a result, she consciously or unconsciously redirects the reader's gaze, encoding much of her grief in the landscape and, as Moskal so beautifully argues, in paintings ("Speaking"). Wollstonecraft, too, projects her suffering onto the landscape but explains for the reader the connection between what she is feeling and what she sees. For example, identifying with seedlings atop a cliff who "brave the elements," Wollstonecraft notes, "I felt 'Like the lone shrub at random cast, / That sighs and trembles at each blast!'" (*WMW* 6:292). Mary Shelley rarely equates the landscape with her present state of mind. Instead, we see her both in pain and healing, but we do not know the details of her internal process. Mary Shelley's representation of her suffering enacts what Caruth describes as the sense of the unknown at the core of the known in trauma (4). She describes remembered landscapes that she associates with her traumatic losses in Italy, but the private

---

6   Shelley also blamed her, at least in part, for his first wife's death (Moskal "Speaking" 206–7, Sunstein 130).

7   She lost an unnamed baby in 1815, Clara at age 1 in 1818, William at age 3 in 1819, and had a nearly fatal miscarriage in 1822. Percy Florence, born in 1819, was the only child to survive.

psychological movement behind these memories remains invisible. This hiding—conscious or unconscious—mirrors the painful experience of her own inability to access these moments of trauma satisfyingly. Precisely because the trauma is not available to her psyche to process consciously, its shape, shadows, and outlines are everywhere present in her visual field.

Surveillance at the Spa

Mary Shelley's account of her 1842 German spa treatment occurs between the narratives depicting her two emotionally charged trips to Italy, yet this experience serves as a useful introduction to the relationships among (in)visibility, trauma, and healing. To put it simply, what Mary Shelley dislikes about her time at the spa negatively correlates with what she finds therapeutic about the act of looking at both landscapes and art. Continental travel and visits to health resorts were practices common to the Shelley circle, yet Mary Shelley had never before visited a German spa.[8] She notes that Dr. A. B. Granville's 1837 travel guide, *The Spas of Germany*, inspired her first visit: "Dr. Granville's book extended our acquaintance with the spas of Germany; and, in particular, gave reputation to those situated in Bavaria" (170).[9] Mary Shelley seems to have chosen spas based in part on Granville's advice. In 1842, she visited two spas—Brukenau and Brocklet—whose waters Granville claimed would "restore lost vigour, or impart a new one to a diseased constitution" (xxix). According to Granville, the waters at the Kissingen spa, where Mary Shelley made her most lengthy stay in 1842, were useful in the treatment of chronic rather than acute or febrile illness and were particularly helpful for "female complaints" (376). Although she relied on Granville's advice initially, Mary Shelley's assessment of the spa experience differs radically from his. This variation arises from differing attitudes toward medical authority. Mary Shelley objects to the physician's surveillance of patients' lives and to being seen within an illness category. In short, Mary Shelley expresses discomfort with the visual scrutiny and categorization to which she feels exposed at the spa.

In his guidebook, Granville lauds the healing power of the mineral waters, but repeatedly emphasizes the dangers of taking the waters without correct medical supervision. In the preface, he discusses English doctors' ignorance of and prejudice against the German spas, outlining the inaccuracies of their recommendations. He describes the complexities of choosing a spa appropriate for a specific illness, distinguishes among a dizzying variety of mineral waters based on chemical composition, and asserts that individual patients may react differently to the waters. In short, without the doctor's guidance through this maze of geographical, chemical, and medical factors, taking the waters is a risky proposition: "It scarcely needs to be stated ... that mineral waters should be used not only in accordance with the advice

---

8   After her husband's death, Mary Shelley visited Brighton in 1826 and 1827. She returned in November of 1836 and again a few months before the first journey described in *Rambles* (*JMS* 549, 564).

9   Granville's travel guide was first printed in two volumes in 1837. The textual references in this chapter are drawn from his second, single-volume edition.

(and only with it) of a physician well acquainted with their nature and effect; but also agreeably to the long-established rules that exist at all the Spas (both of diet and regimen) for their administration or application" (xxix). The spa doctor's authority is broad and deep, reaching into all aspects of the patient's daily life while rooted in "long-established" traditions at the spas.

Granville indicates in his preface that the spa regimen's success depends upon the minute regulation of behavior: "Mineral water should be drunk like other liquids; not gulped down in a hurry, for the sake of the gas or any other reason ... . The warm water should be sipped out of the glass—the cold water should be drunk slowly, and at several draughts" (xxxii). After taking the waters, the spa-goer typically eats breakfast, then Granville recommends "the patient to complete his toilet first, and, above all, never to omit cleaning his teeth with a brush and some proper tincture ... in order to remove all vestige, as well as the taste, of the mineral water" (xxxiii-xxxiv). The breakfast should be one or two cups of coffee and white bread. Between breakfast and dinner, "[e]very severe exertion of the mind is forbidden, and no sleep must be suffered to intrude" (xxxiv). The day continues in this regulated fashion. And, lest readers of the guidebook doubt his assertion that a doctor is needed to navigate the waters, Granville peppers his guidebook with cautionary tales—vignettes of spa-goers who have died because they did not consult a physician and thus used the waters improperly.[10]

Despite the strict regulation of diet and activity, and the professed need to consult a physician interpreter of the mineral waters, Granville positions the German spas as authentic, natural healing sites. Roy Porter explains that appeals to "natural" authority in the competitive rhetoric promoting various medical treatments were common: "Many nineteenth-century irregular medical movements ... boldly declared their outright opposition to ... the corruption of orthodox medicine, advocating instead, a 'return to Nature'" (*Health* 48). Using this rhetorical strategy, Granville promises his readers that upon visiting the German spas they "will have reason to rejoice that [they] exchanged art for nature" (xxxv). Granville seeks to naturalize the structures of authority in which he is so deeply invested. In Granville's view, medical and, as we will see, political authority are essential for transmitting the power of the earth through the human body.

Entering the care of one of the Kissingen spa physicians in June 1842, Mary Shelley finds confirmation of Granville's model of authoritarian medical supervision. In fact, Granville himself was practicing at Kissingen when Mary Shelley underwent her cure (*WMS* 8:174). At first she expresses hope for the spa's healing waters. Echoing Granville's preface and its warnings, she believes the mineral waters "to be very conducive to the restoration of health; but they must only be taken under

---

10 Apparently only the upper classes are sensitive enough for the waters to present a danger, however. Granville notes that at the Maxbrunnen spring, "Labourers, after eating their black bread and small bits of goats cheese, went down in a succession to quaff, out of broken pitchers, this pleasing beverage ... . One of the excellent effects of this practice is, that worms are not known among children at Kissingen, and scrofulous disorders never make their appearance among the inhabitants" (374). The laborers, unlike the fee-paying spa-goers, do not seem to need a physician's guidance to use the waters safely.

a physician's superintendence, as it is dangerous to play with them" (*WMS* 8:170). Even when the cure is most disagreeable, she voices her "great faith in the advantages that accrue" (*WMS* 8:172). In her initial portrayal of the spa treatment, Mary Shelley enthusiastically accepts the medical authority endorsed by Granville.

After three weeks at Kissingen, however, she grows frustrated with the spa physicians' regulation of her daily life. She reports that the Kissingen doctors closely monitor their patients' environment to regulate the influences on both mind and body: "[T]he physicians here discountenance every sort of excitement, and their *malades* are very obedient" (*WMS* 8:172–73). Mary Shelley notices that no one dances in the ballroom: "The cause is the despotic decree of the triumvirate of doctors ... who maintain dancing to be absolutely incompatible with drinking the waters" (*WMS* 8:173). The doctors' authority also reaches into the family structure: "This is another decree of the physicians: children are prohibited, because the mind must enjoy perfect repose, and children are apt to create disturbance in the hearts of tender parents" (*WMS* 8:176). The physicians ignore the diversions and delight of being with children, taking into account only their potential disruptiveness. They also restrict intellectual activity: "We malades are forbidden to exert our intellects; and, to make this prohibition more stringent, the gas one imbibes with the water produces a weakness in the eyes, which has rendered this letter the work of many days" (*WMS* 8:171). Together, the medical surveillance, her own temporarily diminished ability to see, and the restraints on her intellectual activity proved a nightmarish combination for Mary Shelley.

Of all the restrictions, however, Mary Shelley writes with most acerbic wit about the regulation of diet at the spa, the premier example of the spa doctors' control over their patients' lives. Granville concludes his preface with an "alphabetical list of articles of food proper and improper for the patients" undergoing spa treatment (xxxvi–xxxviii). He observes that raw vegetables and fruit should be omitted from the diet as they will cause gas and "incessant rumbling and noise in the stomach" (xxxiv). Mary Shelley expresses frustration with the limited diet: "So many things are supposed to disagree with the waters, that not only everything substantial, but also butter, fruit, tea, coffee and milk are prohibited" (*WMS* 8:170). She offers the reader a comical sketch of her doctor's attempt to police her diet:

> As I was sitting at breakfast this morning I had a visit from my physician. He looked with consternation on the table. "Butter!" he exclaimed; "strawberries! tea! milk!" There was a crescendo of horror in his voice. One by one, these slender luxuries were withdrawn, and I was left with a *little* bread, and water (the staple of the place) *ad libitum*. (*WMS* 8:172, original emphasis).

Mary Shelley positions herself as a misbehaving child, finding humor in the doctor's reaction to her minor rebellion against the bread and water diet, standard fare at storybook prisons. Although Granville asserts that dietary regulations are among the spa's "long-established rules," the rules actually change frequently, requiring a sign to be posted in the Kissingen dining hall listing "the articles of forbidden diet" (Granville 382). Mary Shelley notes, "Every now and then a new article is struck out from our bill of fare, notice being sent from this council, which is stuck up for our benefit at the door of the *salle-à-manger*, to the effect that, whoever in Kissingen should serve at any table pork, veal, salad, fruit, &c. &c. &c., should be fined so many florins" (*WMS* 8:170). Many of the spa rules exceed medical justification, reflecting instead the influence of politics.

Preceding Foucault's argument that modern institutional control is implicitly state control, Mary Shelley explains the apparent arbitrariness of the spa rules by establishing their connection to political authority: "The King of Bavaria is so afraid that his medicinal water may fall into disrepute if the drinkers should eat what disagrees with them, that we only eat what he, in conjunction with a triumvirate of doctors, is pleased to allow us" (*WMS* 8:170). With the word "triumvirate," Mary Shelley recalls one of the most powerful political structures in Western history—the Roman Republic—and thus equates medical authority with political authority. Far from obscuring the connection between medical and state authority, Granville boasts in the second edition of *The German Spas* that the first edition was praised both by spa doctors and by the sovereigns of several German states. He shows respect for Germany's regional kings by organizing the spas in his guidebook into four "geographical groups" composed of the states in the German Confederacy established by the 1815 Congress of Vienna: the Baden and Wurtemburg spas, the Salzburghian spas (Tyrol), the Bohemian spas, and the Bavarian and Nassau spas. He advises his reader that he could have organized the book by illnesses treated at each spa, but chose instead to focus on regions. Mary Shelley describes the state's response to Granville's work: "The King has perceived the flow of money brought into other states by the resort of strangers to the baths, and is very anxious that his should be celebrated. For this reason, he decorated Dr. Granville's button-hole with a bit of ribbon" (*WMS* 8:174). As a practicing physician at Kissingen, Granville augments his power by aligning himself with state authority. His deference to the political organization of German geography resonates with his recommendation that spa-goers should submit themselves to the medical "map" that spa doctors impose on their patients' bodies. In striking contrast to Granville, Mary Shelley resists in spa life the recapitulation of the state's tyranny over the individual.

In fact, Mary Shelley wonders that the doctors do not behave even more like dictators: "It is surprising that, to forward the cure, all letters are not opened first by the doctors, and not delivered if they contain any disagreeable news ... . Kissingen will not be perfect, until the post is put under medical *surveillance*" (*WMS* 8:176, original emphasis). Mary Shelley's speculation gains significance in light of her own experience with postal surveillance. Towards the end of the 1840 trip, she was delayed in Milan waiting for letters containing necessary travel money; the letters were probably being held for inspection by local government authorities who were likely monitoring her communications due to her connection to the Carbonari.[11] Mary Shelley's statement may be interpreted as a sharp criticism of the intrusive authority exercised by the spa doctors, a resistance to both medical and political surveillance.

---

11 The reviewer for *The Literary Examiner* explains that Mary Shelley's letters were probably retained because she wrote to a friend that she wanted to meet a member of the Carbonari (468).

Mary Shelley uses military images to draw another parallel between state power and medical authority. She observes her fellow patients' deference to the medical regulation of their bodies, using words that connote the minute physical regulation of soldiers. She comments on the synchronicity of their movement: "All the Germans get up at four, and parade the gardens to drink the waters till nearly eight; I contrive to get there soon after five" (*WMS* 8:170). One meaning of the verb "parade" is to move as in regulated fashion, as military troops might parade. This military vocabulary pervades Mary Shelley's descriptions of her fellow spa-goers: "I am in the midst of my *cur*, and we are all in the midst of a general cure of a regiment of sick people" (*WMS* 8:169, original emphasis). Mary Shelley observes that the modernization of the state, including military and medical institutions, demands the submission of the individual body to the disciplined behavior of the group. In associating medical prescription with military discipline, she describes what Foucault would identify in *Discipline and Punish* as the emergence of "docile bodies" in the eighteenth century, a phenomenon involving, among other things, control of the "modality" of individual bodies in multiple institutional settings: "[I]t implies an uninterrupted, constant coercion, supervising the processes of the activity rather than its result, and it is exercised according to a codification that partitions as closely as possible time, space, movement" (*Foucault* 181). This discipline increases simultaneously the individual's power to produce and willingness to obey; in other words, it may increase an individual's physical strength and competence, while decreasing his or her political power.

Mary Shelley's repeated resistance to being categorized with this "regiment of sick people" may seem an unsympathetic response to her fellow sufferers, yet is also a significant rejection of "medical colonization" (Frank 10). At Kissingen she expresses discomfort with "being surrounded by the rheumatic, the gouty, the afflicted of all sorts" (*WMS* 8:169–70). Although she hopes "to receive benefit in the end," she regrets that she and her companions must "live, as they say, surrounded by *lepers*" (*WMS* 8:172, original emphasis). She escapes when she can: "I leave the gardens after each glass, and stroll beyond into the meadows bordering the Saale, away from ... the saddening sight of the sick" (*WMS* 8:170). Visiting Brocklet four miles away, she again imagines fleeing the group of ill spa-goers: "I wish we had our little Welsh ponies to scamper over the hills away from the *malades*" (*WMS* 8:175). Leaving Kissingen, she admits: "[I]t is a great blessing to escape from the saddening spectacle of a crowd of invalids assembled *en masse*" (*WMS* 8:176). She describes her fellow spa-goers as the afflicted, the sick, *malades*, invalids, and lepers, thus strongly distancing herself from these groups, and from the categorization of her own suffering by medical authorities.[12]

---

12 This resistance is consistent with her warning to readers not to judge the Italians based on false impressions and generalizations, which Moskal describes as "discourses of race and national manners" ("Mary Shelley's" 205). Mary Shelley explains the challenge of describing another culture in visual terms that resonate both with medical surveillance and with *Frankenstein*: "A stranger can only glance at the surface of things—often deceptive— and put down the results of conversations, which ... by no means convey the whole truth, even if they are free from some bias, however imperceptible, either in speaker or hearer, the result

Arthur W. Frank identifies surveillance and categorization as features of modern medicine that developed in the eighteenth century. Referring to the work of Claudine Herzlich and Janine Pierret, he explains that the condition necessary for the emergence of the "sick person" as a type in the eighteenth century was that "the diversity of suffering be reduced by a unifying general view, which is precisely that of clinical medicine" (Frank 10–11). Individual suffering is thus subsumed in medicine's need to make generalizations and predictions based on categories (Frank 11). Frank describes this state as "medical colonization": "Just as political and economic colonialism took over geographic areas, modernist medicine claimed the body of its patient as its territory, at least for the duration of the treatment" (10). This colonization, he adds, requires that the patient cede control over her life and over the narrative of her illness and healing: "The ill person not only agrees to follow physical regimens that are prescribed; she also agrees, tacitly but with no less implication, to tell her story in medical terms" (6). In addition to her stated awareness of the close ties between spa and state, Mary Shelley's political savvy would have made obvious to her the connection between the surveillance of the sick and political oppression. Esther Schor identifies the link between the cure and politics in *Rambles*: "Surveillance, regime, tyranny; for all its wryness, Shelley's politics of the false cure of Kissingen launches the central concerns of her second journey: the tyranny of Austrian and French imperialism, and the abuses of papal and priestly authority" (244). These objectionable aspects of both cure and government also predict her desire for healing in the landscape—that is, her wish to see without being scrutinized, to imbibe the landscape without regulation, and to express suffering without exposing the details to mischaracterization, or colonization, by someone else's potentially unsympathetic narrative.

Distressed by the powerlessness she feels as a patient and disappointed with her worsening health at the end of the spa regimen in Kissingen, Mary Shelley begins to emphasize the picturesque setting of spas—formerly a kind of "added attraction"—as the most crucial element of healing: "I am heartily tired of the waters ... and the surrounding scenery is by no means interesting enough to *compensate* for our disagreeable style of life" (*WMS* 8:172, my emphasis). Mary Shelley's portrayal of the scenery as "compensation" for her boredom and frustration with the treatment establishes a contrast between spa healing and picturesque healing. She compares the baths of Brukenau, the spa the group visits next, with Kissingen in terms of the picturesque setting: "[A]bove all, the country around was, without being striking from crag and precipice, far more picturesque than at Kissingen" (*WMS* 8:178). "The hills round Brukenau are much higher and more romantic than at Kissingen ... . [E]verything invites the wanderer to stroll on, and to enjoy in fine weather Nature's dearest gifts, shady woods, open lawns, and views of beautiful country; loitering beside a murmuring stream, or toiling on a while, and then resting as you gaze on a wider prospect" (*WMS* 8:177). By comparing the two spas in terms of their picturesque prospects, Mary Shelley links the spas' healing effects with the

---

of which is a false impression—a false view" (*WMS* 8:324). Basing one's assessment of a group on "a glance at the surface of things," "a false view" is dangerous.

surrounding landscapes, implying that these natural scenes may have a more positive effect on her health than does the spa regimen.

Following her mother's example, Mary Shelley suggests that the stimulation derived from the movement of travel and exercise can positively influence an individual's health.[13] In her account of the 1840 visit to Baden-Baden, a spa known for its beautiful natural setting, Mary Shelley portrays the picturesque excursions often available at spas as more crucial to health than the official spa treatments. She observes that Baden-Baden "lies picturesquely yet snugly in the valley, on the banks of the Oes" (*WMS* 8:95). However, she notes that most of the spa-goers seem uninterested in exploring the countryside: "[T]o wander, and ramble, and discover new scenes does not form a portion of their amusements; and yet this is the only real one to be found in such a place" (*WMS* 8:96). The words "ramble" and "wander" connote a less purposeful, less predictable, more leisurely progression than the step-by-step spa regimen. Mary Shelley suggests that healing at the spa may result from the holistic effect of the spa setting.

Although Granville discounts the idea that healing at the spa results from multiple causes, noting that travel, a vacation from work, and a change of air are not responsible for one-tenth of the cure (xxvii), medical writers not employed at spas thought differently. In 1733, George Cheyne recommends that melancholics undertake a combination of spa therapy, mental diversion, and exercise (181). Similarly, in 1786, William Buchan recommends that patients exercise and amuse themselves as they undergo the spa regimen ("Cautions" 18). In his *View of the Nervous Temperament* (1812), the physician Thomas Trotter suggests that the trip to the spa might be more advantageous than the spa treatment itself: "I do not presume to decide whether the natural thermal waters, such as Bath or Buxton, or the water heated by artificial means have the preference. But it ought to be remembered, that a journey to and from these places of public resort, must be advantageous to an invalid" (289). Trotter observes that while some physicians argue over the effects of the temperature or the chemical composition of spa waters, he knows that travel itself will always be effective. Dr. Julius Braun suggests in 1875 that the successful spa *cur* results from multiple causes, including "traveling, country and mountain life, air, and bodily exercise" (10). Although travel to the spa, walking excursions, landscape viewing, and mountain air were not the focus of the spa regimen, these activities may have contributed to the spa-goers' recovery. In contrast to the spa regimen, which puts Mary Shelley under politically motivated medical surveillance, the healing she derives from looking at picturesque scenes lies more in her control. Her accounts of seeing in *Rambles* emphasize the physicality and even agency of the eye itself, drawing on metaphors of eating or incorporation to convey her visual pleasure. In

---

13 While almost all of *Rambles'* seventeen reviewers refer to Mary Shelley's descriptions of picturesque landscape, only one locates healing in these scenes: "She goes abroad to be made happy in the contemplation of scenes and objects congenial to her tastes" (*The Morning Chronicle* 3). In total, only seven reviews mention her search for health at all. The reviewer for *Tait's Edinburgh Magazine* offers an unfavorable comparison of *Rambles* with Wollstonecraft's travel narrative. He complains, "we miss throughout the earnestness, the impulsive movement which dictated Mary Wollstonecraft's *Letters from Norway*" (729).

addition, she frequently relies on the words of those she has lost to depict natural scenes, and alludes to past trauma through its displacement onto the landscape.

Visual Perception and the Landscape of the Mind

Mary Shelley's interest in the salutary picturesque recalls her mother's depiction of health travel and the healing landscape in *Letters from Norway*, a book she deeply admired.[14] Like her mother, Mary Shelley links traveling in pursuit of health with traveling in pursuit of picturesque scenery. Elsewhere I argue that Mary Shelley rejects spa healing, embracing, instead, some aspects of picturesque convention while revising others in order to formulate a theory of self-healing.[15] While I maintain that Mary Shelley contrasts spa healing with the salutary picturesque, in this chapter I take a closer look at the profound difference between the picturesque tradition's emphasis on novel scenes and Mary Shelley's tendency to view the immediate landscape through the lenses of memory and history. Like Wollstonecraft, she explicitly associates the picturesque aesthetic with health: "Travelling is occupation as well as amusement, and I firmly believe that renewed health will be the result of *frequent change of place*. Besides what can be so delightful as the perpetual *novelty* – the exhaustless current of new ideas suggested by traveling?" (*WMS* 8:157, my emphasis). Similarly, she expresses in picturesque terms her hope that the journey will dissipate her nervous illness: "Travelling will cure all: my busy brooding thoughts will be scattered abroad; and ... my mind will, amidst *novel and various scenes*, renew the outworn and tattered garments in which it has long been clothed, and array itself in a vesture all gay in fresh and glossy hues, when we are beyond the Alps" (*WMS* 8:76, my emphasis). Mary Shelley draws on the picturesque tradition in this passage, especially the highly valued qualities "novelty" and "variety." Yet, as Moskal notes, these sentences also echo William Godwin's description of Wollstonecraft's recovery in the Scandinavian landscape (*WMS* 8:76n). Paradoxically, then, Mary Shelley's comments about the salutary effects of picturesque novelty are rooted in memory and in loss. While this paradox is not necessarily consistent with eighteenth-century conceptions of health travel, it is consistent with trauma theory.

Mary Shelley responds with more enthusiasm to the mountains in Saxony than to any other scenes that would have been new to her on these journeys (Nitchie 34). This enthusiasm, I argue, results not only from the novel features of the landscape, but also from the landscape's resonance with Mary Shelley's representation of suffering. She depicts the terrain of Swiss Saxony as a dreamscape that oddly conveys both sublimity and a sense of interiority:

---

14 Wollstonecraft's *Letters from Norway* was one of the few books that Mary Shelley brought with her on her elopement journey in 1816; she and Shelley took turns reading it aloud on their trip down the Rhine (*WMS* 8:34).

15 See Elizabeth A. Dolan (as Beth Dolan Kautz), "Spas and Salutary Landscapes: The Geography of Health in Mary Shelley's *Rambles in Germany and Italy*," *Romantic Geographies: Discourses of Travel 1775–1844*.

[T]he portals of the mountains opened before us, and we plunged into their recesses. It is difficult to describe the peculiarity of this region; it differs so much from every other ... . Generally, when you see mountains, they seem (as they are) upraised above the plains which are the abodes of men; lifting their mighty heads towards heaven. In Saxony, the impression is as if the tops of the hills were the outer circumference of the globe, strangely fissured and worn away by the action of water. We plunge into the depths of the earth; we might fancy some sprite of upper air had forced a passage so to reach the abode of subterranean spirits. (*WMS* 8:212)

Her description of this unusual landscape is emblematic of her larger project. She wishes to plunge into her own emotional recesses—"the abode of subterranean spirits"—during her "pious pilgrimage" to scenes of past suffering, yet to remain out of the view of those who might unsympathetically scrutinize her.

Her continued account of this landscape reads like a post-Freudian understanding of the mind, with some of its knowledge "open to the sky" and some "dark and deep":

There is a charm of novelty in the scene quite inexpressible. We penetrate Nature's secret chambers, which she has adorned with the wildest caprice. Various ravines branch off from the main one, and become numerous and intricate, varied by huge caverns of strange shapes; some open to the sky, some dark and deep; there are little verdant spots in the midst, too, where the turf was green and velvety, and invited us to rest. (*WMS* 8:212)

The "secret chambers" are "wild," "numerous and intricate," yet some areas of this internal landscape provide a restful feeling. This description resonates with an 1823 journal entry written four months after her return to England following the deaths of Shelley and their children. Mary Shelley longs for Italy and reflects on her memories of the natural scenes and on her own state of mind during the period of time she spent recovering in Genoa immediately after Shelley's death: "Then my solitary walks and my reveries—They were magnificent, deep, pathetic, wild, and exalted—I sounded the depths of my own nature; I appealed to the Nature around me to corroborate the testimony that my own heart bore to its purity ... my grief was active, striving, expectant" (*JMS* 470–71). Mary Shelley suggests that both her walks and her reveries are "magnificent, deep, pathetic, wild, and exalted." Although she does not explicitly connect her deep grief and desire for privacy with her descriptions of the Saxon landscape in 1843, she encodes these remembered feelings into her portrait of the landscape, using language that connects the landscape with the grief following her previous, traumatic sojourn in Italy. The structure of this natural vista—difficult to access visually from above, but fascinating and complex from within—reflects Mary Shelley's presentation of her emotional experiences during her journeys.

In an argument that strongly influences my understanding of *Rambles*, Moskal explains that Mary Shelley's passionate descriptions of Italian art in the travel narrative both express and encode emotional pain. Mary Shelley employs her "art criticism as autobiographical dream work, simultaneously revealing and concealing those unspeakable portions of her autobiography that disrupt her roles as the beloved wife and faithful widow of the poet Percy Bysshe Shelley, the editor of his works, and the mother of his son" ("Speaking" 189–90). Based on Mary Shelley's letters, journals, and other biographical material, Moskal argues that the paintings silently express Mary Shelley's desire for vindication at death, her suicidal thoughts, her pain about Shelley's feelings for Emilia Viviani, her grief for her dead children, and her guilt about Harriet Shelley's suicide: "[P]aintings speak what is, as yet, unspeakable about the heroine's life, by performing a kind of dream-work in which a disruptive truth about that life is presented in figural language, partly revealed, partly concealed, rising to visibility just below the surface of consciousness, but not yet breaking the surface to demand full recognition" ("Speaking" 189). In *Rambles*, Mary Shelley does not explain, and is perhaps not fully conscious of, the autobiographical resonances in the paintings to which Moskal argues she responds. Reading Mary Shelley's narrative of suffering in these instances is similar to looking at the Saxon landscape from the mountaintop. Just as a person viewing this unusual landscape from above would be aware of, but unable to see, the depth and intricacy that lies below, so nineteenth-century readers of *Rambles*—who would not, of course, have had access to her letters and journals—observe Mary Shelley looking at landscapes and paintings, but are not able to perceive the details of the interior emotional process her looking ignites.

Mary Shelley invites the reader, then, to imagine and sympathize, rather than to survey and scrutinize. Although she makes abundantly clear her resistance to surveillance in her comments on her spa experience, she finds equally uncomfortable the scrutiny of the ordinary people she encounters during her travels:

> The Germans have a habit of staring quite inconceivable—I speak, of course, of the people one chances to meet traveling as we do. For instance, in the common room of an hotel, if a man or woman there have nothing else to do, they will fix their eyes on you, and never take them off for an hour or more. There is nothing rude in their gaze, nothing particularly inquiring, though you supposed it must result from curiosity; perhaps it does; but their eyes follow you with pertinacity, without any change of expression ... the starers ... do offend grievously, and one has a full right to get rid of them at almost any cost. (*WMS* 8:233–34)

Mary Shelley's frustration with German staring serves to caution her readers not to scrutinize her as if she were an object of curiosity, but rather to imagine her emotional responses to what she sees during her journeys. She notes that the experience of traveling cannot be conveyed fully in words, and thus understanding depends on the reader's participation: "[T]here is a zest in all this ... which is lost in mere words:—you must do your part, and feel and imagine, or all description proves tame and useless" (*WMS* 8:87). Similarly, she invites the reader to sympathize with her feelings about the paintings she describes: "I try in some degree to convey the impression they made, so as to induce you to sympathise in my feelings with regard to them" (*WMS* 8:132). She does not urge the reader to find intellectual inspiration in her art criticism, nor does she solicit sympathy by expressing her emotions directly. Instead, she invites her reader to understand her feelings through comments about external objects. And yet, looking at Raphael's painting of the adoration of the Magi in the Berlin gallery, she observes that "words can never show forth the beauty of which painting presents the living image to the eyes" (*WMS* 8:190). There is a gap between the effect of the image on her and her description of the image to readers—and in this gap she approaches and circles the psychic absence, or what remains of traumatic experience.

Mary Shelley describes the mechanism of this psychological work in physiological terms that resonate with David Hartley's philosophy of association. Hartley argues that "all sensations and ideas are conveyed to the mind by means of the external senses," and posits that vision is the strongest of the senses (ix). He calls the "sensations impressed on the eye" "visual ideas" (9, 12–13). In several passages of *Rambles*, Mary Shelley depicts healing as the transfer of these "sensations impressed on the eye" to what she variously terms the imagination, soul, or heart. Looking at Ghirlandaio's *Adoration of the Magi* in Florence, she explains: "[T]o see [this picture] is to feel the happiness which the soul receives from objects presented to the eye, that kindle and elevate the imagination" (*WMS* 8:304). The images the eye transmits—the "visual ideas"—create happiness in the soul and elevate the imagination. Similarly, looking at the gates of the Batistero in Florence, she enthuses: "Look at these, and a certain feeling of exalted delight will enter your eyes and penetrate your heart" (*WMS* 8:313). Delight is conveyed physically; the visual idea of the paintings enters the eyes and penetrates the heart. Hartley notes that the doctrine of association dictates that a mature eye will receive more pleasure from looking than will the eye of a child: "And thus the eye approaches more and more, as we advance in spirituality and perfection, to an inlet for mental pleasure, and an organ suited to the exigencies of a being, whose happiness consists in the improvement of his understanding and affections" (69). For Hartley, the eyes become "an inlet of mental pleasure"; likewise, for Mary Shelley, delight "enters" the eyes.

The Agency of the Eye

In accordance with the Hartlian philosophy that informs the above passages, Mary Shelley repeatedly emphasizes the physicality and what might be called "the agency of the eye" in her descriptions of both landscape and art. In some cases, the landscape seems to act on the eye. For example, in Salzburg "the indescribable variety of the landscape, *enchant[s] the eye*" (*WMS* 8:245, my emphasis). Similarly, she describes her delight in gazing as the group travels down the Rhine from Cologne to Koblenz: "We gazed ... with eager curiosity, as at each succeeding mile the river became more majestic, its shores more picturesque; and every hour of the day *brought its store of delight to the eye*" (*WMS* 8:161, my emphasis). In other passages, she grants the eye more agency. In the Tyrol, for example, she notes that "*the eye dwells* on the unimaginable variety of grouping which this picturesque and majestic region presents" (*WMS* 8:260, my emphasis). Depicting the eye as adventurous in Amalfi, she declares: "*[T]he eye plunged down* from the height of the myrtle-clothed mountain on which we stood" (*WMS* 8:379, my emphasis). Whether the eye acts or is acted upon, the visual images that enter it affect Mary Shelley's imagination and emotions. In Germany she observes: "Though I skim its surface without having any communication with its inhabitants, still the eye is gratified, the imagination excited, and curiosity satisfied" (*WMS* 8:186). She confesses her superficial understanding of Germany, but, nonetheless, invokes the Hartlian transfer of visual ideas from the eye to the imagination in order to describe the pleasurable experience of seeing this unfamiliar landscape.

Looking at art has the same restorative effect on the soul and heart as does looking at the landscape. Mary Shelley's and her companions' eyes move through the Berlin gallery: "First we saw the Io, of Correggio, a most lovely picture, and near it Leda and the Swan by the same artist; and then *our eyes were attracted* to one still lovelier in its chaste and divine beauty—A Virgin and Child by Raphael" (*WMS* 8:189, my emphasis). She sees in Raphael's earliest work a "beauty not found on earth—inspiring as we look, a deep joy, only felt in such brief moments when some act of self-sacrifice exalts the soul, when love softens the heart, or nature draws us out of ourselves, and our spirits are rapt in ecstacy, and enabled to understand and mingle with the universal love" (*WMS* 8:191). Like love and the finest scenes in nature, this painting draws the self into communion with the divine. Once again, the image the eye consumes brings a healing balm to the heart.

Mary Shelley frequently invokes gastronomical metaphors to depict the eyes' consumption of natural scenes and art. Just beyond the Simplon pass, she chooses to walk rather than ride in a carriage, desiring "to *gaze my fill* on the mighty and glorious shapes around" (*WMS* 8:146, my emphasis). The picturesque drive between Budweis and Linz is so "delightful," "picturesque," "fertile and agreeable" that, she explains, "[m]y heart had *filled to the brim* with delight" (*WMS* 8:237–38, my emphasis). Describing the abundantly beautiful landscape again in terms of food, she relays that "One of our party climbed the heights above Linz, to *feast his eyes* on the view" while she "stood long on the bridge, *drinking in the beauty of the scene*; till the *soul became full to the brim* with the sense of delight" (*WMS* 8:239, my emphasis). Viewing art is apparently equally satisfying. In Venice, she reports: "[We] *feast our eyes* on the finest works of Titian" (*WMS* 8:276, my emphasis). Touring the Vatican collection, she notes: "From room to room the *eye is so fed* by sights of beauty, 'that the sense aches at them'" (*WMS* 8:343, my emphasis). Visual ideas feed her eyes, thus "filling" and nourishing her soul. Although "feast your eyes" and other phrases Mary Shelley uses are common figures of speech, in some instances these gastronomical metaphors serve to contrast directly the pleasures of landscape and art with the disappointment of bad food. Immediately after an unsatisfying meal ("German cooking is very bad") and stultifying company at a table d'hôte in Saxony, the group looks from a highly elevated mass of rock to take in the breathtaking view of the Elbe below (*WMS* 8:213). Still hungry, the travelers enjoy the visual feast: "We indulged, as well we might, in gazing delightedly from this battlement of nature on the magnificent scene around" (*WMS* 8:213). Indulging herself in the landscape compensates for the lack of sustenance she receives from food while traveling and while at the spa. In contrast to the unpredictable offerings at wayside inns or the overly regulated diet at the spa, these visually nurturing scenes rarely disappoint. Her delight in looking at the responsive and changing landscape differs radically from her discomfort with being scrutinized at the spa and elsewhere.

Even more significantly, the language of food signifies incorporation in Mary Shelley's narrative. Hartley argues for physical sympathy between visual and gastronomical pleasures: "The imagery of the eye sympathizes also remarkably with the affections of the stomach. Thus the grateful impressions of opium upon the stomach raise up the ideas of gay colours, and transporting scenes, in the eye" (74). Mary Shelley modifies Hartley's formulation, suggesting that, even as it grows in the fields, food is beautiful and satisfying to consume visually. She compares the earth's abundance to a mother's care. Looking at the landscape near Metz, she effuses:

"I never remember feeling so intimately how bounteous a mother is this fair earth, yielding such plenteous store of food to her children, and this food in its growth so beautiful to look on" (*WMS* 8:81). Mother earth feeds both stomach and vision. As this association suggests, Mary Shelley strives to bring into her body, literally to incorporate, visual pleasure. In the Berlin gallery, for example, she explains, "I desired to learn by heart—to imbibe—to make all I saw a part of myself, so that never more I may forget it" (*WMS* 8:192). Disgusted with a young Englishman who seems to travel only to say he has done so, Mary Shelley insists: "We must become a part of the scenes around us, and they must mingle and become a portion of us, or we see without seeing and study without learning. There is no good, no knowledge unless we can go out from, and take some of the external into, ourselves" (*WMS* 8:213). Mary Shelley's insistence on the incorporation of visual sensation—that is, the desire to "go out from, and take some of the external into, ourselves"—evokes sexual intercourse. Nora Crook argues for the association between hunger, aesthetic beauty, and sex in Mary Shelley's writing. Rather than directly describe sex, Mary Shelley creates "an atmosphere in which danger, hunger, tenderness, a couple in love, darkness, fire, passionate poetry, physical contact and reverie converge in a room containing a bed" ("Pecksie" 10). Mary Shelley associates hunger, Crook argues, with a period in 1814 when she and Shelley would meet to spend the night in inns near London, visits that probably involved physical intimacy, and, as their own accounts of these nights attest, certainly offered them the pleasure of eating inn food during a time in which they had little money. The consumption of beautiful objects, food, and sex, then, pleasurably commingle and overlap in Mary Shelley's writing.

When Mary Shelley wishes in the Berlin gallery "to imbibe—to make all I saw a part of myself, so that never more I may forget it," she depicts memory as a physical creation that begins in the eyes. Visual memories, like food, occupy a limited space in the body: "Some of the forms of beauty on which I gazed, must last in my memory as long as it endures; but this will be at the expense of others, which even now are fading and about to disappear from my mind ... still my mind was full before, the rest can but overflow, ... leaving distinct only a few images that can never be effaced" (*WMS* 8:192). Mary Shelley describes herself as hungry to fill her eyes with beautiful images that will inevitably replace less remarkable visual memories. Her appetite for looking at beauty reflects a desire to displace or lessen the pain of the scenes associated with trauma that are stored in her eyes and memory.

Looking, then, can also trigger sadness. In language that evokes both sexual generation and food, Hartley argues that "the disagreeable impressions on the eye, have some small share in generating and feeding intellectual pains" (69–70). These negative visions occur most often for Mary Shelley on thresholds or borders. Traveling through the Alps to reach Lake Como in 1840, she expresses weariness with the mountains, noting, "the eye longs for space" (*WMS* 8:108). Sad to leave Italy a few months later, she quotes *Romeo and Juliet*: "'Eyes, look your last!' Soon the curtain of absence will be drawn before this surpassing scene" (*WMS* 8:128). Looking back at Italy, she reveals that "With a heavy heart I gazed, till a turn in the road shut out Lago Maggiore and Italy from my sight" (*WMS* 8:143). She grows tired of the dry landscape in the transitional space between Leipzig and Berlin: "The sense the eye received of nakedness was in no way relieved—no hedge, no tree, no meadow, no bush" (*WMS* 8:187). Mary Shelley's often painful movement over thresholds invokes the transitions of birth and death, the fluctuation between love and loss, and the alternation between invisibility and visibility.

Approaching the edge of Venice in 1842, among the most painful of thresholds for Mary Shelley, she again distinguishes between visual memories that dissolve with time and those that will not fade: "Many a scene, which I have since visited and admired, has faded in my mind, as a painting in the Diorama melts away, and another struggles into the changing canvass [sic]; but this road was as distinct in my mind as if traversed yesterday" (*WMS* 8:269). The road to Venice remains distinct in her mind because of its association with the traumatic loss of her daughter Clara on 24 September 1818, just as the Shelleys arrived in Venice. Describing her response to this memory in *Rambles*, Mary Shelley speaks in general terms: "I will not here dwell on the sad circumstances that clouded my first visit to Venice. Death hovered over the scene. Gathered into myself, with my 'mind's eye' I saw those before me long departed; and I was agitated again by emotions—by passions—and those the deepest a woman's heart can harbour—a dread to see her child even at that instant expire—which then occupied me" (*WMS* 8:270). Mary Shelley does not mention Clara's name or the events that led to her death, but focuses instead on vision. By framing the memory as a "scene," Mary Shelley distances herself from it and expresses the importance of the eyes in creating memory. Her "'mind's eye'" "gather[s] into [her]self" a vision of all those she has lost. And, although she mentions this intimate, incorporated vision of her loved ones, she then moves on to generalize the excruciating grief "a woman" experiences when she witnesses the moment of her child's death. This scene is written on the eye; those she has lost are incorporated into her body. The intensity of grief, however, is cast out to general experience. Mary Shelley directs the reader to observe her looking at scenes both past and present, yet defies witness of exactly what she sees and feels. Here the narrative is, as Mary Shelley promised her publisher, "personal to myself." The core traumatic moment is closed within an emotional recess, a structure mirrored in the "numerous and intricate" ravines in Saxony, depths not accessible from an external prospect. Unable or unwilling to describe the exact content of the remembered scene (e.g., Clara laid her head against me, etc.), she wishes to convey to the reader that she both suffers and sees.

Continuing this passage, Mary Shelley explains the phenomenon of traumatic memory, citing Shakespeare as well as her father's friends William Wordsworth, Samuel Taylor Coleridge, and Thomas Holcroft to confirm her own experience[16]:

It is a strange, but to any person who has suffered, a familiar circumstance, that those who are enduring mental or corporeal agony are strangely alive to immediate external objects .... Holcroft, who was a martyr to intense physical suffering, alludes to the notice the soul takes of objects presented to the eye in its hour of agony, as a relief afforded by nature to permit the nerves to endure pain. (*WMS* 8:270)

---

16 Clarissa Campbell Orr argues that Mary Shelley's references to these writers "assimilates three personal friends of her father's circle to the level of England's greatest writer, and by implication suggests that a mother's grief is a species of sublime" (24).

The eye conveys images to the soul, where they then rest. In this example, Mary Shelley suggests that directing attention to the scene is the mind's way of distracting the viewer from pain, the unconscious process of creating what Freud would later term "a screen memory."[17] And yet, once these scenes that distract the person in the moment of trauma become seared into the memory, they become inextricable from the pain which deflected one's attention toward them in the first place. Hartley explains this connection between visual memory and emotion: "[T]here are many ideas, i.e. internal feelings, which have no names, and which yet, by attending our several visible ideas, get this power of introducing them" (72). The visible ideas one associates with pain become the language for inexpressible feelings, which "have no names."

Mary Shelley attests to having had several experiences with traumatic visual memory. Arriving in Italy on the 1840 trip, the familiar physical objects in her room open her emotions to painful associations: "Window-curtains, the very wash-hand stands, they were all such as had been familiar to me in Italy long, long ago. I had not seen them since those young and happy days. Strange and indescribable emotions invaded me; recollections, long forgotten, arose fresh and strong by mere force of association, produced by those objects being presented to my eye, inspiring a mixture of pleasure and pain, almost amounting to agony" (*WMS* 8:107). The objects presented to her eye allow "indescribable emotions" to "invade" her. In the passage alluding to her life-and-death rush toward Venice, she describes the process similarly:

> In both states [mental or corporeal agony] I have experienced it; and the particular shape of a room—the progress of shadows on a wall—the peculiar flickering of trees—the exact succession of objects on a journey—have been indelibly engraved on my memory, as marked in, and associated with, hours and minutes when the nerves were strung to their utmost tension by the endurance of pain, or the far severer infliction of mental anguish. Thus the banks of the Brenta presented me a moving scene; not a palace, not a tree of which I did not recognize, as marked and recorded, at a moment when life and death hung upon our speedy arrival at Venice. (*WMS* 8:270)

For Mary Shelley, indelible memories of physical objects are most often associated with the traumatic loss of her children. In June 1822, shortly before Shelley died, Mary Shelley suffered a nearly fatal miscarriage, a brush with mortality that she recalls in 1839 in visual terms: "My [feeling] ... was—I go to no new creation—I enter under no new laws. The God that made this beautiful world (& I was then at Lerici surrounded by the most beautiful manifestation of the visible creation) made that into which I go" (*JMS* 562). The beauty of the landscape at Lerici consoles her as she faces the loss of a fourth child and anticipates her own death. Children that once grew in her body are lost and then replaced with enduring visual ideas of physical objects. The mother's body, then, is the location where life is given and taken, as well as the place where loss is both displaced and marked by "indelibly engraved" visual memories.

---

17   Schor suggests that each of Mary Shelley's "screen memories" signals less a specific traumatic moment than a more general "traumatic loss of self which she associates with her extended sojourn in Italy" (243).

Making the Inexpressible Visible

In Mary Shelley's narrative, the visual memories that accompany trauma express to the self what is inexpressible in words. The remembered landscape at Lerici, "the exact succession of objects on a journey," and the palaces and trees on the banks of the Brenta all stand in for traumatic loss and inassimilable emotion. These scenes in the visual memory both mark and disguise the original trauma. They simultaneously demand and defy witness. This tension between visible objects and the invisible world of love and loss also informs Mary Shelley's responses to art. In her descriptions of several paintings, Mary Shelley praises Italian painters' ability to make visible what is nearly inexpressible or inconceivable, particularly the divine. Looking at Titian's *Assumption of the Virgin*, she notes: "The Italian painters drank deep at the inspiration of [Dante's] verses when they sought to give a *visible image of Heaven* and the beatitude of the saints on their canvass" (*WMS* 8:277, my emphasis). Of the Italian painters who seek to give "a visible image of Heaven," none succeeds as completely as Raphael, who alone is able "to paint the superhuman, and convey to the eyes the image of that which surpasses the might of visible objects, and can scarcely be conceived by the strongest effort of the imagination" (*WMS* 8:345). She repeatedly marvels at the depiction of the baby Jesus—the invisible God made visible in the mortal form of his son, a nearly unimaginable historical figure made visible again by artists. She praises Florentine painters who, "gifted with pictorial powers, turned their talents to representing bodily to the eye, the Saviour of the world" (*WMS* 8:303). Mary Shelley's focus on Christ's embodiment in life and in art aligns painters with mothers. Julia Kristeva observes in "Stabet Mater" that "Christ, the Son of man, when all is said and done is 'human' only through his mother;" the body of the mother makes the spirit visible (162). And with motherhood comes suffering—the Holy Mother's inevitable loss of the Christ child and Mary Shelley's repeated loss of children. The Virgin mother becomes the *Mater Dolorosa*. Kristeva notes that the representation of Mary as the Virgin avoids (and thus invokes) the connection between sexuality and death. As the child whose birth killed her mother, the mother who birthed three children who died, the woman who lost another child in a miscarriage that nearly killed her, too, Mary Shelley is the physical seat of a death-inducing sexuality.

Rather than invite the reader to scrutinize the body in which these traumatic losses originated, Mary Shelley wishes the reader to see the scenes onto which she has displaced her pain. Rather than remember the details of these traumatic losses, she imagines that her loved ones live around her still. Describing her visit to the Lake of Gmunden during the 1842 tour, she notes that she is drawn to scenes that inspire thoughts of the invisible realm: "Now for another scene, which will ever dwell in my memory, coloured by the softest tints, yet sublime—the lake of Gmunden" (*WMS* 8:241). She quotes Milton's *Paradise Lost*: "'Millions of spiritual creatures walk the earth / Unseen, both when we wake and when we sleep.' It is easier for the imagination to conjure such up in spots untrod by man, so to people with love and gratitude what would otherwise be an unsentient desert" (*WMS* 8:242). She describes herself as one "born to look beyond the grave" and she "yearn[s] to acquire knowledge of spiritual essences" (*WMS* 8:242). She wishes that her sensation of spiritual beings would not end: "I cannot tell you the sacred pleasure with which I brooded over these fancies, which were rather sensations than thoughts, so heartfelt and intimate were they. I scarce dared breathe, and longed to linger on our way, so not so quickly to put from my lips the draughts of happiness which I imbibed" (*WMS* 8:242). As in her description of the landscape, she does not share with the reader the content of her response, or sensations, but relies instead on the metaphor of drinking to describe her incorporation of these visions.

In a similar passage, a paragraph from an 1840 journal entry that she revised to include in *Rambles*, Mary Shelley presents the beauty of the world and invisible presences as coexistent with each other and as equally comforting and influential to her:

> It has seemed to me—and on such an evening, I have felt it,—that this world, endowed as it is outwardly with endless shapes and influences of beauty and enjoyment, is peopled also in its spiritual life by myriads of loving spirits; from whom, unawares, we catch impressions, which mould our thoughts to good, and thus they guide beneficially the course of events, and minister to the destiny of man. Whether the beloved dead make a portion of this holy company, I dare not guess; but that such exists, I feel ... . Surely such gather round me this night, and make a part of that atmosphere of peace and love which it is paradise to breathe. (*WMS* 8:123–24)

Surrounded by the beautifully visible world and guided by invisible presences that she hopes include "the beloved dead," Mary Shelley is invigorated and comforted by both external and internal vision.

In keeping with her sense that the "the beloved dead" are present with her, Mary Shelley looks out of her body—the mother's body, the seat of trauma—often through the eyes of those she has lost, particularly the two people she would have associated most closely with maternal loss. She refers to a wide range of English, German, American, and Italian authors in *Rambles*, but she speaks most often through the words of her mother and her husband to describe landscapes. She looks then not only through her own eyes—embued with the maternal losses she inevitably conflates with the loss of Shelley—but also through the eyes of the lost maternal body, her mother. In *Letters from Norway*, Wollstonecraft muses as she looks at the frontier in Sweden, describing it as "[t]he bones of the world waiting to be clothed with everything necessary to give life and beauty" (*WMW* 6:262, *WMS* 8:145n). Mary Shelley looks through her mother's eyes at the sublime landscape as she crosses the Simplon pass on foot: "There was a majestic simplicity that inspired awe; the naked bones of a gigantic world were here: the elemental substance of fair mother Earth" (*WMS* 8:145). Significantly, she does not identify as a source Wollstonecraft's narrative—a text that she had probably long before incorporated into her unconscious—but she does use the word "mother" in her description. Pointing out the beauty of the lake of Gmunden, one of the primary locations in which she feels invisible presences, Mary Shelley's words again resonate with Wollstonecraft's, in this case Wollstonecraft's repeated praise for Scandinavia's sheltering landscapes: "a lake amidst mountains must always exceed a grassy valley: there is a magic charm in the notion of a cot on the verdant, wooded banks of a lonely lake—the boat drawn up in a neighbouring cove—the sheltering mountains gathering around" (*WMS* 8:242–43). Feeling the presence of others, Mary Shelley sees as they would see. The daughter, like her mother, also responds to the fleeting pleasure of the landscape as music. In an ebullient mood, Wollstonecraft says of herself: "Let me catch pleasure on the wing—I may be melancholy to-morrow. Now all my nerves keep time with the melody of nature" (*WMW* 6:294). At Amalfi, Mary Shelley echoes: "It was a scene,—and hour,—when Nature imparts a quick and living enjoyment akin to the transports of love and the ecstacy of music—it touches a chord whose vibration is happiness" (*WMS* 8:381). On a walk near Menaggio, Mary Shelley watches the "shadows of evening climb the huge mountains": "With what serious yet quick joy do such sights fill me; and dearer still is the aspiring thought that seeks the Creator in his works, as the soul yearns to throw off the chains of flesh that hold it in, and to dissolve and become a part of that which surrounds it" (*WMS* 8:123). As Moskal points out in a footnote, this passage also echoes Wollstonecraft's *Letters from Norway*: "With what ineffable pleasure have I not gazed—and gazed again, losing my breath through my eyes—my very soul diffused itself into the scene" (*WMS* 8:123n). Mary Shelley absorbs into her vision some of the most hopeful, even joyous, moments of *Letters from Norway*, a text that is not on the whole uplifting, but rather is marked by dramatic lamentation and longing. Looking through her mother's eyes, Mary Shelley seems to answer Wollstonecraft's plea for a sympathetic gaze. And, looking with and through (rather than *at*) her mother brings healing pleasure to this daughter.

Unlike the unacknowledged, even unconscious, resonances with Wollstonecraft's *Letters from Norway*, Mary Shelley's invocations of her husband's texts are more direct. They are memories of a shared vision, of actual views—a material reality that was impossible to share with her mother. She quotes "Julian and Maddalo," for example, to extol "the view from the sea near Leghorn" that they both enjoyed (*WMS* 8:341). And, entering Italy in 1840, she remembers a view that Shelley praises in "Lines Written Among the Euganean Hills": "I remembered once how the sense of sight had felt relieved when I exchanged the narrow ravine, in which the Baths of Lucca are placed, for the view over the plains of Lombardy, commanded from our view among the Euganean hills" (*WMS* 8:108, 108n). Although she does not mention Shelley directly, she portrays her time with him in the Euganean hills, melting the words "I remembered" and "I exchanged" into "our view." Distressed in Milan on the 1840 trip as she waited alone for letters ("I am miserable" *WMS* 8:135), she "takes refuge in solitary walks and country rambles" to soothe herself (*WMS* 8:136). Her favorite overlook near Milan was also Shelley's favorite (*WMS* 8:136n): "The influence of this spot soothes my mind, and chases away a thousand grim shadows, prognosticating falsehood, desolation, and hopeless sorrow ... . The Resegone is there, reminding me of the ecstasies I felt on the Lake of Como, which I remember as dreams sent from heaven, vanished for ever" (*WMS* 8:136). Remembering her life with Shelley in Italy is both painful and restorative.

Looking through her mother's and Shelley's eyes, Mary Shelley suggests that trauma, as Caruth explains, elaborating on Freud's *Moses and Monotheism*, "is never simply one's own" (24). In her vision, Mary Shelley brings to life those closest to her own traumatic losses. Her responses to art help illustrate how "the beloved lost" become present again in shared vision. In Dresden, she is awed by the depiction of Jesus in Raphael's *Sistine Madonna*: "And he, the Godhead (as well as feeble mortals can conceive the inconceivable, and yet which once it is believed was visible) sits enthroned on his brow, and looks out from eyes full of lofty command and conscious power" (*WMS* 8:198). Just as Jesus' eyes see with God's vision ("the Godhead" "looks out from [his] eyes"), Mary Shelley's physical eyes see as Wollstonecraft and Shelley saw. Part of her work of mourning is to find meaning in loss. She incorporates her mother and Shelley into her vision and then sees through the most positive aspects of their subjectivity, pushing down, displacing, or at least not articulating the more unsettling memories of lost children, Shelley's marital infidelity, and the unfulfilled desire to know her mother's physical presence. However, the closeness of Wollstonecraft and Shelley to these unsettling memories remains; the focus on joyful views may screen, but does not erase, the trauma. She re-approaches the site of trauma in the company of those she has lost, signaling their incorporation by looking with their best vision.

Mary Poovey asserts that after publishing *The Last Man*, Mary Shelley largely abandoned the public commitment to radicalism that she inherited from Wollstonecraft and shared with Shelley, embracing instead a complex version of the proper woman writer. Poovey concedes that Mary Shelley never relinquished Shelley's idea that true poetry invites the audience to participate: "It strengthens the individual's moral sense because it exercises and enlarges the capacity for sympathetic identification, that is, for establishing relationships" (Poovey 130). In *Rambles*, Mary Shelley expresses a desire to cultivate a friendship with the landscape: "One longs to make a familiar friend of such sublime scenery, and refer, in after years, to one's intimate acquaintance with it, as one of the most valued among the treasures of recollection which time may have bestowed" (*WMS* 8:89). Using the language of visual memory, Mary Shelley asserts that travel, like Shelley's poetry, invites sympathetic identification with others. Citing Mary Shelley's description of the self as "'the undiscovered country,'" the "'noblest of terrae incognitae,'" Schor argues that Mary Shelley recognizes "travel writing as an exploration of the self through an encounter with the other" (237).[18] Mary Shelley's rapturous description of the traveling self recalls Wollstonecraft's and Shelley's ways of looking:

> [T]o fly abroad from the hive, like the bee, and return laden with the sweets of travel—scenes, which haunt the eye—wild adventures, that enliven the imagination—knowledge, to enlighten and free the mind from clinging, deadening prejudices—a wider circle of sympathy with our fellow creatures;—these are the uses of travel, for which I am convinced every one is the better and the happier. (*WMS* 8:157)

Although the scenes one encounters when traveling may "haunt the eye," they also widen "the circle of sympathy with our fellow creatures," a vision of sociability that resonates with Wollstonecraft's longing for "fellow feeling." Mary Shelley also echoes Shelley's activist hopes for poetry—the desire to "enlighten and free the mind from clinging, deadening prejudices." The "others" Mary Shelley encounters during travel, then, include her lost mother and husband, others who have become nearly inseparable from any sense of self. However, she also introduces into this

---

18 Schor cites Mary Shelley's 1823 essay "Giovanni Villani" in *The Mary Shelley Reader*, eds. Betty T. Bennett and Charles E. Robinson (New York: Oxford University Press, 1990) 331–32.

shared vision her own desire. She hopes that the displaced trauma one encounters in particular landscapes might invite a sympathetic identification with the political struggles and suffering that others experienced there.

History, Landscape, Trauma

The invisible presences that Mary Shelley senses populate the landscape, then, are not only her own "beloved dead," but are also historical figures who suffered for righteous causes. The written account of her journeys invites readers to establish a relationship with the landscape that honors the courageous political suffering marking specific locations. She wishes to experience not only the picturesque beauty of the landscape, but also the history of suffering written on it. She has "seen enough of the Rhine as a *picture*," and would like "to penetrate the ravines, to scale the heights, to linger among the ruins, to hear still more of its legends" (*WMS* 8:163, original emphasis). In a passage about the Tyrol, she is more interested in the political history that saturates the landscape than in the standard picturesque view. She refers to William Beckford's 1780 celebration of the landscape's "'picturesque wonders,'" but suggests that recent history has rendered the landscape more historically interesting than beautiful: "The Tyrol is now endowed with a higher interest: it is hallowed by a glorious struggle, which gifts every rock, and precipice, and mountain-stream, with a tale of wonder" (*WMS* 8:248–49). She refers to the Tyrolian people's heroic revolt in 1809 against Napoleon's transfer of the region's rule from the Austrians to the Bavarians. In Mary Shelley's view, this revolutionary act of collective courage suffuses the natural landscape: "Every portion of the route we traversed had been the scene of victory or defeat, and rendered illustrious by the struggle for liberty" (*WMS* 8:250). Focusing especially on the biography of Andreas Hofer, the revolutionary who led the Tyrolese uprising against Bavarian rule, she concludes: "Such are the deeds, such the name, that shed glory over the rugged and romantic passes of the Tyrol" (*WMS* 8:259). In order to shed glory, Hofer also had to shed blood. He was assassinated in 1810, refusing, as Mary Shelley carefully points out, to wear a blindfold as he was executed (*WMS* 8:259). Instead he looked back at his prosecutors, fully implicating them in his suffering. Caruth argues "that history, like trauma, is never simply one's own, that history is precisely the way we are implicated in each other's traumas" (24). In her representation of the Tyrolian landscape and of Hofer, Mary Shelley encourages her readers to identify with these historical examples of courageous suffering displaced onto the rocks and soil, a displacement that is not so much a form of psychological protection as it is a marker of the common ground of suffering.

Directly implicating her British readers in historical trauma, Mary Shelley laments the much "overlooked" suffering of the Hessians as she gazes at their home landscape. Although her fellow Britons would have been well aware that George III relied on "mercenary sons" to fight the war against the American colonies, they may not have considered the suffering this policy visited upon the Hessians themselves:

> We censure the policy of government, we lament the obstinacy of George III, who, exhausting the English levies, had recourse to "the mercenary sons of rapine and plunder;" and "devoted the Americans and their possessions to the rapacity of hireling cruelty." But

our imagination does not transport itself to the homes of the unfortunate Germans; nor is our abhorrence of the tyranny that sent them to die in another hemisphere awakened ... . [W]hen first the order was given out for the enlisting of the soldiers, hundreds deserted their homes and betook themselves to the neighbouring mountains of Franconia, and were hunted down like wild animals, and starved into surrender. (*WMS* 8:179–80)

Seeing the homes that the Hessians fled and the mountains in which they hid makes visible previously unseen suffering. Mary Shelley consistently uses the word "suffering" when describing landscapes associated with the fight for liberty. Celebrating Protestant German towns, she proclaims, "Hail to the good fight, the heart says everywhere; hail to the soil whence intellectual liberty gained, with toil and suffering, the victory—not complete yet—but which, thanks to the men of those time, can never suffer entire defeat! In time it will spread to those countries which are still subject to papacy" (*WMS* 8:182). The very soil is a parchment on which the history of political suffering is written. The liberty gained by this suffering predicts hope for the cause of nationalism in Italy, the country most directly "subject to papacy" (*WMS* 8:182).

Just as she points out that the Hessians' suffering has not been seen by the English, so Mary Shelley argues in her introduction that the Italians, too, are suffering from English misperception, and suggests to her countrymen that they take "another view":

We have lately been accustomed *to look on Italy* as a discontented province of Austria, forgetful that her supremacy dates only from the downfall of Napoleon. From the invasion of Charles VIII till 1815, Italy has been a battle-field, where the Spaniard, the French, and the German, have fought for mastery; and *we are blind indeed, if we do not see* that such will occur again. (*WMS* 8:68, my emphasis)

As the examples of Tyrolese and Hessian suffering illustrate, Mary Shelley depicts this social trauma as simply manifest in the natural setting, threatening repetition as it seeks a sympathetic eye. One would have to be "blind indeed" not to see it. In her account of the landscape outside Rome, Mary Shelley asserts that it would be impossible not to see the traumatic history infusing the land: "No one can look on this country as merely so much earth—every clod is a sacred relic—every stone is an object of curiosity—every name we hear satisfies some desire or awakens some cherished association" (*WMS* 8:342). The visual metaphors in these examples connect displaced personal trauma—evident to Mary Shelley in specific natural scenes and objects—with the encryptment of social trauma in the landscape. As in her response to her son's love of sailing—"I can bring no help, except constant watchfulness"—her depictions of the suffering evident in the land call for vigilance to prevent a repetition of trauma (*WMS* 8:113). Visual ideas are written on the mind during trauma, and when those visual ideas resurface, they trigger the feelings of that suffering. Similarly, the objects in these historically suffused landscapes, Mary Shelley hopes, will invite the sympathy and vigilance—both emotional and political—of the armchair travelers who accompany her. Thus, by re-enacting the creation of traumatic memories in the structure of her travel narrative, Mary Shelley turns personal suffering into political argument. She is what Kaja Silverman terms a "world spectator"—"not just someone to whom the past returns, but someone who holds [her]self open to the new form it will take—who anticipates and affirms the transformative manifestation of what was in what is" (25). Displacing her own suffering onto the landscape, she invites the reader to look at similarly expressive landscapes in order "to regard with greater attention, and to sympathise in the struggles" of Italy as it seeks to become whole (*WMS* 8:70).

In the Romantic era, subjectivity, as I explain in the introduction, was signaled by both vision and suffering. Romantic-era writers such as Wordsworth and William Blake explicitly equate vision with subjectivity. Concurrently, one strand of the late-eighteenth-century animal rights debate cited suffering as evidence of subjectivity—especially where, as with animals, speech is not possible. In Mary Shelley's resistance to physician surveillance and categorization at the spa, she demands to own the vision of her suffering, rather than be told by an authority that she does not see it accurately and must trust the doctors to see it for her. She insists on retaining her subjectivity—that is, both her sense of the borders of her "self" and this self's unique point of view—even though it feels at times quite fragile (e.g., "I am torn to pieces by Memory" *JMS* 559). She takes note of objects and scenes that both mark and displace trauma. She is drawn to locations in which she feels the dead around her. These interactions are transmitted through her body—her womb, her eyes—a body that resists the scrutiny of outside authority. Thus, seeing her own suffering in the landscape, while a displacement, allows for the working through of mourning that helps reconstitute subjectivity.

Mary Shelley's resistance to categorization contrasts with Smith's faith that categories of comparison would retain the alterity of individual suffering while making that suffering visible to others. As I argue in chapter 4, however, knowing who establishes these categories is crucial for understanding their effect. Mary Shelley resists an increasingly powerful medical authority that dispenses nomenclature along with prescriptions for behavior. Smith's faith in the power of naming, categorizing, and comparison would not have included this kind of sweeping authority from above; she relished too much her own and others' ability to name and compare experiences, and thus to make suffering visible. In contrast, categorization was particularly painful to Mary Shelley. As her multiple displacements of pain reveal, she was not willing to expose her body—the seat of trauma—to unsympathetic scrutiny. Mary Shelley understood such univocal, scrutinizing authority to be dangerous to the body politic as well. Like *Frankenstein*, then, *Rambles* is a collaborative text. Mary Shelley sees through the eyes of the lost and echoes their words in her descriptions of the landscape. She feels "the beloved dead" around her, and, as Moskal notes, she "incorporates the voices of others into the narrative," including Gatteschi's account of the Ancona uprising, Percy Florence's friend's letter, and numerous literary quotations and references to historical sources (*WMS* 8:50). Mary Shelley trusts the voices of others most in the context of collaboration, be it co-editing or a kind of otherworldly channeling. These voices urge her and her readers to shift their point of view, to see differently. For Mary Shelley, the most ethical kind of authority rests finally in our own (shared) vision—that is, in what we together are and are not able to see either literally or with "our mind's eye."

In this spirit of collaborative vision, Mary Shelley drew on her own experience with trauma in order to express her long-standing support for the unification of

Italy.[19] In *Rambles*, Mary Shelley presents her own losses as resonant with the trauma involved in the struggle for liberty in Italy. Moskal observes that Mary Shelley cleverly recasts the origins of Italian nationalism as rooted in English, rather than in Napoleonic, ideals in order to make the Risorgimento more palatable to her readers ("Gender" 195, "Travel" 248–49). Mary Shelley proclaims, "Englishmen, in particular, ought to sympathise in their struggles: for the aspiration for free institutions all over the world has its source in England" (*WMS* 8:67). Telling the foundational story of Italy in terms of English history is both politically canny and also helpful to Mary Shelley as she works through the loss of people in her life who were most invested in cultivating "the seed" of freedom all over the world (*WMS* 8:67). In her support of Italian nationalism, she extends her mother's commitment to developing free institutions in France and interest in the Scandinavian countries' progress toward liberty; additionally, she continues to express the hopes she shared with Shelley for Italy's success as a nation. She carries on their work, and thus her own work of mourning, in her engagement with Italian politics.

Even as she positions herself as a secondary witness to political suffering for the cause of liberty (i.e., she is not there in the moment of trauma, but witnesses it as evident in the landscape), she resists objectifying the suffering she would have her readers see. She depicts Hofer looking back at his executioners, retaining his subject position as she/we "see" him. In a slightly different mode, she corrects historians for seeing the Hessians only as pawns of King George III and not as human beings who also suffered. Her hope for Italian nationalists, then, is to protect them from an entrapping, draining objectification and persecution. Crook notes that while Mary Shelley's support for the Risorgimento in her accounts of Italian history and culture is quite direct, she imparts her experience with politically touchy situations (such as the Austrian authorities' surveillance of her mail in Milan) as "knowledge from behind a veil" ("Meek" 79). As in *Frankenstein*, Mary Shelley endorses strategic invisibility when it is necessary to escape the dismantling gaze of authority. She supports the Carbonari's cloak of invisibility because it is necessitated by political and papal surveillance:

> Do not think that I advocate any secret society: the principle is bad. The crown of every virtuous act and feeling is, not to fear the light of day. But it must be remembered with what fearful odds the Italians have to contend [i.e., both Austrian rule and the Catholic church] .... Can it be wondered that men who wished to regenerate their country in the face of so penetrating, so almost omnipotent a power, should cloak themselves in impenetrable secrecy, and strive to check the influence by counter terrors,—equally awful? (*WMS* 8:321)

Veiling, displacing, recasting, cloaking—all responses to trauma—serve Mary Shelley well in her attempt to help readers see and sympathize with Italy's struggle. Her appeal to readers to support Italy's reunification is resonant, if not parallel, with her concomitant desire for and resistance to the witness of her own suffering. Both struggles are written on the land, both threaten to repeat themselves, both call for

---

19 For the details of her support for the Risorgimento, see Crook "Meek," and Moskal "Gender" and "Travel."

vigilance, and both occasionally require strategic invisibility. Mary Shelley's final publication enacts the transmission of knowledge around a crisis marked by both its defiance of and demand for witness. We do not need to know all the details of the trauma, nor do we need to assimilate fully our own or others' trauma in order to sympathize, to see the outline, to feel the shadow, to sense the shape of trauma. But we do need to be alive to the presence and power of these crises in order to understand the ways in which they implicate us all.

PART 3
Social Justice

Chapter 6

Seeing Poverty:
Smith's *Rural Walks* and
Wollstonecraft's *Original Stories*
as Fictional Ethnography

"[W]e are more deeply affected by one single tale of misery, with all the details of which we are acquainted, than by the greatest accumulation of sufferings of which the particulars have not fallen under our notice. Could I but separate this immense aggregate into all its component parts, and present them one by one to your view, in all their particularity of wretchedness, you would then have a more just impression of the immensity of the misery which we wish to terminate."

William Wilberforce

In his *A Letter on the Abolition of the Slave Trade* (1807), William Wilberforce notes how difficult it is to help readers understand the suffering of slaves when one talks about the enslaved as an "immense aggregate," that is, in terms of statistics or general descriptions. Following his extensive discussion of the evils of slavery based on numbers, eyewitness reports, and explanations of general conditions and trends, Wilberforce wishes also to present individual cases of suffering under slavery "one by one to [his readers'] *view*, in all their particularity of wretchedness" in order to convey a "just impression of the immensity of the misery" (340–41, my emphasis). Although he does not follow through on his desire to present cases "one by one," Wilberforce identifies such a visually based innovation in narrative form as crucial for helping his fellow British citizens and parliamentarians apprehend the suffering of slaves and move toward social action. However, at the moment Wilberforce alludes to the power such an innovation *might* have, this very narrative form already exists in children's literature to address another major social issue. Mary Wollstonecraft's *Original Stories from Real Life* (1788) and the first of Charlotte Smith's six children's books *Rural Walks* (1795) collect fictional portraits of impoverished people—"one by one"—in order to expose the causes of poverty in England as socially rather than individually based. Wollstonecraft and Smith develop aspects of eighteenth-century didactic children's literature to create what might be thought of as a fictional ethnography of the poor.

Creating episodic narratives in which child characters, with the guidance of a female teacher, learn from the people, animals, and plants they encounter, Wollstonecraft and Smith explore the social power of seeing—and of teaching children to see—ethnographically. Both Wollstonecraft and Smith were practiced in the kind of narrative innovation needed to make complex social problems visible.

As I argue in chapter 3, Wollstonecraft transformed the typical travel narrative to describe both the social conditions of countries she visited and her own emotional suffering in *Letters from Norway*. Chapter 1 explains that Smith modified and thus revived the sonnet tradition in order to express her suffering from both chronic illness and chronic worry about finances. Most relevant to this chapter, in her references to the practice of botany (the subject of chapter 4), Smith worked to invent a language that would make individual suffering socially recognizable, a language dependent on comparisons and context and practiced by collecting, naming, and contextualizing. Similarly, Wollstonecraft's and Smith's fictional ethnographies for children collect and juxtapose stories of people struggling with poverty in late-eighteenth-century England.

It may seem anachronistic to label Wollstonecraft's and Smith's innovative narrative form "ethnography." It is, though, more ironic than anachronistic. As Mary Louise Pratt explains, the practice of ethnography emerged in the eighteenth century, overlapping with the endeavors of scientific exploration and colonial conquest. Ethnographers such as John Barrow, author of *Travels into the Interior of Southern Africa* (1801), contrasted Europeans with Africans, "relegating the latter to objectified ethnographic portraits set off from the narrative of the journey" (59). This kind of ethnography works to "other" the subjects through temporal distancing—that is, by erasing the observer's participation in the temporal moment of the lives that he observes, and fixing the subject in an eternal present (Pratt 64). The narrative further removes evidence of the observer's agency by focusing on what he sees rather than on what he does: "[T]he travelers are chiefly present as a kind of collective moving eye on which the sights/sites register; as agents their presence is very reduced" (Pratt 59). While Wollstonecraft and Smith both collect portraits of the poor, their methods diverge from the masculine practice of ethnographers such as Barrow, a practice that would dominate what was thought of as legitimate ethnography (and by 1874, anthropology) for well over a century.[1] The irony, then, is that these authors of eighteenth-century children's books put forward an alternative ethnographic method—a way of seeing cultural practices and social structures—well before the field was codified and required the corrective theorizing that unfolded in the second half of the twentieth century. Unlike ethnographers from Barrow to those practicing in the early twentieth century, many current ethnographers explicitly acknowledge the mutually constitutive nature of the experience of the observer and the observed. Smith's and Wollstonecraft's narrators, then, are ethnographers who look and write in a way that anticipates twentieth-century "participant observation" in anthropological field work, a practice that requires and acknowledges "simultaneous emotional involvement and objective detachment" (Tedlock 465).[2] My use of the word

---

1   Buzard notes that anthropology became a "recognized academic subject" when it "earned its own section in the British Association for the Advancement of Science (BAAS) in 1874" (5).

2   The writing up of this the participant observation experience, Tedlock explains, led to a splitting between the "objective" study and the personal memoir. She notes that the field has attempted to heal this breach with alternative ethnographic forms that are dedicated to "the observation of participation" (465), or an explicit description of the "unsettling of the boundaries that had been central to the notion of a self studying an other" (461). These

"ethnography" implies an explicit and expressed mutual constitution of observer and subject. In his analysis of the autoethnographic work of nineteenth-century British novels, James Buzard uses the term "ethnography ... in the twentieth-century sense of a people's way of life centering on the method of 'immersion' in extensive fieldwork and raising the issue of how, and how far, the outsider can become a kind of honorary insider in other cultures" (8). In this chapter and the next, I will explore the degree to which Smith's and Wollstonecraft's social activism requires identification across insider and outsider positions.

The highly influential anthology *Writing Culture: The Poetics and Politics of Ethnography* (1986), edited by James Clifford and George Marcus, announces the importance of understanding both the poetics and politics of ethnography, that is, exploring the power differentials encoded in the hybrid genre of ethnography—"a strange cross between the realist novel, the travel account, the memoir, and the scientific report" (Behar and Gordon 3). In their revisionist anthology *Women Writing Culture* (1995), Ruth Behar and Deborah A. Gordon reveal *Writing Culture* as both belated and sexist. They demonstrate that women have had a long tradition of writing in hybrid genres with an awareness of both poetics and politics, a sense of the personal and the ethnographic, as well as a consciousness of the power dynamic between observer and subject.[3] I regard Wollstonecraft's and Smith's mingling of fiction and fact, identification with the subjects they describe, and social observation as an early contribution to this tradition. To be specific, I argue that Wollstonecraft and Smith develop three aspects of eighteenth-century children's literature in order to train readers to see the social structures that create and exacerbate poverty. They 1) feature a teacher figure who serves as an ethnographer, 2) represent experiential learning through dialogue, and 3) create an episodic narrative structure. These three qualities of late-eighteenth-century didactic literature resonate to differing degrees with three aspects of ethnography: 1) "reciprocity of perspectives (that is, seeing others against a background of ourselves and ourselves against a background of others)," 2) "emphasis on dialogue and discourse," and 3) "comparison through families of resemblance" (Harrison 235).

First, Wollstonecraft and Smith create a teacher figure who becomes an ethnographer, collecting and commenting on individual people's stories so that others might apprehend the relationships among gender, class structure, illness, and poverty. Unlike other children's literature that uses impoverished characters

---

forms work "to bridge the gulf between self and other by revealing both parties as vulnerable experiencing subjects" (467). Other terms for this approach include the new ethnography, autoethnography, literary ethnography, alternative ethnography, and narrative ethnography. In addition to the anthology by Behar and Gordon, discussed below, see essays by Harrison, Wolf, and Ellis and Bochner on this subject.

3   In her introductory essay to the anthology, Behar notes: "In an act of sanctioned ignorance, the category of the new ethnography failed to take into account that throughout the twentieth century women had crossed the border between ethnography and literature—but usually 'illegally,' as aliens who produced works that tended to be viewed in the profession as 'confessional' and 'popular' ... The *Writing Culture* agenda, conceived in homoerotic terms by male academics for other male academics, provided the official credentials, the cachet, that women had lacked for crossing the border" (4).

as props for teaching gentry-class children how to give charity, Wollstonecraft's Mrs. Mason and Smith's Mrs. Woodfield place themselves on a continuum with the poor people they encounter. Furthermore, like their teacher figures, Smith and Wollstonecraft experienced financial pressures and health problems that helped them understand poverty, illness, and women's oppression as interdependent social problems. Accordingly, their narratives teach child readers to practice a "reciprocity of perspective" in their interactions with the poor (Harrison 235).

Second, Wollstonecraft and Smith portray learning as experiential by creating an in-the-present-moment dialogue between teacher and children. This formulation emerges from Jean-Jacques Rousseau's novel *Emile* (1774), in which Emile is educated by carefully controlled experiential learning rather than by books. He learns from what he sees, and one of the major goals of this education through observation is to cultivate his compassion: "Emile's first observations of men are directed to the poor, the sick, the oppressed, and the unfortunate" (Bloom 17–18). In a woman-centered variation of Rousseau's pedagogical vision, late-eighteenth-century didactic children's literature generally depicts a strong female teacher who instructs her pupils in dialogues that occur largely outdoors. The teacher and students follow a curriculum driven by daily events that inspire the children's curiosity and reason. When the children encounter an unfamiliar person, object, or situation, the teacher steps in to offer an interpretive context for the experience. This literature recreates a peripatetic "classroom," in which visual experiences initiate learning and questions are pursued in dialogue. As in the "new ethnography," observers construct representations of others through "dialogue and discourse" (Harrison 235).

Finally, Wollstonecraft and Smith structure their narratives episodically. This narrative form reflects that of three other vastly popular books for children— Caroline-Stéphanie-Félicité de Genlis's *Les Veillées du Chateau* (1784), Sarah Trimmer's *Fabulous Histories. Designed for the Instruction of Children, Respecting their Treatment of Animals* (1786), and Anna Letitia Barbauld's and John Aiken's *Evenings at Home* (1792–96). Offering homage to Trimmer, Wollstonecraft has the teacher in *Original Stories* assign *Fabulous Histories* to her pupils to read.[4] Although their children's books differ in their political message, Wollstonecraft clearly admired Trimmer's strong teacher figure and her representation of experiential learning in fictional episodes. Like Wollstonecraft, Smith situates her narrative in the emerging tradition of popular children's books. In a 1794 letter to her publishers, Smith proposes *Rural Walks* as a variation of Barbauld's and Aiken's *Evenings at Home*, describing her book as "A Work less desultory than Mrs. Barbauld's 'Evenings at home' (which have had & still have an amazing sale) & calculated for young persons three or four years older" (*CLCS* 131). Whereas the lessons in *Evenings at Home* take place as unconnected episodes—miscellaneous stories told in the evenings—Smith proposes a less "desultory" text, organized by walks and an active and consistent

---

4   Wollstonecraft's publisher Joseph Johnson introduced her to both Barbauld and Trimmer, whose children's books, along with those of Madame de Genlis, she regarded as models for *Original Stories*. She was particularly drawn to the strong women teachers in Genlis's and Trimmer's works (Todd 125–26).

cast of characters.[5] She notes that her proposed book "shall give an opportunity of discoursing on Landscape on the simple parts of botany, and natural history, with short stories of suppositious persons ... such as may be at once interesting and moral" (*CLCS* 130–31). Although Smith does not claim that her children's books will contain social commentary, the "interesting and moral" fictional stories in *Rural Walks* serve as Trojan horses for social criticism. Smith presents repeated fictional portraits of people whose lives illustrate the interdependence of gender, illness, and poverty, as well as the duties of the charitable and of the state to help those in need.[6] These stories broaden readers' understanding of what might seem without the episodic context to be individual problems, encouraging readers to make "comparisons through families of resemblance" in order to understand the social structures underlying poverty (Harrison 235).

The Problem of Poverty

Social historian John Roach notes that "the overmastering concern in men's minds [in England] between 1780 and 1830 was the problem of poverty" (66). In late-eighteenth-century England, the rural laborer was gradually losing his ability to survive due to the losses caused by the Enclosure Acts, the constraints of the long-standing Act of Settlements, and the rising cost of food during the war against France. While almost all historians writing about eighteenth-century poverty explain that the complexity of local systems of poor relief make it difficult to generalize about the lived experience of poverty, they agree that these three conditions—enclosure, settlement, and the rising cost of food—adversely affected the lives of many cottagers and rural laborers, if to varying degrees.[7] Between 1761 and 1801, the number of successful Acts of Enclosure increased by a factor of ten compared with the previous forty years (Hammond 17). When a large farmer or landlord gained permission to enclose land through a successful petition to Parliament, his land size, farming efficiency, and thus wealth, increased. However, these enclosures meant that small farmers, cottagers, and squatters lost access to common pasture land in which they might keep a cow or other livestock, common garden space in which they might grow food for their family, common waste land on which they were accustomed to gather furze or branches for fuel, and common woods on which they might hunt for small game (Hammond 73–81). As land was consolidated under larger farmers, the working poor were also prevented from "gleaning" leftover wheat or beans from the fields after harvest (Hammond 83–85). In addition, the Act of Settlements, which required that the poor live in their legal parish in order to receive aid or medical

---

5   Although not organized by a central teacher figure, the miscellaneous stories in *Evenings at Home*, as Fyfe notes, are ordered according to a "gradual progression in difficulty" (457).

6   For contemporaneous works on urban poverty that also mingle fact with fiction, see the first volume of *The Metropolitan Poor: Semifictional Accounts, 1795-1910*, eds. John Marriot and Masaie Matsumura.

7   See especially Steven King's study for more on the ways in which the variations among local approaches challenge the construction of an intelligible history of poverty in this era.

care, prevented them from moving to search for work or assistance (Hammond 88). Although this law was inconsistently enforced, parishes tended to become stricter when they experienced "worries over spiraling costs" such as food (King 23). The more than doubling of public expenditure on poor relief between 1786 and 1803 is a measure of the distress caused by these limitations and by rising food prices during the war against France (Andrew 200).

Significantly, 1795, the year Smith published *Rural Walks*, was the first of several years of "scarcity": "The harvest of 1794 was short, and in the autumn wheat prices began to rise. In January the average was 7s. a bushel, the highest since 1790; by August it had almost doubled, and the new harvest was not good enough to remedy the scarcity" (Poynter 45). As a result, 1795 was marked by "food riots all over England" in which the poor seized grain and other food from farmers not to steal it, but to demand that it be sold at a fair price (Hammond 96). This 1790s crisis inspired British citizens to discuss a variety of reforms to the 1601 "Act for the relief of the poor." The 1601 Poor Act implemented a local tax system that enabled each of more than 15,000 parishes to provide relief for its own poor, but, as many historians point out, it was a system characterized more by the variety of ways in which it was implemented than by its consistency. In most parishes, however, an impoverished person would apply for relief to an overseer—an unpaid official, usually a large farmer or landlord, who collected and distributed the money raised by the poor rates. Two kinds of relief were possible: outdoor relief of a few shillings a week (the amount depended upon the parish, the overseer, and the individual case), or indoor relief in the workhouse. In some parishes, if the poor refused to enter the workhouse, they gave up their right to receive public relief of any kind. In addition to providing relief, the overseer was to establish apprenticeships for pauper children, jail the idle, and return vagrants—especially pregnant women—to the parish of their birth in accordance with the 1662 Act of Settlements and its later revisions (Newman 564). In most parishes, the overseer's decisions were regulated by the justices of the peace or county magistrates by the 1790s.

Proposed reforms to this system in the 1790s included a minimum wage;[8] wage supplements tied to the price of food and family size during times of scarcity;[9] several systems to help the poor save money;[10] allotments of land and livestock meant to

---

8   In the winter of 1795, Samuel Whitbread brought his proposal before Parliament for minimum wage. He argued that regulation of wages would be a dignified alternative to the charity of the rich (Hammond 117–19).

9   In 1795, a group of Berkshire magistrates met to create a scale that tied relief to the cost of bread and shortfall in wages for families of various sizes in order to guide overseers in their administration of relief. This Speenhamland Scale was only one of several attempts to regularize local practice, but it was made famous in Sir Frederick Morton Eden's account of it in *The State of the Poor*, published in 1797 (Michael Rose 33–35).

10   Poynter describes three types of proposals to encourage savings. First, Francis Maseres unsuccessfully proposed an annuity plan to which the poor would contribute in 1772. Second, politicians tried to harness the grassroots development of friendly societies—collaborative groups of workers that established a kind of mutual insurance—in a series of proposals that led to the Friendly Societies Act of 1793. And, third, several plans for savings banks appeared, beginning in 1795 (35–39).

restore these means of subsistence taken by enclosure acts;[11] the employment and training of children in Schools of Industry;[12] and the replacement of public relief with private charity alone. Although major changes to the 1601 Poor Law were not implemented until 1834 with the more centralized (and ultimately more harmful) New Poor Law, the system did begin to modulate in the 1790s, and the discussion about the issues mid-decade reveals a variety of strenuous opinions about how to respond to poverty. The historians whose work I draw upon in the paragraphs above focus on the origins of poverty in the 1790s, yet "English poor law administrators [of the period] consistently failed to address the causes rather than consequences of poverty" (King 40). Likewise, while there were numerous works published about the problem of poverty in the last two decades of the eighteenth century—including religious tracts recommending charity to the poor; sermons dictating proper behavior for the poor; census-like documents listing the poor by name, number in household, and age; and political proposals for the relief of the poor—compilations of the stories of the poor were rare and rarely designed to expose the social structures underlying poverty.[13] For example, although Thomas Burgess's collection of anecdotes about the poor, *Moral Annals of the Poor, and Middle Ranks of Society, in Various Situations of Good and Bad Conduct* (1793), would seem ethnographic, it is rather designed to teach the poor who attended Sunday schools in Durham proper behavior and values such as "honesty," "gratitude," "fidelity," and "good citizenship." A fictional ethnography that directs attention to the lives of the poor and to the causes of their poverty, then, was a significant intervention in the national discussion in the eighteenth century and continues to be an important resource for the historical reconstruction of the lives of the poor from our perspective.

Activist Children's Literature

By creating fictional ethnographies in the tradition of didactic children's literature, Smith and Wollstonecraft herald education's crucial role in effecting social change, and present the education of children as women's most powerful site of influence on political and social issues.[14] As several critics have argued, late-eighteenth-century readers expected to find social commentary and criticism in children's literature (Clarke, Fyfe, Myers "Little Girls," Robbins). Norma Clarke notes that "women who wrote rational literature for children were consciously or inadvertently offering those children, and the adults they would grow into, tools for reappraising their

---

11 See especially J. L. and Barbara Hammond on this point (130–37).

12 This was a favorite idea of Prime Minister Pitt's that was shot down—primarily by Jeremy Bentham—along with the rest of Pitt's 1796 proposal. The schools were designed to train children in employable skills after age 5. The profit from the work they completed while in training would pay for the cost of the school (Hammond 125–26, Poynter 69–70).

13 To some degree, Sir Frederick Morton Eden's *The State of the Poor* (1797) and Robert Malthus's *Essay on the Principle of Population* (1798, 1803) are important exceptions to this statement.

14 In her discussion of Wollstonecraft's *Original Stories*, Myers notes: "Barred from participation in Georgian sociopolitical life, the tales suggest, women can redefine power ... as pedagogic and philanthropic power" ("Impeccable" 43).

social and political situations" (93). Mitzi Myers argues that "Georgian maternal pedagogy, linking private and public spheres, insists on the communal consequences of domestic instruction" ("Impeccable" 37). However, it is also true that rather than educate children about social causes and institutional solutions to poverty, most didactic children's narratives instead instruct children in charitable giving. M. O. Grenby asserts that in children's literature published between 1770 and 1830 "neither the Poor Law, nor ... other kinds of institutional informal relief ... makes any appearance" (186). Furthermore, he notes that didactic children's literature offers "an increasingly narrow understanding of the properties of charitable behavior" (185). Although perhaps overstated, Grenby's argument holds for the narratives he includes in his study—children's books by Edmund Butcher, Arnaud Berquin, Mary Belson, W. F. Sullivan, Jane West, Eleanor Finn, Mary Budden, Thomas Day, and a number of anonymous authors. Representing major exceptions to Grenby's assertion, Wollstonecraft's *Original Stories* and Smith's *Rural Walks* teach children a rather broad approach to charity that focuses on the social causes of poverty. In addition, Smith's narrative educates children about political reform and institutional relief for the poor.

Charity, as Grenby points out, was a common feature of didactic children's literature, yet one must analyze the power dynamic encoded in charitable scenes in order to determine the political message.[15] Offering charity was often a deeply conservative gesture. Edmund Burke's *Thoughts and Details on Scarcity* (1795), for example, maintains that the suffering of the poor is exaggerated and that to offer them further public relief or to create a minimum wage would endanger the well-being of farmers and tradesmen who would be burdened with higher rates (Poynter 52–55). He asserts that appropriately distributed charity will solve any problem that might exist. In 1799 Hannah More writes that the upper classes must first *see* poverty in order to relieve it: "In a sequestered, though populous village, there is, perhaps, only one affluent family: the distress which they do not *behold*, will probably not be attended to: the distress which they do not relieve, will probably not be relieved at all" (195, my emphasis). Like Wilberforce, Wollstonecraft, and Smith, More articulates the pressing need to make suffering visible if one wishes to provide succor. However, More attributes the problem of rural poverty to individual affluent families vacationing at the spa and other resorts while they should be staying at home to fulfill their class-based duties. She does not paint a picture of a systemic

---

15 For example, one of the first popular books for children, *The History of Little Goody Two-Shoes* (1765), begins with an introduction meant primarily for adult readers that outlines the ruin of Goody Two-Shoes' family due to the greedy actions of the Lord of the Manor and a large farmer—who also serves as parish overseer and church warden. The introduction to this children's book, then, depicts the ways in which the Enclosure Acts allowed a hard-working family to be driven off their land and into poverty. However, the text itself displays the orphaned Little Goody Two-Shoes responding to adversity with good humor, fortitude, and perseverance. Rising up through poverty by her own wits and hard work, Goody Two-Shoes is rewarded near the end of the narrative by marrying into money, a situation which allows her to become a philanthropist within her community. Although the narrative begins with the suffering of Goody Two-Shoes' family due to the Enclosure Acts, the book is meant to inspire good deeds in children rather than to incite social reform.

crisis in the social structures that offered rural laborers sustenance or—in the case of disability or old age—relief. She suggests that when affluent families return to do their philanthropic duty in their own communities, the problem of rural poverty will be solved. In this statement and elsewhere, More assumes that there will always be poverty, and that it will always be the duty of the wealthy to offer the poor charity. Thus, the poor are objects to be seen and aided by the dutiful wealthy, rather than speaking subjects who themselves are perceptive agents.

Like Burke and More, leaders of charitable organizations were concerned about escalating need and thus worked to develop methods of "further discrimination" to separate the undeserving from the deserving poor (Andrew 200). Public appeals for individual charity inevitably highlight the most readily accepted characteristics of the "deserving" poor, including the poor person's legitimate residency, and "impotence" (or inability to work due to age, illness, or injury). Consider, for example, representations of the poor in solicitations for charity, taken from the 16 January 1794 issue of *The Bath Chronicle*:

> Sarah Taylor a Poor Woman who is well known to many creditable persons in this city, and who has lived in and been respected by some of the principal families in the kingdom, is reduced by Old Age, and still more by a violent Paralytick Stroke, to extreme indigence. She humbly solicits the bounty of the well-disposed, as her distresses are very great, being in want of every comfort and every necessity of life. Donations received at Mr. Roubel's, in the Grove, at Mr. Meyler's, and by the printer of this paper.—She gratefully acknowledges the following Benefaction: *At Mr. Cruttwell's*, a Clergyman 5s

> To the Charitable and Humane
> The humble Petition of Mary Ford, widow of John Ford, of the parish of St. James's, in the city of Bath, who has carried on her business as Laundress in the same dwelling in the Full-Moon-Yard, Horse-Street, 50 years: She is now at the age of 84, has been afflicted these five years with the dead palsy, which has rendered her incapable of assisting herself, for which reason she has lost the greatest part of her work, and now finds it impossible to pay her rent, so that she is daily in expectation of her few goods being seized for rent, and she sent to the workhouse, unless by the kind benevolence of some Ladies or Gentlemen whom Providence may direct to her deplorable situation. The above case is attested by the Churchwardens of St. James's.—The smallest donations will be thankfully received at Mr. Hazard's Library, Cheap-Street. She returns thanks for the following donations: *Mrs. Metbold 1£. 1s. A Lady 10s. 6d. Mrs. Bennett ?s. 6d.*

Sarah Taylor, an elderly long-term resident of Bath, has been struck by a paralytic stroke; Mary Ford, a laundress who has lived and worked in the same house in Bath for fifty years, is afflicted with palsy. These advertisements exemplify solicitations in *The Bath Chronicle* between 1794 and 1800 in that they identify illness as the cause of poverty, describe an impoverished woman rather than a man, carefully establish that woman's legitimate residency in the community, and portray the poor person as grateful for help. The person who wrote these advertisements assumes that potentially charitable readers need evidence of the worthiness or deservingness of these poor women.

In this culture of "reading" or visually identifying poverty, then, how can one interpret charity as anything other than disciplinary? Michel de Certeau's definition of "place" and "space" in *The Practice of Everyday Life* offers a vocabulary for evaluating charitable acts, or more specifically, for analyzing the movement of power in scenes that depict encounters between members of different classes:[16]

> A place ... is the order ... with which elements are distributed in relationships of coexistence. It thus excludes the possibility of two things being in the same location ... . The law of the "proper" rules in the place: the elements taken into consideration are beside one another, each situated in its own "proper" and distinct location ... . It implies an indication of stability. (117)

In the context of characters' visits to the poor, a clear and stable differentiation between the charitable, gentry-class character's status and the impoverished, working-class character's status would create a "place." The "proper" interaction between giver and receiver reifies their class distinction. More's assertion that it is the duty of affluent families to offer charity in their home villages, for example, fortifies a "place" that stabilizes class distinctions.

Further illustrating the qualities of "place," the painting *Portrait of Sir Francis Ford's Children Giving a Coin to a Beggar Boy* (Figure 7) by Sir William Beechy (1753–1839) places a crippled beggar boy and gentry children in balanced and opposite planes.[17] The charitable children are sheltered by the tree framing their side of the painting, while the beggar boy is exposed to the elements and to the scrutinizing gazes of the children. The well-dressed gentry children and even the dog look directly at the young beggar, while the crippled boy's eyes are downcast, demonstrating his humility rather than his empowerment or ability to look back at his benefactors. Beechy presents a stable and well-defined relationship between the poor and the charitable in this painting, a compelling visual example of de Certeau's "place."

As in Beechy's painting, the way in which characters look at one another largely determines the construction of "place" with regard to class. In contrast, de Certeau explains:

> A *space* exists when one takes into consideration vectors of direction, velocities, and time variables. Thus space is composed of intersections of mobile elements ... . Space occurs as the effect produced by the operations that orient it, situate it, temporalize it, and make it function in a polyvalent unity of conflictual programs or contractual proximities ... . In contradistinction to the place, it has thus none of the univocality or stability of a "proper." (117, original emphasis)

When texts depict overlapping concerns among characters of different classes, slippages between their "proper" roles, disruptions or reversals in the prescribed pattern of giving and receiving, or contextually and temporally dependent definitions of social power among characters, the author constructs a non-reifying "space." In

---

16 Constance Relihan's argument in *Cosmographical Glasses* about the fictional elements of Elizabethan ethnography and the ethnographic elements of Elizabethan fiction led me to de Certeau.

17 I am indebted to Gerald Newman (in whose *Britain in the Hanoverian Age* I first encountered this image), N. Merrill Distad (whose entry it illustrates), my colleague Scott Gordon, and especially M. O. Grenby for help in identifying this image.

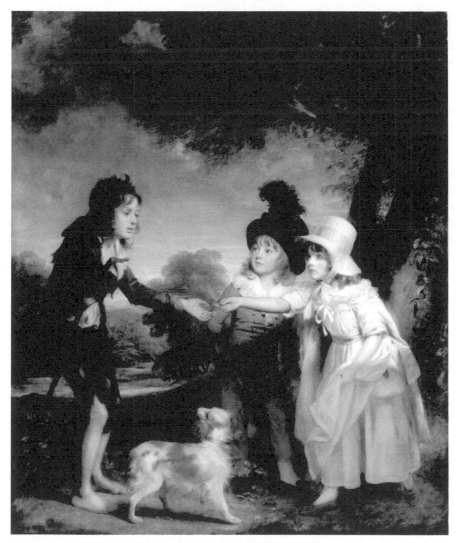

Fig. 7.   **Sir William Beechy.** *Portrait of Sir Francis Ford's Children Giving a Coin to a Beggar Boy*

this sense, participant observation creates "spaces" rather than "places" because the roles of observer and observed are fluid and share the same temporal moment. De Certeau notes that stories "carry out a labor that constantly transforms places into spaces or spaces into places" (118). Stories can alternatively create the "tableau" of "place," or "organize [the] movements" of "space" (119).

Evaluating the ways in which stories construct de Certeauan "places" or "spaces" (that is, the ways authors depict the teacher/ethnographer interacting with the poor) is crucial for understanding the political work attempted by the texts considered below. To suggest the ways in which Smith and Wollstonecraft draw on the tradition of activist children's literature and also diverge from it, I will briefly take up moments in Trimmer's *Fabulous Histories* and Barbauld's and Aiken's *Evenings at Home* that address poverty, illness, and charity. The ways in which these authors portray encounters between middle- or gentry-class narrators and more impoverished characters are crucial for understanding the degree to which each episodic narrative engages the ethnographic imagination without reasserting the power differential between the observer and the observed.

In Trimmer's *Fabulous Histories*, the mother Mrs. Benson repeatedly reminds her children to direct their compassion and charity more toward the poor than toward the animal kingdom, thus establishing a clear hierarchy of creatures that situates animals at the bottom, the poor in the middle, and those who can give charity at the top (9). Furthermore, she instructs the children to remain consistent in their generosity toward the robins they have rescued, ultimately a lesson in the practice of charity. When the children oversleep and feed the robins much later than usual, Mrs. Benson tells them: "[F]or the future, whenever you give any living creature cause to depend on you for sustenance, be careful on no account to disappoint it; and if you are prevented from feeding it yourself, employ another person to do it for you" (17). Similar to the quotation from More above, this scene speaks to the traditional duty of landowners to care for the poor in their neighborhood, and is consistent with what Moira Ferguson describes as the text's reification of the social hierarchy during a time of "anxiety of people in Trimmer's class about potential disorder throughout England, [and] threats to the sanctity of private property" (7). Doing one's traditional duty, then, promised to preserve the landed class's traditional privileges during a time of ominous class unrest.

In a scene that addresses poverty more directly, Mrs. Benson and her daughter Harriet encounter a poor woman whose pleas for help have been ignored by their wealthy neighbor Mrs. Addis. Rather than treat her poor neighbor with charity, Mrs. Addis directs all her attention to her menagerie of animals. When Mrs. Benson and Harriet meet the poor woman, she "entreat[s] them to give her some relief, as she had a sick husband and seven children in a starving condition; of which, she said, they might be eye-witnesses, if they would have to goodness to step into a barn hard by" (110). The poor woman's offer to allow Mrs. Benson and Harriet to be "eye-witnesses" teaches the child reader that the visual verification of poverty is a necessary component of charitable giving. And, indeed, when she enters the "mansion of real woe," Mrs. Benson describes the scene as a kind of painting: "she beheld a father, surrounded with his helpless family, whom he could no longer supply with sustenance; and he himself, though his disease was subdued, was almost on the point of expiring for want of some reviving cordial" (111). This scene, then, fulfills de Certeau's definition of "place" as a two-dimensional tableaux composed of the charitable observer in one plane and the poor family in the other. Mrs. Benson's gaze fixes the two groups in this interaction as "properly" separated by class standing. When Mrs. Benson asks why the family has not obtained relief, the poor woman replies that they have always been hard workers and had been ashamed to ask for help until that day. Having found the family to be deserving of her help—hard working and not in the habit of asking for aid—Mrs. Benson offers immediate charity and promises more. In these examples, the child reader of Trimmer's book sees a mother instruct her children how to offer charity correctly: to remain consistent in one's duty to the poor and to give charity only when it is clearly deserved. The reader's focus, however, remains on the act of giving correctly rather than on the suffering of the poor. Seeing in Trimmer's text, then, is figured more as surveillance than as sympathy or social criticism. In spite of its conservative values, however, the peripatetic, episodic, and woman-centered structure of Trimmer's popular children's book strongly influenced both Wollstonecraft and Smith.

Barbauld's and Aiken's *Evenings at Home* offers a critique of several social issues, including a dissenting view on the problem of poverty.[18] While Trimmer celebrates the charitable child, Barbauld and Aiken draw attention to the industry and worth of the impoverished person. Aileen Fyfe comments:

> Unlike Trimmer's rural parish society ... the poor in *Evenings at Home* were to be treated not as objects of charity, but as respectable workers performing tasks which were necessary to society. While Trimmer could argue that philanthropy to the poor helped the rich to be distinguished "by their benevolence and greatness of mind," Aiken argued that impoverished workers deserved better treatment by society, not out of charity but due to the natural rights which they possessed as much as the next man. (462)

The two narratives from *Evenings at Home* that take up the issue of poverty most directly—"Perseverance Against Fortune" and "Humble Life; or, The Cottagers"—emphasize a small farmer's and a cottager's abilities to persevere under distressing circumstances.

In the first, the gentry-class father, Mr. Carleton, observes his son Theodore abandoning his new garden when it is trampled by runaway pigs. Rather than comment on his son's lack of tenacity, Mr. Carleton takes the boy to visit a resilient and hardworking small farmer, appropriately named Mr. Hardman, who lives in the neighborhood. Mr. Carleton asks Mr. Hardman to tell Theodore about his extraordinary life, which includes enough adventure, disaster, and financial worry to fill a novel. Mr. Hardman and his family bounce back repeatedly from these challenges through hard work and occasional charity. Although the farmer's story is certainly designed to be an object lesson for Theodore, it is not primarily a lesson in charity, but rather a lesson about perseverance. Most important, Mr. Hardman narrates his own story and he, rather than Theodore's father, articulates its moral to Theodore: "This, Sir, is my history ... if it impresses upon the mind of this young gentleman the maxim, that patience and perseverance will scarcely fail of a good issue in the end, the time you have spent in listening to it will not entirely be lost" (iv:28). Thus, Barbauld and Aiken present the farmer as self-aware, in control of his own narrative, and fully able to teach his values to members of the landed gentry.

---

18 Fyfe notes that *Evenings at Home* "recommend[s] serious education for girls, promot[es] science and manufactures, argu[es] against war, and rank-based distinctions, and suggest[s] a moral code of conduct based on reason" (458). Grenby explains the dissenting view on poverty: "It was almost a principle of their rational dissent that any institutional form of charity, and the Poor Law in particular, should be regarded with deep skepticism" (187).

In "Humble Life; or the Cottagers," a different father, Mr. Everard, attempts to teach his son Charles respect and compassion for poor cottagers when Charles speculates about how horrible their lives must be, how much better his own is in comparison. Although this is an ostensibly sympathetic observation, it serves to reassure Charles of his own privilege. During their visit to the cottage, Jacob, a weaver, describes the tasks his family undertakes—spinning, weaving, cutting pegs for shoemakers, and basket-weaving. In addition to practicing these arts, the cottagers know quite a bit more than does Charles about botany. Mr. Everard gives this deserving family a piece of his own land to help them prosper. In this story, the gentry father offers the tale's moral, noting that the cottager's family "may, from untoward accidents, be rendered objects of our compassion, but they never can of our contempt" (v:134). The child learns respect as well as charity, and quite radically, charity in this story means sharing one's own land with the poor rather than offering them a few coins.

However, while both narratives from *Evenings at Home* emphasize the hardship the impoverished characters face, in both cases the suffering of the poor is temporary and never as dire as that portrayed by Smith or Wollstonecraft. In "An Inquiry into Those Kinds of Distress Which Excite Agreeable Sensations" (1774), Barbauld and Aiken echo Adam Smith's assertion that people are less likely to sympathize with the suffering of a beggar than with that of a middle-class character who has fallen on hard times (Richey 428): "Poverty, if truly represented, shocks our nicer feelings; therefore, whenever it is made use of to awaken our compassion, the rags and dirt, the squalid appearance and mean employments incident to that state, must be kept out of sight, and the distress must arise from the idea of depression, and the shock of falling from higher fortunes" (99). They further observe that "deformity is always disgusting" in life and in literature (98). Yet, they argue, "we ought to remember, that misery has a claim to relief, however we may be disgusted with its appearance; and that we must not fancy ourselves charitable, when we are only pleasing our imagination" (104). In *Evenings at Home*, Barbauld and Aiken represent the impoverished or formerly impoverished with a great deal of dignity. They give Mr. Carleton control over his own story and its moral, represent Jacob as a teacher rather than a dependent, and depict Mr. Everard's act of charity as the redistribution of property. However, the reader does not feel the weight of repeated portraits of suffering, and understands poverty to be best alleviated by the hard work of the poor and occasional charity from neighbors.

In other words, while this text does its own political work, it does not function ethnographically in the way that *Original Stories* and *Rural Walks* do. Wollstonecraft's and Smith's texts feature an ethnographer figure who, like the people she interacts with, is much more vulnerable to poverty and suffering than are Trimmer's Mrs. Benson and Barbauld's and Aiken's father characters. Wollstonecraft's and Smith's narratives position the teacher as an insider, rather than as a charitable and dutiful outsider; they create charitable characters who are vulnerable to the same social problems that cause the suffering they encounter in others. If characters see in one another a part of their own experience—past, present, or possible future—there is a much better chance that the depiction of their interaction will constitute a "space" of possible reform, rather than a "place" of traditional class relations. Furthermore, with their linked, episodic format, Wollstonecraft's and Smith's texts teach child readers to consider multiple causes of and solutions to poverty, even as the characters offer charity to the poor people they meet.

Original Stories

In his introduction to Smith's *The Romance of Real Life* (1787), Michael Gamer identifies *Original Stories from Real Life* as part of a "fictional sub-genre" that presents "real life" incidents in story form (*WCS* 1:10). In this sense, *Original Stories* announces its ethnographic intentions in its title. While each incident in the book is not identifiable as "real," certainly the circumstances the narrative depicts reflect Wollstonecraft's work as a governess for the three daughters of the Kingsborough family in 1786–87. Because Wollstonecraft found the children's education in compassion to be deficient, she determined that she would take the oldest daughter, Margaret, to visit the poor in order to develop the young woman's capacity to empathize with others (Gordon 94). Wollstonecraft named her characters in *Original Stories* after the younger Kingsborough daughters and recreated her curriculum for the girls in the children's book. Lyndall Gordon refers to Wollstonecraft's *Original Stories* as the record of "an education in seeing—seeing, for instance, that the lower classes and all lower forms of life were no less alive than aristocrats" (95). Although the teacher Mrs. Mason sermonizes the girls in order to correct their bad habits—Caroline is too proud of her beauty and is a gluttonous eater, while Mary procrastinates and is habitually tardy—she also exposes the girls and her readers to a series of portraits of the poor that offers a utopian vision of an egalitarian society.

It is true that the ostensible purpose of the text is to teach wealthy children to give, but it is also true that the stories of the poor they encounter shift the focus away from the "place" of stratified society to imagine a society built upon more fluid and mutually dependent relationships. Even Wollstonecraft's stories about negligent members of the gentry do not end as one might expect. Inspired by a visit to "a mansion house in ruins," Mrs. Mason shares with her students the story of Charles Townley, heir to this establishment (*WMW* 4:402). Townley's repeated failure to repay debts and catastrophic delays in offering aid to those in distress create a cascade of suffering reaching from his immediate friends to their children. Most dramatically, his friend's daughter Fanny marries badly in order to escape poverty, and then goes mad from the treatment of her "vicious" husband who locks her in a madhouse (*WMW* 4:405).[19] After suffering a series of disasters himself, Charles visits Fanny in the asylum. He asks her if she remembers him:

> Fanny looked at him, and reason for a moment resumed her seat, and informed her countenance to trace anguish on it—the trembling light soon disappeared—wild fancy flushed in her eyes, and animated her incessant rant. She sung several verses of different songs, talked of her husband's ill usage—enquired if he had lately been to sea; and frequently addressed her father as if he were behind her chair, or sitting by her. (*WMW* 4:405)

---

19 This character not only rewrites the mad Maria of Laurence Sterne's *A Sentimental Journey* (1768), but also prefigures the singing woman confined in the madhouse in *The Wrongs of Woman*, discussed in chapter 7.

Charles looks at Fanny, but Fanny also "look[s] at him." The repentant Charles not only sheds tears for Fanny, but also takes her home and cares for her until the end of his life. Thus, Wollstonecraft shifts the focus from the man of sensibility's emotional experience to the dire need of the woman in the asylum. While tragic, this story functions to transform a "place" of stable difference, constructed by neglect and selfishness, into a "space" of interactive care and mutual suffering, created by the alternation and confluence of characters' class identities.

Wollstonecraft depicts several well-intentioned parents and grandparents who are unable to care for their families because they are exploited by the wealthy. In the story of Crazy Robin, the title character is reduced to poverty and homelessness by an unkind landlord who throws him in debtor's prison, leaving his wife to die and his children to beg. This poverty eventually causes his malnourished children to die as well, and Robin's grief for them leads to his insanity (*WMW* 4:375). This series of tragic events exposes the toxic power of greedy and unregulated landlords. In another chapter, the girls and Mrs. Mason encounter a London shopkeeper in "visible distress" (*WMW* 4:441). Her son is imprisoned for debt and has turned to alcohol in his despair, leaving the shopkeeper to care for her grandchildren on her own. Unfortunately, she has many wealthy clients who buy from her on credit and never pay their bills; thus, she is on the verge of having to send her grandchildren to the workhouse. The shopkeeper comments, "If the quality did but know what they make us poor industrious people suffer, surely they would be more considerate" (*WMW* 4:442). When Mrs. Mason acknowledges the shopkeeper's "visible distress," "place" begins to shift into "space." Because Mrs. Mason is both widowed and frugal, the teacher and the shopkeeper identify with one another in spite of their class difference. Mrs. Mason pays the struggling shopkeeper in cash and offers her charity, but the woman's precarious financial position is nonetheless palpable. Her son's torment continues to unfold in debtor's prison, and the workhouse threatens her grandchildren's future. Wollstonecraft, unlike Trimmer, does not allow the reader to feel that doing one's charitable duty will permanently alleviate the suffering of the poor or resolve potentially disruptive class discontent. This "space is composed of intersections of mobile elements," including the moment of identification between Mrs. Mason and the shopkeeper and the ominous certainty that the shopkeeper's urgent financial crisis—relieved for the moment—will return (de Certeau 117). Together with the tale of Crazy Robin, the shopkeeper's story exposes the ways in which "the quality" prey upon the working classes, making it impossible for them to care for their loved ones.

Upsetting the hierarchy between giver and receiver, Wollstonecraft depicts the poor both gazing back at and giving back to their benefactors. In a way, of course, this reciprocity demonstrates the value of charitable giving for the wealthy (Grenby 190). Mrs. Mason teaches the girls that giving is a virtue that will make their lives more meaningful: "When we squander money idly, we defraud the poor, and deprive our own souls of their most exalted food" (*WMW* 4:445). However, the recipients of Mrs. Mason's charity do more than demonstrate her virtue and their gratitude; they enter into a mutually caring relationship with her and others. Taking refuge in a fisherman's cottage during a storm, the girls learn that the fisherman, who was shipwrecked, lost an eye, and was confined in a French prison, "might have been begging about the streets, but for [Mrs. Mason]," who took care of him after his return to England (*WMW* 4:398). He supplies Mrs. Mason with fish and keeps a watch for shipwrecks so that he may be "as kind to a poor perishing soul as she has been to me" (*WMW* 4:398). Similarly, an "old Welsh harper," another person Mrs. Mason has "rescued ... out of distress," comes to Mrs. Mason's neighborhood during harvest time each year to play his harp. Mrs. Mason met him in Wales, where she found him persecuted, unable to care for his family, and rendered homeless by his tyrannical landlord. Mrs. Mason asked a wealthy friend in Wales to let the harper lease a farm on his estate and she "gave him money to buy stock for it, and the implements of husbandry" (*WMW* 4:420). She thus restores to him two basic means of sustenance that were gradually removed by the Enclosure Acts of the late eighteenth century—keeping livestock and having common land to cultivate. Myers notes that "Mason's lessons ... in cultural responsibility not only envision social melioration, but actually bring it about in miniature" ("Impeccable" 43). Because Mrs. Mason offers each man not simply charity, but the means by which to become self-sustaining, Wollstonecraft also criticizes the ill effects of the Enclosure Acts. *Original Stories* imagines a society not based on hierarchy but rather on a flat web of social and financial interdependence, a "space" in which the giver may become impoverished and the impoverished may wish to give.

Unlike the charity of Trimmer's Mrs. Benson, Mrs. Mason's sympathetic giving derives from identification with the distressed people she encounters rather than from a sense of superiority to them. She attributes her ability to sympathize with Peggy, an orphaned child who lives with her, to her own loss of husband and child. Grieving over the deaths of her family members, Mrs. Mason runs into Peggy's father, who is too hopeless even to beg and is on the verge of suicide. His despair resulted from his inability to provide for his starving daughter, who had lost her mother. When Peggy's father dies, Mrs. Mason takes Peggy into her home. This story offers another example of de Certeau's "space" rather than "place," a moment when the ethnographer/teacher interacts on the same dynamic plane with the sufferers she observes. Indeed, Mrs. Mason explicitly situates the story about Peggy's family within the context of her own experience of suffering, allowing their story and their lives to intertwine with hers.

Still, there is in all this charity an awareness of the disciplinary nature of giving. Mrs. Mason encourages the girls to listen to the stories of the poor, to give the most to those who seem to have the greatest need, but never to refuse to help a person in distress: "I would have you give but a trifle when you are not certain the distress is real, and reckon it given for pleasure. I for my part would rather be deceived five hundred times, than doubt once without reason" (*WMW* 4:441). And yet, when she teaches the wealthy children to give charity to poor tenants, Mrs. Mason is quite aware of the effect of her visits: "These visits not only enabled her to form a judgment of their wants, but made them very industrious; for they were all anxious that she should find their houses and persons clean" (*WMW* 4:399). Like her predecessor Rousseau, Mrs. Mason also conducts surveillance of her students. Going to bed one night, Mary remarks to her sister: "I am afraid of Mrs. Mason's eyes—would you think, Caroline, that she who looks so very good-natured sometimes could frighten one so? I wish I were as wise and good as she is" (*WMW* 4:389). Myers describes Mrs. Mason's consciousness of her good deeds and her tendency toward surveillance as "constructive fantas[ies]" ("Pedagogy" 204): "Through the histories and assorted moral tales that she relates and through the educational and charitable activities that she carries on, Mason interprets, orders, and heals not just the girls but the whole little community. Her hegemony caters to female fantasies of heroism. She is a dream of strength and power, even omnipotence" (206). Although this fantasy of power makes Mrs. Mason overbearing for some readers, her identification with people in distress and the intensity of the individual stories of the poor work together to figure *Original Stories* as social criticism. Wollstonecraft's form of social criticism teaches children to respond charitably to the poor, but also to allow their lives to intermingle with those they help. More radical than suggesting that the state restructure the way it offers relief, Wollstonecraft re-imagines the nature of society.

Rural Walks

Smith's *Rural Walks* intervenes more directly than does *Original Stories* in a heated public debate about how to address poverty, a difference that reflects the increasing acuteness of the problem during the war against France. Like Wollstonecraft, Smith uses the episodic unfolding of experiential learning in order to emphasize the importance of seeing the suffering caused by poverty. Smith's Mrs. Woodfield becomes an ethnographer as she instructs her daughters Henrietta and Elizabeth, along with her niece Caroline, to aid the distressed people they encounter on their walks, including a cottager who has lost his job due to illness, a disabled vagrant, an orphaned boy made sick by his relentless but financially imperative work as a clerk, and a grandmother who cannot support her grandchildren on the relief she receives. In addition, they learn about a series of middle-class women whose well-being proves to be precariously dependent upon their fathers or husbands. With these portraits of financial struggle, Smith creates a fictional ethnography that depicts the connections among work, illness, poverty, and gender that she experienced in her own life and expressed in letters and prefaces that were not as warmly received as was this children's book.

Smith wrote her fictional ethnography *Rural Walks* both to help teenage girls understand the turbulence of 1790s England as they approached adulthood and also to support her own struggling family. The author was in the midst of an ongoing financial and health crisis as she ventured into the genre of children's literature. The long-standing emotional and financial pressures under which Smith struggled were particularly intense as she wrote *Rural Walks*. In 1793 Smith's third son Charles lost his leg in the Siege of Dunkirk, a loss that she blamed on his having to serve in the Army because the trustees of her father-in-law's estate would not pay for his education and she could not afford to keep him at Oxford herself. As she finished *The Banished Man* and began to write *Rural Walks* in 1794, Smith was in Bath, not in the midst of a holiday, but struggling to pay for expensive spa treatments for her daughter Anna Augusta's difficult pregnancy and consumption. While she was writing, Smith sought additional advances from her publishers to obtain medical help for her own worsening rheumatism and for Anna Augusta's illness.

The repetition of Smith's complaint alienated her publishers and some of her reviewers, putting her in danger of experiencing what David Morris describes as "the silence of chronic pain patients who discover that months of complaint finally just exhaust caregivers and even family" (197). In August of 1794, for example, Smith wrote to her increasingly disgruntled publishers: "I am very sorry to be compelled to ask all these favours of any Bookseller ... I should not have wanted any [advances], but that my own and my daughter's illness has put me to such immense expences" (*CLCS* 190). In the next few months, she made several requests for advances on partial manuscripts (including the first two thirds of *Rural Walks*), apparently pushing Cadell and Davies to the limit by September when she asked them to cover bills totaling ten to fifteen pounds (*CLCS* 220). Their blunt refusal did not stop her from asking for five pounds in November, but it did inspire a more lengthy description of her troubles:

> [I]f there is [money from subscriptions in excess of publication costs] & it is possible for you to spare me a note of five pounds, it would be doing me the greatest favor in the World, as it is impossible to describe how cruelly my daughters very long illness—who is still attended constantly by a Physician twice or thrice a week—and my being oblig'd to have her at a separate lodging out of the Town has [sic] distress'd and harrass'd me .... [I]t is quite impossible that the most incessant labor on my part can entirely support a family of seven persons in the requisites of existence, & my daughters four months illness, & five Medical Men, who have continually attended her have really reduced me to more cruel exigencies than I have ever yet known, & in a place where not being near my own friends, I find it more than I can do to supply my family with the means of existence from one day to another ... . [the conflicts over the will] hav[e] now for eleven years unceasingly oppress'd me with [a] severity that has nearly destroy'd my intellects and entirely my health. (*CLCS* 232)

In spite of this letter's impassioned description of the "cruel exigencies" that threatened her health and intellect, it is unclear that Cadell and Davies complied with her request. Smith's repeated requests for early payment and her description of the interdependence of financial and physical deterioration put an enormous strain on her relationship with her publishers.[20] As I explain in chapter 1, Smith experienced a similar disintegration of sympathy in the critical reception of her novels and poetry. Simply put, her complaints about chronic illness became tedious in their repetition, whereas her series of portraits of the impoverished ill in *Rural Walks*—a different kind of repetition in narrative—was well received.[21] Smith's fictional ethnography, then, functions as an experiment in the expression of suffering, a struggle against silence.

---

20 See Judith Phillips Stanton's "Charlotte Smith's 'Literary Business'" for more on Smith's relationship with her publishers.

21 *The New Annual Register* reviewer notes: "Mrs. Charlotte Smith's Two volumes of 'Rural Walks, in Dialogues, for the Use of Young Persons,' contain pleasing information on subjects in natural history, and instructive lessons on manners, accompanied with some elegant pieces of poetry. They are well adapted by their form, in which Mrs. Smith has united the interest of the novel with the instruction of the school book, to engage the attention of the young, and to introduce them into acquaintance with what are called *les petites morales*" (283). *The Monthly Review* and *The Analytical Review* both defer to Smith's account of the book: "We cannot, perhaps, give a more fair and just view of this pleasing performance than by a few extracts from the lady's own preface" (*MR* 349) and "In announcing to the public this first attempt of the ingenious and indefatigable Mrs. Smith, to write a book for the use of children, it is proper that she should be allowed to speak for herself, concerning her design. It is thus modestly and sensibly expressed in the preface" (*AR* 548). The *Critical Review* also quotes extensively from Smith's preface in order to praise the work.

Given the circumstances of the book's production, one might expect from *Rural Walks* an account of life and health care in late-eighteenth-century Bath. However, *Rural Walks* is set in the countryside rather than in Bath. Despite the touted virtues of the spa regimen, some potential spa goers discovered that the financial demands of life in Bath either affected their health adversely or prevented them from obtaining spa treatment at all. Smith felt this paradox in her personal life and used *Rural Walks* to expose the more general problem of illness's impoverishing effects across all classes and, conversely, the deleterious effect of financial worries on one's health. This series of fictional portraits of the ill and impoverished takes Smith's observations out of the realm of individual complaint and emphasizes the social basis of the problem of poverty. While firsthand experience with financial hardship would seem to give Smith more credibility than others writing on this topic, her experience also left open the possibility that her observations about poverty would be regarded as self-interested whining. Resisting this classification, the portraits in *Rural Walks* do not only fictionalize aspects of Smith's own suffering, but also portray the suffering of people quite different from Smith.

Smith's depictions of the poor in *Rural Walks*, then, emerge not simply as object lessons in charity and proper conduct, but as political opinions in a heated national discussion about how to offer the poor private charity and public relief. Her descriptions of sufferers and the aid they receive illustrate the need for social change rather than the worthiness or unworthiness of the poor. She does not, however, exclude from her fictional ethnography portraits of those who would fall in the most widely accepted category of the "deserving" poor, including those rendered "impotent" by illness or age. In "The Sick Cottager," the group visits a "poor family" whose father has fallen ill. Mrs. Woodfield notes that the father's illness has put the family "in a situation to want even the little assistance we can give them" (*WCS* 12:8). The narrator observes that his "pale emaciated figure presented too strong an image of disease and famine" (*WCS* 12:8). Smith emphasizes that laborers impoverished by lost wages due to illness are deserving of charity. The cottager explains: "[T]ill I got this fever and ague last barley harvest, I never have left work one day since I was married" (*WCS* 12:9). Smith's cottager is hard-working, unfortunate, and from almost any political point-of-view, deserving of charity. This portrait of a sick cottager whose family suffers from his inability to work is very similar, for example, to the poor family encountered by Trimmer's Mrs. Benson.

Several of Smith's portraits of working-class characters, however, directly counter classifications and stereotypes emerging from the rhetoric of the debate about the poor. For example, out on a botanical excursion, Mrs. Woodfield and the girls meet a recovering laborer whom Mrs. Woodfield congratulates on being healthy again. This encounter with the recovering laborer, along with the portrait of "the sick cottager" discussed above, portray disease as the *cause* of extreme poverty, showcasing these men as deserving examples of the temporarily "impotent" poor. Having seen this example of a recovered working man, the group then meets a crippled beggar. Mrs. Woodfield's daughter Elizabeth comments that one does no charity in giving a common beggar money. While other authors might have juxtaposed the ill and recovered laborers with the beggar to illustrate the distinction between the deserving and undeserving poor, Smith has Mrs. Woodfield reply: "I have not, for my part, sagacity enough to distinguish what are called common beggars, from poor men disabled by illness from working, or accidentally distressed in a strange country, where they have no claim to parochial relief" (*WCS* 12:19). Smith's comment is remarkable in light of historian R. P. Hastings's description of "vagrants" in the 1790s as "expensive and unwanted outsiders ... the least sympathetically treated of all paupers" (26). Although Mrs. Woodfield encounters these men while teaching the girls to classify plants on a botanical excursion, she refuses to classify or "distinguish" among the impoverished ill. As I argue in chapter 4, Smith is interested in categories derived from the complex material circumstances of a person's life, not in un-contextualized binaries such as "deserving" and "undeserving" poor. In resisting easy distinctions, Mrs. Woodfield reflects what Donna Andrew describes as the medieval-period attitude that offering private charity was an innately good act that, even if it misdirected resources, would never be wasted in its glorification of God. In the late eighteenth century, though, Mrs. Woodfield's readiness to aid a crippled immigrant is extraordinary, as he would have had no right to relief in any English parish and, therefore, according to popular opinion, little right to charity either. For example, the Reverend Joseph Townsend, a vocal critic of public relief for even legitimate residents of parishes, argued in 1786 that "indiscriminate private charity was as unnatural as the Poor Law" (Poynter 42). In contrast, Smith teaches her children that all people in need are worthy of aid.

Mrs. Woodfield and her children, like the perambulating learners in children's books by Wollstonecraft, Trimmer, Aiken and Barbauld, not only encounter the poor on walks, but also enter into their houses, thus revealing the degree to which the poor are vulnerable to surveillance. However, during these visits in *Rural Walks*, Smith (like Wollstonecraft) creates a de Certeauan "space" in which the poor might gaze back at and return the judgment of their more financially stable neighbors. Out on a walk, Mrs. Woodfield and the children stop in a shepherd's hut on the Downs, where they find the shepherd's twelve-year-old daughter dining alone on "some crusts of bread, and two or three half boiled potatoes" (*WCS* 12:20). When Henrietta reports that the girl is one of five children and her mother is dead, Mrs. Woodfield offers her money and asks to meet with her father the next day with the intention of "doing him some more permanent service, than bestowing on him mere present relief" (*WCS* 12:25). Mrs. Woodfield also asks the shepherd's daughter to bring a bench outside the hut so that she and the girls might sit down. This bench, the poor family's only piece of furniture, provides both rest and a vantage point from which Mrs. Woodfield can point out two houses of wealthy men "of different characters," whose stories provide a lesson on the "use and abuse of riches" (*WCS* 12:20). The bench, which does double duty as the only table and place to sit for the shepherd's family, represents the Bench from which justices of the peace made quarterly decisions about the distribution of relief, decisions that would certainly affect what appeared on this family's own table/bench. Smith has Mrs. Woodfield and the girls borrow this symbolic bench in order to legitimize any judgments the poor might make about those who have the means to help them.

The first wealthy man whose house they view from the bench is Sir Herbert Harbottle, an exemplar of gluttony and greed, who makes himself known to his poor neighbors primarily through his oppression of them: "Poverty and misery surround him; for his tenants are at rackrent, and the peasants are, at many seasons of the year, without employment. The consequence is that he is continually complaining that his game is destroyed by poachers, and his farm-yard robbed by thieves" (*WCS* 12:20). He exacerbates the suffering caused by an enclosure that has turned once common hunting grounds into his private land by vigorously prosecuting as poachers the poor who hunt for dinner on his property. In addition, he refuses the poor the right to "glean" after his crops are harvested and charges his tenants exorbitant rent. Furthermore, he pays his sister-in-law's jointure with "infinite reluctance," sometimes compelling his brother's widow and her two daughters to "wait many months" (*WCS* 12:20). In spite of these abusive and neglectful behaviors, Sir Herbert, nonetheless, is well received in society. Smith paints a portrait of irresponsible, yet socially and legally sanctioned, upper-class male power over both the poor that surround him and the women in his own family. Thus, she criticizes from the viewpoint of the poor family's bench not just one man, but members of the enfranchised, upper classes who condone and thus facilitate his actions.

Sitting on the bench, the group can also see the house of Mr. Somerville, a wealthy man who does not have a title, yet takes exceptionally good care of the people living within ten miles of his estate:

> [N]ever did he see anguish impressed on the countenance, even of a common acquaintance, without attempting to relieve it. Is a farmer distressed by bad seasons, or accidental losses? Mr. Somerville will assist him with his purse, or his credit. Is a labourer sinking under sickness and poverty? It is by Mr. Somerville he is ordered medical advice, and from his kitchen comfortable nourishment. (*WCS* 12:21)

In spite of his good deeds, Mr. Somerville has suffered the loss of his wife, the disappointment of wayward sons, and concern about his only daughter who married a wealthy man only to be rejected by his family when she was not able to bear children: "She lost her health and now passes almost all her time with her father, who endeavors, by tenderness and attention, to heal the wounds of a broken heart, which are, I fear, slowly, but certainly, condemning her to an early grave" (*WCS* 12:22). Although the daughter suffers much less deservedly than do the irresponsible sons, all three children interrupt the cycle of inherited wealth in England—the sons by gambling or otherwise squandering their inheritance, and the daughter by failing to produce an heir for her in-laws. In addition to demonstrating in the father's story that suffering is not tied to one's moral choices and in the daughter's story that emotional distress can cause illness, Smith suggests that a wealthy man's resources are more productively distributed among the local poor than bestowed upon his sons. Her implicit observation that Mr. Somerville's money has done more good as charity than it did when passed on to his children challenges the principle of the accumulation of wealth that underlies the "duty" of the wealthy to help the poor. As these stories told from the symbolic bench suggest, Smith portrays the limitations of charity as an effective method of relieving poverty and thus quietly supports the mandatory poor rates.

However, Smith offers criticism of the arbitrary nature of the parish relief system as well. The girls see a "poor old woman" who is gathering faggots as her grandchildren collect strawberries to sell. Mrs. Woodfield speaks to her, gives her "a small present," then explains:

So very old and so very poor;—the spectacle is indeed humiliating and painful. Yet this poor old woman, whose figure has almost lost the traces of humanity, was the daughter of a rich farmer, and was, as I have heard other women of the neighborhood relate, a great beauty in her time, and a celebrated horsewoman. When the mind is carried back to those days, it is difficult to imagine how such a change can have taken place. (*WCS* 12:61)

This portrait of the character Sarah Hobloun is the sort of "fall from riches" story with which it was easy for middle- or upper-class readers to sympathize (Richey 428-29). However appealing the narrative of Sarah Hobloun might be to middle-class readers, it does not inspire the charity of the wealthy characters in this narrative. Instead, the story decries the lack of financial security available to women in the period and cautions readers against stereotyping the poor. Furthermore, the story gains power in its placement in a series of portraits that together anatomize the 1790s poverty crisis. As this dialogue unfolds, the story of Sarah Hobloun does not merely invite the sympathy of readers, but reveals problems with the social mechanisms of both charity and the relief system in 1790s England.

Moved by the cause of Sarah Hobloun, Elizabeth wonders how she might help "such a poor old woman as we have just seen" by appealing to the wealthy Mrs. Wadford for charity on her behalf. She imagines interrupting a card game with a petition for help that includes a factual description of Sarah Hobloun's suffering:

Mrs. Wadford, I am glad to see you have won a good deal tonight, and I am come to beg some of it for a poor old distressed woman, who is incapable of procuring any of the comforts of life, though her great age makes them so necessary to her. She lives in a miserable cottage, which does not keep out the weather;—she has only a few rags instead of clothes, and no nourishing food;—she has nobody to help her, for all her children are dead; and, what is yet more distressing, she has three of her grandchildren, whom the parish have sent to her to take care of, when she had more occasion to have some person hired to take care of her. (*WCS* 12:62)

Speculating that Mrs. Wadford would refuse her request, Elizabeth shifts tactics. Next she imagines appealing to Mrs. Wadford's ability to sympathize and "bid her think, that she herself is old, and has the gout and the rheumatism, which she finds bad enough to bear, even with all manner of comforts about her; how hard then, I would say, must be the sufferings of a poor desolate creature, older and more infirm than you are, Ma'am, and who has not the necessaries of life?" (*WCS* 12:63). Mrs. Woodfield guesses that Mrs. Wadford would reply, "if people were poor, there was a provision made for them by the parish" (*WCS* 12:63). As Elizabeth's speech illustrates, the uncharitable wealthy used the existence of the Poor Laws to excuse themselves from seeing suffering and relieving it directly.

Intervening to help, Elizabeth's cousin Caroline suggests that they appeal to Mrs. Wadford's sensibility with some of Robert Burns's poetry about poverty, but Mrs. Woodfield fears that a poetic plea would not work either: "I am afraid that your project of affecting her feelings in prose, or that of Caroline to address her in verse, would be equally fruitless; and we must have some more certain method, if we would do any good to the ancient grandmother of our little Strawberry Girls" (*WCS* 12:64). This imaginary game, like the portraits of the wealthy men Sir Herbert Harbottle and Mr. Somerville, illustrates that charity is inconsistently given and cannot be depended upon as the only means of aiding the poor. The discussion is also a commentary on the goals of Smith's own ethnography. The imaginary, uncharitable Mrs. Wadford is as unmoved by Elizabeth's dispassionate description of Sarah Hobloun's suffering—exactly the sort of portrait Smith provides in *Rural Walks*—as she is both by the attempt to arouse her sympathetic identification with the elderly and ill woman, and also by poetry meant to appeal to her refined sensibility. With this discussion, Smith signals to readers that her fictional ethnography is not designed so much to inspire charitable giving as to reveal the limitations of all structures available to relieve the suffering of the poor in the 1790s.

Seeking additional parish relief rather than charity for Sarah Hobloun, Mrs. Woodfield takes the girls to the house of the parish overseer Mr. Goosetray to request more aid for the impoverished and ill grandmother.[22] Finding this proprietor of a large farm busy in his fields, Mrs. Woodfield tells his wife, "I wished to have seen Mr. Goosetray, as he is overseer and church-warden, to have asked him to allow some farther relief to poor old Sarah Hobloun" (*WCS* 12:68). Mrs. Goosetray unsympathetically shrieks, "that artful old jade ... wants for nothing ... . I'd be glad to know whether we be to keep the paupers to live better than ourselves" (*WCS* 12:68). Mrs. Woodfield observes that "the parish allow her no more than three and sixpence a-week" (*WCS* 12:68), but "seeing it in vain to contend with ignorance and avarice so invincible, silently determine[s] to speak in favour of the unfortunate poor creature (whom she could not herself help to the extent of her wishes) to a magistrate in the neighbourhood" (*WCS* 12:68). This interaction reveals the extent to which the mechanism of parish relief was dependent on special pleading rather than a consistent and fair system, and shows the additional suffering caused when one must ask for aid from a self-interested or corrupt overseer. The sick cottager's wife sums up the situation: "[A]ll goes by favour in our parish!" (*WCS* 12:9). Smith does not share the outcome of Mrs. Woodfield's subsequent visit to the magistrate with readers, but we do learn from this portrait that some poor women like Sarah Hobloun needed an advocate to obtain relief; additionally, even more well-to-do advocates such as Mrs. Woodfield had to work their way up the chain of command in the structure of parish relief in order to secure aid for the poor.

Smith presents the parish overseer as unhelpful in his official office and as actively contributing to the suffering of the laborers he employs. Upon approaching Mr. Goosetray's large farm, Mrs. Woodfield and the children see "the farmer ... an immense fat man" mistreat his laborers, "urging his men to exertion" (*WCS* 12:67). None of the laborers "appeared to serve him with pleasure ... but executed their task, though with alacrity, yet without that delight with which labourers work at the harvest home of a good and considerate master" (*WCS* 12:67). Seeing his workers only as a means of increasing his own wealth, Mr. Goosetray represents the ways in which the interests of the large farmer coincided with the traditional "lord of the manor." In fact, when Mrs. Woodfield and the girls first meet Mrs. Goosetray, "they [are] received with as much state by the mistress of the mansion, as if she had been

---

22   This dialogue is the most obvious exception to Grenby's assertion that the Poor Laws make no appearance in children's books: "[T]hough these books are populated by a cast of orphans and beggars, disabled paupers and gentlewomen fallen on hard times, not one has recourse to the Poor Law" (189).

the lady of the manor, instead of the tenant of the manor-farm" (*WCS* 12:67). In her portrayal of Mr. Goosetray's treatment of his laborers and her criticism of Mrs. Goosetray's class pretensions, Smith registers her objection to the way in which the Enclosure Acts create a gulf between, on the one hand, landed gentry and large farmers, and on the other, laborers and cottagers. Passing by another large farmer's field, the group witnesses the completion of the wheat harvest. When "groups of children and old persons" begin to glean the scattered remains, the farmer drives his "herd of hogs [into the field], before these unhappy people had gathered the scanty refuse that was left them" (*WCS* 12:67). Here Smith illustrates problems with the distribution of relief through the parish system and describes the economic and legal structures that cause or exacerbate financial distress among the working poor. As with the portraits of Sir Herbert Harbottle and Mr. Somerville, Smith indicts not just one corrupt overseer, then, but an entire economic system that makes the poor more vulnerable to suffering.

Smith also suggests that this suffering was increased by negative assumptions about the poor informing proposed solutions to poverty. Smith's portrait of the Bennison children, Fanny and Billie, who are orphaned and left destitute by their parents' death, criticizes one of the most prevalent assumptions—that the poor were simply idle and improvident. Fanny explains the decline of her family's financial situation to Mrs. Woodfield:

> [T]he long illness of my poor father, who, though only about forty years old, was struck with the palsy many months before we lost him, and the languishing illness my dear, dear mother fell into immediately after his death, and which ended in our being deprived of her too, naturally exhausted their little savings. (*WCS* 12:71)

The illness and death of Fanny's father, a curate, address the common assumption that poverty was exacerbated by the poor's general lack of discipline and specific failure to save money. By presenting her readers with a financially stable family who lose their savings to illness, Smith comments on the absurdity of chastising the impoverished ill for irresponsible saving habits, an attitude implied in the 1790s proposal that the state create a national system to help the poor save money (Roach 70, 182–83). Smith illustrates her views on the proposal that the poor save money in another scene that involves animals rather than people. The girls encounter a dormouse who saves only a bit of food for the winter, and Mrs. Woodfield compares him to the squirrel who stashes a large supply. While for many children's authors this would be an opportunity to anthropomorphize the animals, vilifying the lazy dormouse who does not save and praising the industrious squirrel who does, Smith has Mrs. Woodfield explain instead that both are protected by nature: the dormouse by hibernation and the squirrel by the ability to gather. Although their "savings habits" differ, both animals survive in an environment designed for these differences. The political lesson, then, is that laborers must be allowed rights, such as property ownership or the right to common land, in order to weather difficult times in accordance with the specific conditions of their actual lives.

Most crucially, like Wollstonecraft, Smith places herself, her middle-class characters such as the Bennisons, and by extension, her readers, on a continuum with the impoverished ill. Smith's narrative portrays Mrs. Woodfield as an ethnographer who identifies with the poor as much as she understands herself to be temporarily more fortunate than they are. Unlike earlier eighteenth-century characters such as the eponymous hero of Thomas Bridges' *The Adventures of a Bank-Note* (1770–71), whose circulation among many sorts of people Diedre Lynch classifies as more illustrative of society than of any individual self, Mrs. Woodfield's circulation among the poor in *Rural Walks* not only illustrates the social networks that cause and alleviate suffering but also offers the reader a central character with psychological development (Lynch 7). Just as we learn that Mrs. Mason's own losses lead her to sympathize with the suffering of others, so we find out that Mrs. Woodfield's personal struggles resonate with those of the characters she aides.

Mrs. Woodfield's husband suffered a reversal of fortune and died, leaving Mrs. Woodfield with recurring health problems and the constant financial worry of raising her children. Embodying the interdependence of financial security and health, or conversely financial strain and illness, Mrs. Woodfield's story presents a version of Smith's own lifelong struggle to support her family while her own health deteriorated. The narrator informs readers that "[a]nxiety for a brother [Mrs. Woodfield] loved [who has sustained an injury in the war against France], with other domestic uneasiness, had at length so far affected Mrs. Woodfield's health, that it became absolutely necessary for her to follow the advice of a medical friend, and to go for a few weeks to the sea" (*WCS* 12:74–75). Mrs. Woodfield, like Smith, understands her class position to be as precarious as that of the terribly impoverished and sick people she encounters. However, as long as there is someone "in a situation to want even the little assistance [she] can give them," Mrs. Woodfield happily does what she can (*WCS* 12:8). The narrator describes the salutary effect of charity on Mrs. Woodfield's mental state: "The success of her benevolent exertions in favour of the unfortunate, was a balm to the heart of Mrs. Woodfield, and consoled her for many vexations which sometimes weighed heavily on her spirits" (*WCS* 12:74). Although Mrs. Woodfield demonstrates real compassion for those who suffer, her ability to help the poor also reassures her of her own class status (just as Smith's repeated references to her birth into the gentry class compensated emotionally for her financial distress). Ultimately, however, the financial problems that Mrs. Woodfield and Smith experience make them better able to see the suffering of the poor. Situated as a "participant-observer," the teacher helps the reader to see sociologically, thus transforming "place" into "space."

Diffusing her own struggles through the portrait of Mrs. Woodfield, as well as through depictions of other characters, Smith demonstrates that the financial stability of women and children is dependent on the health of the male bread-winner, thus challenging any sense that "the poor" exist in a social category from which her readers are entirely protected. In the dialogue "Fanny Bennison," which I mention above, the protracted ailments and eventual deaths of the Bennison parents leave their nearly grown children orphaned and destitute. As Smith was acutely aware, poor health imperils not only the ill individual's financial standing, but also the socioeconomic position of family members. Well-educated until their father's illness, the Bennison children are not able to pursue the marital and educational opportunities usually available to members of their class. Instead, family financial troubles that originate in illness force the children to work in menial jobs. This labor, in turn, ruins the children's health. When Mrs. Woodfield offers Fanny employment in her home, Fanny explains that she is reluctant to leave her brother who slaves away in a clerical job: "[T]he constant toil he now undergoes ... the doctors say, was the cause of his illness at first, by obliging him to sit so much, and to lean with his breast against a desk" (*WCS* 12:72). Fanny's brother's job has caused him to suffer from consumption, yet he cannot stop working. Smith's grief for the loss of her son's leg during his financially necessitated service in the army haunts this portrait as does Smith's own relentless struggle to support her family by writing while suffering from chronic rheumatism in her hands. Smith demonstrates both that illness can cause financial ruin, and also that financial woes and strenuous work can cause illness. Mrs. Woodfield finds alternative employment for both Fanny and her brother. When their financial situation improves, so does their health.

In the final narrative of the first volume of *Rural Walks*, Smith depicts another woman whose class status has fallen and whose health has suffered due to the decisions made by the men in her life. The only child of a "very good family"—that is, of a father who became rich in the West Indies and mother who was "a young woman of fortune"— Miss Harley was raised in an affluent household (*WCS* 12:50). When Miss Harley became engaged to a young nobleman, her father settled a great deal of property on the couple, but then committed suicide the day of the wedding. His suicide note confesses that his own "imprudence and infatuation," combined with "the villany of others" led to the loss of his assets (*WCS* 12:51). Miss Harley's fiancé deserted her once it was clear that she had no money, and her mother died "unable to bear such a cruel reverse in fortune" (*WCS* 12:52). Left "absolutely destitute" and dependent on her relatives, Miss Harley falls ill after having to watch her former fiancé marry her insensitive but wealthy cousin (*WCS* 12:52). Miss Harley's illness and her mother's death demonstrate how a woman's financial status and thus health are tied to the well-being and benevolence of men. Furthermore, the noble fiancé's choice to marry for wealth rather than for love reveals that upper-class women are valued primarily as signifiers of and conduits to their fathers' fortunes.

Although *Rural Walks* might seem a standard educational book designed to instruct young women in codes of behavior, an examination of the social context in which Smith wrote the work makes clear that *Rural Walks* does more: it provides young readers with powerful political commentary on English attitudes toward the ill and impoverished in the 1790s. With her assertion that ill health can lead to poverty for both working- and middle-class individuals, Smith urges her fellow Britons to widen their definition of the deserving poor to include vagrants and immigrants as well as residents, and men as well as women. More radically, Smith's suggestion that financial hardship can actually cause illness adds a new element to the national debate about poverty. And finally, the repeated portraits of women who are exposed to danger and ill health by their fathers' and husbands' choices, offer a critique of the laws that create a detrimental hierarchy in England based on gender and class.

Three specific aspects of eighteenth-century children's literature make possible a coalescence of instruction and social critique—the dialogic structure of experiential learning within the stories, the episodic organization of stories, and the powerful teacher figure(s). The communal/dialogic interactions and the focus on vision/experiential learning invite the reader to see the social context of suffering. Because the domestic scene of this genre—a teacher and her students exploring the local community—explicitly represents social interdependence, it serves as a productive ground for social criticism. William McCarthy's comment about Barbauld's *Lessons for Children* applies to Wollstonecraft's *Original Stories* and Smith's *Rural Walks* as well: "There is no question, in *Lessons* as in Marx, of the Romantic individual glorying in some transcendental solitude; people always live together, in some form of mutual dependence" (211). Furthermore, the mutual dependence represented is not simply that of the nuclear family. Neither book represents an exclusive mother/ child relationship—as a governess (who has also adopted a child), Mrs. Mason educates other people's children; Mrs. Woodfield teaches her niece as well as her own daughters. Their ties with one another and with the local community are strengthened by dialogue and interaction. Living together, the characters in children's literature also explicitly learn from what they see. The depiction of hybrid family structures distinguishes Wollstonecraft's and Smith's imagined communities from the communities portrayed in didactic children's literature by Trimmer or Barbauld and Aiken.

The episodic organization of stories is also a powerful tool for social commentary. Representing not just one person's struggle but many variations of the individual experience of poverty, the experiential text becomes ethnographic. Each individual struggle enters a social context. Collecting narratives of suffering under poverty, the teachers and children begin to speak what I describe in chapter 4 as Smith's language of suffering. In her references to botany, Smith recommends a language of suffering that would attend to the particularity of individual experience as well as aspects of that experience that are shared or reflected in others. Likewise, the works I discuss here both create a social body and also anatomize the individual stories that constitute this body. Just as physician James Wardrop argued that anatomy (the structure of individual organs) and physiology (the actions of these organs and sympathetic interactions among them) were best understood in relation to one another, so Smith and Wollstonecraft present individual people as unique, yet as constituted by their interactions and socially-dependent material circumstances (Wardrop xxi). As in botanical collecting, each new case of suffering that the group encounters can be named and understood most fully only in the context of other cases. And, each time a variation on suffering enters the lexicon, the structure of the language changes; the meaning of those previous cases of suffering under poverty shifts.

The quality of didactic literature most crucial for exposing the social structures that underlie suffering is the development of a teacher figure. Functioning as an ethnographer, the teacher negotiates the space between the authors' own experiences of suffering and the broader social structures that underlie that suffering. However, as my analysis of Trimmer's *Fabulous Histories* demonstrates, a three-dimensional teacher character does not guarantee a reformist perspective. The essential difference between Trimmer's Mrs. Benson (or even Barbauld and Aiken's fathers) and the teachers in Wollstonecraft's and Smith's narratives is the identification between the teacher and those she aids. This identification allows ethnographic seeing to challenge the basic assumptions of sentimental literature, a genre concerned with seeing suffering, but in a quite different way. Mrs. Woodfield's and Mrs. Mason's neighborhood excursions might be thought of as a local version of the eighteenth-century "man of feeling's" journey abroad in which he visits, weeps over, and sometimes offers charity to female objects of pity in insane asylums or work houses. Wollstonecraft's *Original Stories* and Smith's *Rural Walks*, however, challenge this economy of sensibility in which, as Claudia Johnson convincingly argues, female suffering is "the one-thing-needful to solicit male tears" (*Equivocal* 15), and in which the male observer's humanity is confirmed and displayed through his ability to be moved by the suffering of others. In this formulation, the observer's gender, health, class, and (often) nationality distinctly separate him from his female object of pity. In contrast with Sterne's Yorick and Henry Mackenzie's Harley, Mrs. Woodfield and Mrs. Mason do not fetishize, but rather identify with the suffering of others. Seeing poverty is crucial in these experiences, but sympathetic seeing can collapse into surveillance and the reinforcement of class reifying "place" if there is not reciprocal identification between the characters who see and those who suffer. When the sufferers look back or give back, and when the givers understand themselves to be as vulnerable as those they help, surveillance becomes sociability, "place" transforms into "space." Both Mrs. Mason and Mrs. Woodfield teach children that they are as vulnerable as the poor people they encounter, though far more fortunate. To put it simply, the fictional ethnographies the teachers present are versions of reality created by women who are also marked by that reality. Furthermore, Wollstonecraft and Smith not only use ethnography to expose social problems, but also teach children the methodology of ethnography as a way of understanding social structures.

Wollstonecraft's Mrs. Mason and Smith's Mrs. Woodfield invite us into a world in which humans are each bound to one another. Wollstonecraft depicts both the way these ties can lead to suffering—one man's bad decisions can cause his entire network of family and friends to suffer. Yet she also explores the way in which a recognition of our mutual dependence can lead instead to mutual care. Mrs. Mason, then, teaches children to offer charity not in order to enact and secure their class standing, but rather to forge connections across and in spite of class. Although the narrative acknowledges the suffering caused by the Enclosure Acts, Wollstonecraft's *Original Stories* is less concerned with specific political solutions to poverty, such as reforms to the Poor Law, than is Smith's *Rural Walks*. In part this may reflect, as Grenby argues, Wollstonecraft's distrust of government. However, it is also true that in 1788, institutions designed to alleviate poverty were less at the forefront of the discussion than they would become in the mid 1790s, when Smith wrote *Rural Walks*. In her first children's narrative, Smith exposes the limits of both charity and the Poor Law as they are practiced in England in 1794. She also highlights the problem of women's financial dependence on men. Her ethnography removes the question of whether or not individuals are deserving of aid, suggesting instead that social structures must change to accommodate need indiscriminately and to offer all people—including women—more opportunities for self-support. The final chapter of this book deepens the exploration of ethnography's challenge to the sentimental plot that I mention above, particularly with regard to the oppression of women.

Chapter 7

Unsentimental Seeing:
Wollstonecraft's *The Wrongs of Woman* and Didactic Children's Literature

> "Yes, Jemima, look at me—observe me closely, and
> read my very soul; you merit a better fate."
>
> Mary Wollstonecraft's Maria

Mary Wollstonecraft began *The Wrongs of Woman* in 1796, a year of great personal turmoil. She was not long returned from the emotionally fraught trip to Scandinavia recorded in *Letters from Norway* and the suicide attempt that followed. In addition, she was entering into a new relationship with William Godwin, even as her circle of friends and the public incorrectly understood her to be deserted by, yet still married to, Gilbert Imlay. Wollstonecraft and Godwin kept their relationship a secret until they were forced by Wollstonecraft's pregnancy to marry. Not marrying would reveal that her expected baby was illegitimate; yet marrying publicly meant acknowledging her daughter Fanny Imlay's illegitimacy. Trying to ameliorate both negative outcomes, as well as to protect Godwin (an outspoken critic of matrimony) from ridicule, they kept their marriage on 29 March 1797 secret for a time (Todd *Mary* 417). As their union gradually became public, Wollstonecraft endured censure from those who criticized her for posing as a married woman and from friends who resented the couple's secrecy about their relationship. Addressing these upheavals in her intimate and friendly relationships while undergoing a second pregnancy, Wollstonecraft also worried a great deal during the writing of *The Wrongs of Woman* about finances, including a significant debt to her publisher Joseph Johnson (Todd *Mary* 415) and inconsistent support of Fanny from Imlay (*CLMW* 403). Shortly after they were married and trying to maintain two households, Wollstonecraft writes to Godwin: "I am tormented by the want of money" (*CLMW* 407). Wollstonecraft represents these experiences as well as details from the lives of other women in her novel's fictional characters. If, as I argue in chapter 3, Wollstonecraft portrays health in *Letters from Norway* as an exchange between solitude and sociability (that is, a state of wellness based on the interdependence of individual growth and social improvement), in *The Wrongs of Woman* she examines individual financial, emotional, and physical suffering in the context of corrupt and oppressive legal and social structures. Wollstonecraft develops the three major elements of children's literature that I discuss in the previous chapter—episodic narrative structure, dialogic experiential learning, and a teacher/ethnographer character—in order to present a series of portraits that together convey suffering not just as the author's "personal troubles," but rather as the result of an oppressive and neglectful society. In addition, she acknowledges the appeal of the sentimental plot, yet sharply criticizes its powerlessness to inspire social change.

Mitzi Myers's description of Wollstonecraft's early published works—*Mary, Thoughts on the Education of Daughters*, and *Original Stories*—as "experiments in selfhood," in which she "transforms personal dilemma into alternative images of female selfhood," applies also to *The Wrongs of Woman* ("Pedagogy" 195). As the novel begins, Maria awakens from drug-induced sleep to find herself imprisoned in a madhouse, her four-month-old daughter taken from her by her cruel husband George Venables. She befriends the asylum keeper Jemima and establishes an intimate romantic relationship with fellow inmate Henry Darnford, by whom she becomes pregnant. The three inhabitants of the asylum tell their life stories to one another—Jemima and Darnford in person, and Maria in a memoir she writes to her daughter and shares with her asylum companions. Many critics see in Maria Venables's abusive father, weak mother, and unfairly favored brother Wollstonecraft's own family of origin. Most compellingly, Diane Long Hoeveler reads in this "barely-disguised sociological text" the traumatic narrative of Wollstonecraft's painful childhood, a failure of the nuclear family that she re-experienced as a "second wounding" in her relationship with Imlay ("Reading" 392, 391). Hoeveler observes that Maria's anger toward her husband Venables and illusions about her suitor Darnford reference Wollstonecraft's relationship with Imlay, and thus re-approach the trauma of childhood. Eleanor Ty notes a resemblance between the marriage of Wollstonecraft's sister Eliza and the life story of the "lovely maniac," who is also imprisoned in the asylum (*Unsex'd* 40), while other critics see the reference to Eliza's life in Maria's attempted escape from Venables.[1] Offering the reader autobiographical resonances, Wollstonecraft becomes a participant observer, an ethnographer who situates her own experience within the social structures or culture she describes.

The autobiographical references in the novel are most powerful, then, when considered in the context of women's collective struggle against oppression. Wollstonecraft took care to direct her readers' attention toward the social problems that the novel depicts rather than toward elements of her own life.[2] She identifies as her "main object, the desire of exhibiting the misery and oppression, peculiar to women, that arise out of the partial laws and customs of society" (*MTWW* 73). On the whole, Wollstonecraft insists, the narrative "ought rather to be considered, as [the history] of woman, than of an individual" (*MTWW* 73). Myers points out that

---

   1   See the Oxford edition of the novel, in which editor Gary Kelly makes this connection (*MTWW* n2, 217). See also Matthews (87–89), and Michaelson (250–51).

   2   In spite of her desire to direct readers toward the activist goals of her final work rather than towards its autobiographical content, Wollstonecraft's social critique was drowned out in the storm of condemnation that met *The Wrongs of Woman* upon publication. Godwin published Wollstonecraft's unfinished novel the same year as his scandalous, if honest, *Memoir of the Author of the Rights of Woman*. *The Wrongs of Woman* was immediately and inextricably linked to Godwin's revelation of Wollstonecraft's suicide attempts and unconventional intimate relationships with Henry Fuseli and Gilbert Imlay (Myers "Unfinished" 107). In addition, Wollstonecraft's posthumous works went to press in a political environment in which all things considered French, including avant-garde love relationships, were strenuously condemned in mainstream British culture (Todd *Mary* 426).

Wollstonecraft "knew firsthand all the caretaking occupations that were the only jobs available for a middle-class woman, and she found them all wanting" ("Pedagogy" 198). Yet her social commentary includes the experiences of women who were even more radically marginalized than were governesses. In February 1797, she visited London's Bedlam with Godwin and Joseph Johnson, perhaps to conduct research for her final novel (Todd *Mary* 427). Preparing to write the trial portion of the plot, she read accounts of adultery trials in *The Newgate Calendar* and the anthologized *Trials for Adultery* (*MTWW* 230).[3]

In his preface to the novel, Godwin asserts that Wollstonecraft gave considerable thought to the formal structure of *The Wrongs of Woman*: "The purpose and structure of the following work, had long formed a favourite subject of meditation with its author, and she judged them capable of producing an important effect" (*PW* 1:ii). The connection between purpose and structure is implied when, in her own preface to the novel, Wollstonecraft notes that wise readers will understand that the narrative is not limited to her own life experience: "[S]urely there are a few, who will ... grant that my sketches are not the abortion of a distempered fancy, or the strong delineations of a wounded heart" (*MTWW* 73). The aim of her project is not to voice an individual complaint, but rather to present a range of suffering in order to expose a social problem. Godwin appended to Wollstonecraft's preface an excerpt of a letter she wrote to George Dyson about her manuscript for the novel, which states as her goal "to show the wrongs of different classes of women, equally oppressive, though, from the difference of education, necessarily various" (*MTWW* 74). Multiple portraits of individuals were necessary "to show the wrongs of different classes of women." To achieve that goal, she developed a narrative structure—repetitive "sketches"—based on the episodic form of children's literature.

Significantly, in the *Posthumous Works of the Author of a Vindication of the Rights of Woman* (1798), Godwin annexes to the end of *The Wrongs of Woman* one of Wollstonecraft's children's works—*Lessons*, an unpublished text Wollstonecraft wrote for her daughter Fanny in 1797 (Tauchert 108). Godwin defends the juxtaposition of the two works, directing the reader to note the similarities "between the affectionate and pathetic manner in which Maria Venables addresses her infant, in *The Wrongs of Woman*; and the agonizing and painful sentiment with which the author originally bequeathed these papers, as a legacy for the benefit of her child" (*PW* 2:173–74). The epistolary format of *Lessons*—Wollstonecraft writing to her child— resonates with Maria's letter to her lost daughter in the novel. At the same time, the peripatetic structure of Wollstonecraft's *Original Stories*, discussed in the previous chapter, lays the groundwork for the set of embedded narratives that comprise the fictional ethnography of *The Wrongs of Woman*. Just as Mrs. Mason gathers verbal portraits of the poor, Maria and Jemima incorporate the stories of many other women into their own tales, creating two meta-ethnographies within the structure of a novel that is itself ethnographic. Although critics generally discuss Wollstonecraft's last novel as a revision of her first novel *Mary* (1788) or as a fictional continuation of *A Vindication of the Rights of Woman* (1792), I will argue that the novel is firmly

---

3 See Komisaruk and Jordan for more on Wollstonecraft's knowledge and general public discussions of adultery trials.

rooted both in the prevailing narrative structure of didactic children's literature and also in Wollstonecraft's own works for children that helped shape this tradition.

Genre

Certainly, Wollstonecraft writes *The Wrongs of Woman* with the goals of the Jacobin novel in mind.[4] Godwin and Thomas Holcroft, as Gary Kelly points out, developed the Jacobin novel to inspire "individual moral reform," and thus effect social change by cultivating readers' sympathy for individual characters rather than by presenting abstract arguments (*The English* 11). Kelly notes that the English Jacobin novelists treated "technique as of the utmost importance," creating novels with a unified structure that was designed both to have a radicalizing effect on the reader and also to integrate smoothly the author's own "autobiographical impulse" (*The English* 19). Like other Jacobin novelists, Wollstonecraft integrates her life experience into a panoramic social portrait of "things as they are." However, the multiplicity of experience that her ethnographic mode presents distinguishes *The Wrongs of Woman* from other Jacobin fiction. While Wollstonecraft's final book shares the goals of other Jacobin novels, its narrative structure has more in common with didactic children's literature than it does with works by Godwin or Holcroft.

The novel's twenty-seven portraits of suffering women—including Maria, Jemima, the "lovely maniac," and many women struggling to rise out of the servant class—form the core of Wollstonecraft's modulation of the Jacobin novel. Although scholars discuss the proliferation of portraits in a number of ways, they have not linked the episodic narrative form the portraits create to the episodic structure of children's literature.[5] As in didactic children's literature, these portraits of women's lives are not gracefully woven into the plot, but rather enter the narrative in encapsulated form, or as what Claudia Johnson terms "inset tales" (*Equivocal* 60) and Ashley Tauchert describes as "Chinese boxes of women's stories" (106).[6] Myers refers to the novel as "a feminist anatomy of socioeconomic abuses" and notes that "not just Maria and Jemima, but every minor female character is a case study of oppression" ("Unfinished" 110). Johnson and Ty observe resonances among the inset tales, moments in which these short narratives work together to tell the story of oppression under patriarchy. Ty argues: "In depicting the various 'wrongs suffered

---

    4   *The Wrongs of Woman* also includes characteristics of what Kelly has identified as the "coterie novel": the incorporation of publicly recognizable, autobiographical elements in the fiction, the use of dialogue to invite reader participation and thus transformation, and references to a "reading list" designed to help raise the middle-class reader's political consciousness. In his discussion of the coterie novel, Kelly identifies the need to extend his analysis into, among other areas, an investigation of strategies women writers might have used to "distinguish their work within the genre, creating perhaps a third direction of address" ("Politicizing" 159). This chapter answers that need, but shifts the discussion to the genre of didactic children's literature.

    5   Some critics have noted the similarities between Maria's letter to her daughter and "popular conduct and advice books of the period" (Matthews 95, Tauchert 108). I see didactic children's literature as a clearer model for the novel as a whole.

    6   See also Ty (*Unsex'd* 40).

by women' ... Wollstonecraft makes visible and physical the horrors of subordination which symbolic language and patriarchal culture tend to cover up or ignore" (43). While perhaps violating novelistic conventions, this atomistic narrative technique was Wollstonecraft's explicit goal. Collectively, the ethnographic portraits offer a critique of English marriage law, which allowed men to abuse, rob, rape, and neglect their wives. In addition, they anatomize the relationship between poverty and criminality, the abuse of laws governing private asylums, the lack of opportunities women had to support themselves, the difficulty the poor had in raising "caution money" to cover their burial fees, the unethical experimentation on the poor in hospitals, and the inhumanity of workhouses. Read in the context of the activist children's literature that I discuss in chapter 6, *The Wrongs of Woman* becomes less a failed Jacobin novel than an experimental commingling of Jacobin and didactic literary goals—a text that presents politics as pedagogy.

With this revision of the Jacobin novel, Wollstonecraft sought to meet the considerable challenge of making women's suffering visible. Her friend George Dyson's response to a draft of the novel was particularly discouraging (Myers "Unfinished" 110). He found Maria's story to be too central and her plight to be too detailed and tiresome. Wollstonecraft was frustrated by Dyson's inability to sympathize with her heroine, explaining to him in a letter:

> I am vexed and surprised at your not thinking the situation of Maria sufficiently important, and can only account for this want of—shall I say it? delicacy of feeling by recollecting that you are a man. For my part I cannot supposed any situation more distressing than for a woman of sensibility with an improving mind to be bound, to such a man as I have described, for life ... yet you do not seem to be disgusted with him!!! (*CLMW* 412)

Wollstonecraft attributes Dyson's lack of understanding to his gender, thus suggesting that this man's inability to understand her social critique would be replicated in other male readers. Johnson observes that the failure of "even a well-disposed male reader" to fathom Maria's situation "undermines the premise of the entire novel, that women as a class of persons are systematically 'wronged'" ("Mary" 202). Dyson also seems to have found fault with the style in which Wollstonecraft wrote Jemima's dialogue, a misunderstanding indicative of a troubling disjunction between men's and women's experiences of language. In her letter to Dyson, Wollstonecraft defends her representation of Jemima's voice: "Persons who have received a miscellaneous education, that is are educated by chance, and the energy of their own faculties, commonly display the mixture of refined and common language I have endeavored to imitate" (*CLMW* 413). Dyson's failure to sympathize with either Maria or Jemima enacts the very problem Wollstonecraft sought to remedy with her innovative narrative form: how to make women's suffering visible. Giving Jemima a voice that carries and conveys her life experience is consistent with ethnographic approaches that construct reality through dialogic collaborations between ethnographer and subject. It is not surprising that Dyson would not be able to "see" a character who, speaking in her own voice, was invisible in culture. Because of this significant central challenge, Todd notes that Wollstonecraft was "much concerned with readers' attitudes toward this work" and thought a great deal about how to structure the narrative to convey her ideas most effectively (*CLMW* 343).

Indeed, scholars identify as one of the novel's major themes the difficulty of expressing women's experience in the language of the father. Laurie Langbauer argues that Wollstonecraft addresses this problem by presenting Maria as a writing mother: "Locating the woman writer with motherhood, difference, and division allows her to make sense—and nonsense—within the patriarchal order, to work within it without completely accepting its rule" (5). S. Leigh Matthews observes that Wollstonecraft depicts Maria as a pregnant woman writing to her daughter in order to create a "text which embodies the alternative discourse inherent to her body, the pregnant body, the mothering body" (92). Comparing Godwin's and Wollstonecraft's fictional depictions of the search for justice, Glynis Ridley notes that women's "habitual silencing ensures that, when they do find a voice, their articulation of the injustices which they suffer will be reliant upon linguistic registers entirely alien to the law" (87). In an attempt to overcome these significant barriers to communication, Wollstonecraft models her final novel on the genre of didactic children's literature—a genre that represents women as powerful cultural figures who express themselves, instruct children, and effect social change within and against the confines of patriarchal culture. The pedagogical worlds of Mrs. Mason and Mrs. Woodfield—in which children learn to interpret the social and natural phenomena they encounter with the guidance of an intelligent mother-teacher—offered promising ground on which women might cultivate social change.

The ethnographic features of didactic children's literature provided the tools with which Wollstonecraft might interrupt and thus criticize the structures of desire in the sentimental novel. Mary Poovey argues that Wollstonecraft's third-person omniscient narrator collapses into Maria's sentimentalism, thus draining the power of the novel's critique of this form ("Mary"). In contrast, Johnson, Matthews, and Daniel O'Quinn argue that Wollstonecraft offers an effective critique of the ideology of sentimentalism or, as Johnson puts it, "exposes the concealed logic of sentimentality" (*Equivocal* 61). I agree with the second perspective, but would add that Wollstonecraft not only lays bare the logic of sentimentality—she offers an alternative mode of perception, enacted as I discuss in the final section of this chapter by the major characters' movement from sentimental seeing to seeing a social context. It is worth saying that the critical disagreement about Wollstonecraft's intervention into sentimentalism, however, points to her novel's designs on our desires as readers. By inviting the reader's desire for a sentimental ending, the novel is designed to provoke self-examination, to instruct and reform our ways of reading—one of the major goals of didactic children's literature.

Wollstonecraft's references to children's literature, and the presentation of Jemima and Maria as teacher figures provide additional signals that this novel has a broad pedagogical goal. In a gothic twist on Barbauld's and Aiken's *Evenings at Home*, in which a family sifts through a box of tales in order to select the evening's reading, Jemima tells Maria stories of the other inmates in order to pass the evenings they both must spend in the asylum: "Jemima would labor to beguile the tedious evenings, by describing the persons and manners of the unfortunate beings, whose figures or voices awoke sympathetic sorrow in Maria's bosom" (*MTWW* 92).[7] The first story

---

7   Similarly, Darnford asks to read the memoir Maria has written for her daughter "to beguile the tedious moments of [her] absence," and he promises "Jemima the perusal as soon as he returned them" (*MTWW* 123).

about these "unfortunate beings" is also the only portrait of an oppressed woman that is not embedded within Maria's or Jemima's stories of their own lives, and thus serves as a pedagogical preamble for readers. When Maria has read all of Darnford's books in English, Jemima promises to secure the books in French for Maria, and in the meantime gives "her a new subject for contemplation, by describing the person of a lovely maniac, just brought into an adjoining chamber" (*MTWW* 88). Placing the story before Jemima's and Maria's full narratives, and before the inset tales contained in those narratives, Wollstonecraft refers back to *Original Stories*, the source of her idea for the novel's structure. The "lovely maniac" is a revision of the much more sentimentally portrayed insane daughter of Townley's friend in *Original Stories*.[8] In addition to this reference, the storytelling establishes Jemima as a teacher figure, a characterization that balances the structure of power within the asylum. Jemima's ability to teach implies an educational level parallel to Maria's, an overlapping quality that creates community between the two women despite Maria's higher class status and Jemima's immediate power over her in the asylum. The traditional teacher figure in children's literature was a middle-class or gentry-class woman who reflected the author's own class status; however, in *The Wrongs of Woman*, Wollstonecraft extends the responsibility of teaching to a working-class woman. As a result, Wollstonecraft signals her own willingness to reach across class in order to fight women's oppression, constructing the asylum as a dynamic de Certeauan "space."

Finally, with the lovely maniac episode, Wollstonecraft prepares her readers for the difficulty inherent in seeing suffering unsentimentally, and announces the two major ways in which she will describe women's oppression. In Maria's shifting response to the lovely maniac, Wollstonecraft acknowledges her readers' potential discomfort with the suffering she will present in the inset tales. Maria hears her fellow inmate's beautiful singing and begins "with sympathy to pourtray to herself another victim" (*MTWW* 88). Maria immediately imagines that the bearer of this beautiful voice is unjustly imprisoned just as she is and begins to sympathize through her own experience. But then "the lovely warbler flew, as it were from the spray, and a torrent of unconnected exclamations and questions burst from her, interrupted by fits of laughter, so horrid, that Maria shut the door" (*MTWW* 88). The horrible reality of the maniac's insanity—conveyed in her unintelligible utterances—interrupts Maria's sentimental identification, frightening her so much that she "shut[s] the door." Wollstonecraft acknowledges that seeing human suffering without the lens of sentimentality will be as difficult for her readers as it is for Maria. However, helping readers make the transition from perceiving suffering sentimentally to seeing the social origins of suffering—without shutting the door—is one of Wollstonecraft's major goals for the novel. This shift in seeing depends on the reader's/Maria's interest in learning about the causes of women's oppression, marginalization, and madness. Disturbed by the young woman's suffering, Maria recollects herself and asks what precipitated the woman's madness. Jemima explains: "She had been married against

---

8   Todd suggests that the "lovely maniac" is the fusion of two actual people Wollstonecraft met on her 1797 visit to Bedlam—a singing maniac and a love-sick girl—who both, "when approached, let out an unearthly laugh" (*Mary* 427). Matthews compares the "lovely maniac" to the female inhabitant of Bedlam in Mackenzie's *The Man of Feeling* and to Laurence Sterne's Maria in *A Sentimental Journey* (87).

her inclination, to a rich old man, extremely jealous ... and that, in consequence of his treatment, or something which hung on her mind, she had, during her first lying-in, lost her senses" (*MTWW* 88). Jemima's description illustrates that the cause of women's suffering is both social (in this case, marriage laws that allow the lovely maniac's husband to treat her badly) and physical (here, post-partum depression). With this initial portrait, Wollstonecraft establishes as the novel's primary theme the ways in which women are oppressed both by external power structures and by their bodies' entrapment within these structures. To convey this major theme, Wollstonecraft worked to revise the Jacobin novel's structure and to interrupt the seductive power of the sentimental novel.

Jemima's Ethnography

Just as Jemima presents the first portrait of a sufferer, so she offers the first full ethnography. Her own life story, as many critics have commented, is a veritable catalogue of the suffering to which a late-eighteenth-century female servant was vulnerable. She is orphaned by her unwed mother, beaten by her father, virtually enslaved by her stepmother, raped by her apprentice master, and rendered homeless. She aborts a pregnancy, turns to prostitution to support herself, suffers physically from her work as a washerwoman, persecutes another woman in order to live with a tradesman, is left destitute again when the tradesman dies, sustains a serious injury, struggles to gain admittance to a hospital, turns to stealing, is sent to prison and then to the workhouse, and finally finds employment at the asylum. Although her own life would seem to be an amalgam of many women's stories, within her narrative, Jemima mentions in passing at least eight other women whose interactions with her illustrate two major responses to suffering: a woman's own suffering can induce her to sympathize with others who suffer, or the fear of additional suffering or losing what she has gained can cause a woman to persecute other women. The women Jemima meets who have access to the least power are kindest to her: one woman teaches her prostitution (*MTWW* 109), a girl on the street recommends her to "a house of ill fame" so that she might have shelter while working as a prostitute (*MTWW* 110), and a landlady helps her pay the "caution money," or burial fees necessary for admittance into the hospital (*MTWW* 117). In contrast, several women persecute other women in order to protect the little power they have: Jemima's mother's "virtuous mistress" makes Jemima's unwed mother live in the garret when she is pregnant but doesn't punish the father; Jemima's competitive and favored half-sister never offers her friendship or protection (*MTWW* 103); one of Jemima's mistresses directs her "violent fits of passion" toward Jemima (*MTWW* 110); a condescending nurse in the hospital is helpful only when she is being watched by doctors (*MTWW* 118); and the wife of Jemima's lover's heir turns Jemima out of the house immediately after the wealthy lover dies (*MTWW* 112). With these portraits of women abusing other women, Wollstonecraft illustrates women's complicity in their own oppression under patriarchy, or as Johnson puts it, the way normative heterosexuality requires "female-female violence" (*Equivocal* 66).[9] Rather than explain this phenomenon,

---

9   See also Mellor "A Novel" 415, Hoeveler "Reading" 400.

the novel simply interweaves the stories of women in these two groups, challenging readers to engage with this pedagogical/ethnographic narrative as curious learners. Offering a collection of portraits, the text resists the reading of any single character as evil, pointing instead to the social situation of women as the cause of their treatment of one another.

In addition to these passing sketches, Jemima tells more fully developed stories of at least five women, after which either Jemima or the narrator explains the factors motivating the women's behavior, much in the way that the teacher figure in didactic literature sometimes intervenes to help children interpret what they see. These five portraits are thematically linked, each depicting a different sort of violation of the relationship between mothers and daughters, or what Tauchert describes as interruptions in "Matrilineal exchange" (114). Jemima's mother, dreading the shame more than the poverty that would likely follow the birth of her illegitimate child, tries to starve herself and dies nine days after Jemima is born, leaving her motherless (*MTWW* 102). Jemima's nursemaid, hired when Jemima's mother dies, is incapable of expressing tenderness to the children she nurses because her emotions have been hardened by poverty and by the loss of children (*MTWW* 103). Jemima's stepmother, another potential surrogate mother, mistreats Jemima because Jemima's very presence reminds the stepmother that Jemima's father had an illicit lover. Similarly, her first master's wife treats Jemima as a moral pariah, forcing her to wear labels like "glutton" into town, hitting her and blaming her when the master rapes Jemima (*MTWW* 107).[10] Jemima bears society's unfair condemnation of her mother, who was seduced and abandoned by Jemima's father. Passing on the wound of her mother's own persecution, Jemima pushes a tradesman's pregnant lover out of the house so that she might live with him. When the woman commits suicide by drowning herself in a watering tub for horses, Jemima in effect becomes "the murderess of her own displaced mother" (Hoeveler "Reading" 395). Graphically displaying the suffering caused by women's mistreatment by men, Jemima's gritty "documentary realism" (Jones 211) describes the tragic cascade of suffering that results from the original mistreatment of her mother, both by Jemima's father and also by her mother's master's wife.

Jemima spins an intricate narrative web of persecution and suffering that helps the reader see the interrelationships of women under oppression rather than the sentimental figure of an individual sufferer. The story of her own suffering is deeply intertwined with these "inset tales"; thus, as a participant observer or a pedagogical ethnographer, she both bears her own suffering and bears witness to other women's suffering. Jemima describes three sets of women—sufferers who help one another, women who police their gains in patriarchy by abusing other women, and a group of related mothers and potential surrogate mothers who fail to take care of their daughters. By exposing the difficulty of sustaining healthy and mutually nurturing relationships among women under the economic and legal restrictions of late-eighteenth-century England's patriarchal society, Jemima's narrative calls for a restructuring of that society in order to make mutually supportive relationships possible.

---

10 See Cooper for an insightful discussion of this treatment of Jemima as a "misreading" (765).

Maria's Ethnography

A companion piece to Jemima's story, Maria's memoir outlines the ways in which even relatively well-to-do women are vulnerable to suffering under England's marriage laws. Maria records her narrative on paper with the hope that her daughter will "gain instruction" from it (*MTWW* 124), just as Wollstonecraft wrote *Original Stories* for her pupils, the Kingsborough girls. Thus, Maria (like Jemima) is figured as a teacher in the novel. Maria explains in her narrative that her father and brother dominate both her mother and the rest of the children. However, Maria's uncle favors her and treats her as his own. When Maria's mother dies, her father takes a mistress and forces her to leave the home. She marries George Venables who has misled her about his generosity and sensitivity in order to gain access to her uncle's money. An unfaithful husband, Venables repeatedly pressures Maria to wring money from her uncle to cover his gambling debts and other bills. When her husband tries to prostitute her to his friend, the pregnant Maria announces she will no longer live with him. She escapes from the house but has to stay on the run from Venables, hiding in several different lodgings. When her uncle bequeaths his fortune to Maria's baby, Venables takes the child and imprisons Maria in a private asylum in order to obtain the money willed to his daughter.

Maria embeds within her memoir passing sketches of at least three women whose stories are inextricable from those of the men in their lives—the fiancé who breaks Maria's uncle's heart by marrying his best friend (*MTWW* 127), the woman who takes care of Venables's illegitimate child (*MTWW* 151), and the maid Venables pays to drug and kidnap Maria. Thus, even in these brief references, Maria demonstrates the difficulty of separating women's life stories from men's. In addition, Maria creates fully drawn portraits of eight women. Similar to Jemima's five developed portraits, four of these eight stories depict the suffering of daughters under patriarchy, specifically the disruption of the financial, emotional, and physical aspects of potentially nurturing mother/daughter relationships. On a financial level, Maria's nurse's sister Peggy, like so many characters in *Original Stories*, is widowed and struggles to support her children in a society that offers disastrously few economic options for single mothers. On an emotional level, Maria's mother is unable to nurture her daughter both because she is damaged by her husband's unkindness and because she devotes her emotional energy to her husband and eldest son rather than to her daughters. On a physical level, Venables's mistress is unable to care for her daughter; seduced and then abandoned by Venables when he married Maria, the young servant mother dies in poverty. This orphaned, mistreated, and deformed daughter is perhaps the most painful of all the portraits in Maria's narrative. Maria notices that Venables's daughter "totter[s] along, scarcely able to sustain her own weight ... her complexion was sallow, and her eyes inflamed ... mixed with the wrinkles produced by the peevishness of pain" (*MTWW* 149). Tauchert describes the portrait of Venables's illegitimate daughter as the culmination of the "novel's layered refrain of the fears of mothers for daughters; specifically the fear that a mother will be prevented from caring for her daughter by economic, legal, and moral forces outside of her control" (114). She argues that "the neglected illegitimate daughter ... embodies the damage patriarchy effects on the mother's daughter, as well as the horror faced by a mother of daughters under patriarchy" (115). The resonances among these individual stories offer what Tilottama Rajan describes as "a reading that uncovers what is not actually articulated in the text" (221). Together, the stories reveal a traumatic facet of the everyday oppression of women—the loss of mothers' ability to nurture their daughters, a loss that is rendered invisible by its very familiarity.

In two of the other four major inset tales included in her fictional ethnography, Maria offers a socially based explanation for the suffering of the women discussed. Maria's stepmother is unkind to Maria and to her sisters and tries to seduce Maria's brother. Maria situates her stepmother's behavior in its social context: "By allowing women but one way of rising in the world, the fostering the libertinism of men, society makes monsters of them, and then their ignoble vices are brought forward as a proof of inferiority of intellect" (*MTWW* 137). Although she, in effect, calls her stepmother a monster, she also describes a cycle that encourages women to behave in an "ignoble" or "inferior" manner. In addition, Maria characterizes her sisters' difficult careers as governesses as symptomatic of a widespread problem in women's employment: "[A] well-educated woman, with more than ordinary talents, can struggle for a subsistence; and even this is a dependence next to menial" (*MTWW* 148). She then places the story of her sisters' struggle on a continuum of women's oppression: "Is it then surprising, that so many forlorn women, with human passions and feelings, take refuge in infamy?" (*MTWW* 148). Writing to her daughter after having heard Jemima's dismal account of prostitution, Maria broadens her concern for her sisters' struggles into a criticism of the lack of respectable paid employment available to women. In this portrait and elsewhere, Wollstonecraft depicts the movement of Maria's sympathy across class, the crucial imaginative mechanism that will make women's suffering visible—at least to one another.

Having demonstrated the difficulty of sympathizing across class and beyond one's own troubles through multiple portraits of women oppressing women, Wollstonecraft also portrays ways in which women overcome these obstacles in order to support one another. In Maria's descriptions of the two women with whom she boards during her attempted escape from Venables, Wollstonecraft offers a mirror in which Maria might see the way in which her suffering overlaps with that of working-class women. These landlady episodes occur in the narrative after the reader has encountered Jemima's story, but before Maria has met Jemima in "real" time. This ordering of the narrative allows Wollstonecraft to demonstrate to the reader why Maria, unlike so many other women in Jemima's life, is able to respond to Jemima's suffering sympathetically. Immediately after she escapes from Venables's house, Maria boards with a hard-working woman whose husband takes the money reserved for bills, gets drunk, and beats her—a more physically violent version of Venables's abuse of Maria. When her husband sees Venables's advertisement in the paper threatening anyone harboring Maria with "the utmost severity of the law," he forces his wife to make Maria leave (*MTWW* 172). Maria understands the landlady's decision to follow her husband's orders, but chooses "not to inform [her] landlady where [she] was going":

> I knew that she had a sincere affection for me, and would willingly have run any risk to show her gratitude; yet I was fully convinced, that a few kind words from Johnny would have found the woman in her, and her dear benefactress, as she termed me in an agony of tears, would have to be sacrificed, to recompense her tyrant for condescending to treat

her like an equal. He could be kind-hearted, as she expressed it, when he pleased. And this thawed sternness, contrasted with his habitual brutality, was the more acceptable, and could not be purchased at too dear a rate. (*MTWW* 173)

Wollstonecraft resists criticizing this individual woman's participation in Maria's oppression, citing "the woman in her" and offering examples of other women who respond to the patriarchal power structure similarly. As Maria acknowledges, she herself was guilty of giving in to Venables when she felt affection for him. In short, Maria works to see herself in this landlady and thus to regard the landlady's potential betrayal of her with understanding rather than resentment.

The second woman with whom Maria boards shares the story of her difficult marriage after Venables finds Maria and tries to force her to come home with him. In this case, Maria is an impatient listener, understandably anxious to move on to her next hiding place. This landlady explains that she worked as a servant, saved money to open a lodging house, and married a footman. Her husband had an affair and spent her hard-earned money to impress his mistress with gifts, causing her to lose her lodging house and thus to have to work again as a servant. The husband drinks, steals from her, and finally takes work as a soldier. During the six years of peace that she enjoys while he is fighting in the war, she reopens her lodging house. Because her property is legally his, she loses everything again when he returns in debt. Finally he dies. The landlady comments: "I know so well, that women have always the worst of it, when law is to decide" (*MTWW* 178). Like the previous landlady, this woman's story mirrors Maria's own experience with a husband's theft of his wife's money. What is most instructive about this story, however, is Maria's initial resistance to listening: "I did not attempt to interrupt her, though I wished her, as soon as possible, to go out in search of a new abode for me, where I could once more hide my head" (*MTWW* 177). Maria struggles against her own urgent need for a hiding place in order to listen to her landlady's tale. In this moment of tension, Wollstonecraft acknowledges the struggle to sympathize with another woman's problems when one's own problems feel pressing. Ultimately, though, Maria stays and listens to the landlady, thus demonstrating how crucial it is for women to witness one another's suffering. Without these experiences, Maria might not have been as responsive to Jemima's story, an interaction that becomes the basis of their friendship. And this friendship offers the only potential avenue toward Maria's escape and reunion with her daughter. Rather than rewarding appropriate feminine behavior with marriage, as does the sentimental novel, Wollstonecraft's novel imagines at least one plot line that will reward women's compassionate acknowledgement of one another's experience with shared freedom from oppression.

In addition to these scenes with the landladies, Wollstonecraft presents several moments in which Maria moves from the immediate apprehension of her own suffering, outward to sympathy with other women's experiences, and finally to a more general understanding of women's collective oppression. Two scenes in particular demonstrate Maria's need to move from the self-absorption of sensibility into an understanding of the social context of oppression. As in children's literature, these scenes model desirable behavior in order to instruct readers. After she confronts Venables for prostituting her to his friend, he locks her in her room. While imprisoned in her home, she begins to see her marriage with "the piercing sight of reason" and suddenly feels singled out for persecution: "Had an evil genius cast a spell at my birth; or a demon stalked out of chaos, to perplex my understanding, and enchain my will, with delusive prejudices?" (*MTWW* 165). Maria's thinking then dramatically shifts from this self-absorbed reflection to a more socially based perception: "I pursued this train of thinking; it led me out of myself, to expatiate on the misery peculiar to my sex" (*MTWW* 165). Similarly, when she discovers she is interred in the madhouse, Maria first "writes some rhapsodies descriptive of the state of her mind" (*MTWW* 82). Just as she does when confined within her own home, Maria shifts from melancholic rumination to a consciousness of the social oppression of women:

> [T]he events of her past life pressing on her, she resolved circumstantially to relate them, with the sentiments that experience, and more matured reason, would naturally suggest. They might perhaps instruct her daughter, and shield her from the misery, the tyranny, her mother knew not how to avoid. This thought gave life to her diction, her soul flowed into it, and she soon found the task of recollecting almost obliterated impressions very interesting. (*MTWW* 82)

Having moved from individual feeling (or "sentiment") to social awareness (or "more mature reason"), Maria wishes to educate her daughter about potentially harmful situations. Once in the asylum, Maria is able not only to move from self to social consciousness, but also to contextualize other women's stories in the way that she has framed her own. Maria listens to Jemima's evening narratives about the other inmates and immediately "generalize[s] her observations" into an analysis of the kinds of people who lose their reason (*MTWW* 92). In the middle of Jemima's tale, Maria notes: "[Y]our narrative gives rise to the most painful reflections on the present state of society" (*MTWW* 115). Significantly, all of these examples of seeing the social context occur when Maria is confined—first in her home and then in the asylum. These moments of illumination within confinement illustrate that there is no space of freedom for women in patriarchal culture. More interestingly, they suggest that it is only when women's imprisonment within patriarchy is made explicit that the identification among women required for collective action can begin.

Reciprocal Seeing

If Maria must learn to see beyond self to social context, Jemima must learn to act sympathetically. However, like the landladies Maria encounters, Jemima has more to lose than does Maria in reaching across class to help another woman. Jemima asks an essential question: Why should an oppressed woman take up the cause of other women? She notes that she has been "'the witness of many enormities'" in the four years she has worked in the asylum, but feels unmoved to help other women: "'What should induce me to be the champion for suffering humanity?—Who ever risked any thing for me?—Who ever acknowledged me to be a fellow-creature?'" (*MTWW* 119). Jemima's question suggests that witnessing another's suffering is not always enough to inspire sympathetic action. Witnessing must be accompanied by the hope that one's sympathy and nurturance will be reciprocated. Although the idea of un-altruistic sympathy—that is, a woman expressing sympathy for another's suffering when she desires help from the sufferer—seems unethical, Wollstonecraft presents the desire for reciprocal sympathy as a necessary component of women's collective action. For example, after Maria begins to think about the oppressed state of women, she neither stays in a state of rational reflection, nor collapses in despair, but rather begins to think of how Jemima might help her. Maria expresses sympathy to Jemima in order to obtain Jemima's help in finding her daughter: "She spoke with energy of Jemima's unmerited sufferings, and of the fate of a number of deserted females, placed within the sweep of a whirlwind, from which it was next to impossible to escape" (*MTWW* 55). Followed by Maria's request for Jemima's help, this statement seems ethically unstable at best. However, it conveys both that Maria witnesses and sympathizes with Jemima's suffering and also that she is dependent upon her for help. In short, Wollstonecraft argues that women need both to witness one another's suffering and also to understand themselves as mutually dependent.

To argue, as Julie McGonegal does, that Jemima is "an underdeveloped character whose oppression is simply a repetition with difference of Maria's and Wollstonecraft's own suffering" is to ignore the subtleties of the characters' interaction, including the exchanges of sympathy between them, the unbalancing of class structures in the asylum, and the difficulty they have interpreting each other's stories accurately (357).[11] Maria is aware of both her dependence on and influence over Jemima. Jemima, similarly, is aware of her power to help Maria, yet she remains careful not to "[hazard] the loss of her place" at the asylum (*MTWW* 80).[12] When Maria drops hints that she needs help escaping, Jemima explicitly considers the risks to herself. Jemima cautiously resolves "not to do more than soften the rigour of confinement, till she could advance on surer ground" (*MTWW* 83). Jemima understands the social nature of women's suffering but has shut down her response to it. The narrator explains Jemima's situation: "Jemima ... had felt the crushing hand of power, hardened by the exercise of injustice, and ceased to wonder at the perversions of the understanding, which systematize oppression" (*MTWW* 80). Finally, though, her sympathy for the injustice done to Maria as a mother softens her position: "[W]hen told that [Maria's] child, only four months old, had been torn from her, even while she was discharging the tenderest maternal office ... Jemima determined to alleviate all in her power ... the sufferings of a wretched mother, apparently injured, and certainly unhappy" (*MTWW* 80). As Christine Cooper argues, at the heart of Jemima's sympathy for Maria's loss of her child is her sympathy for herself as an abandoned child (776). In this case, the subtle power of self-interest operates as identification—a crucial feature of a participant/observer ethnography.

Significantly, Maria does not just ask for Jemima's help, but promises to make the recovery of her daughter beneficial to them both:

---

11   In contrast to McGonegal, Myers argues "Eighteenth-century texts participate in distinctive generic traditions, which we may misread as defective forms of what we're familiar with, rather than as significant inflections of a stylized and conventional grammar" ("Little Girls" 137).

12   See Cooper (772) and Kipp (30) on the dangers to which Jemima exposes herself in sympathizing with Maria.

"In the name of God, assist me to snatch her from destruction! Let me but give her an education—let me but prepare her body and mind to encounter the ills which await her sex, and I will teach her to consider you as her second mother, and herself as the prop of your age. Yes, Jemima, look at me—observe me closely, and read my very soul; you merit a better fate;" she held out her hand with a firm gesture of assurance; "and I will procure it for you, as a testimony of my esteem, as well as of my gratitude." (*MTWW* 121)

Maria submits herself to Jemima's scrutiny: "[L]ook at me—observe me closely, and read my very soul." She then, in turn, reads Jemima: "[Y]ou merit a better fate." In addition to this reciprocal seeing, Maria offers Jemima not just gratitude, but esteem. Jemima and Maria's mutual dependence radically disrupts the typical relationship between the charitable gentry woman and the redeemed prostitute in which, as Vivien Jones explains, "charity is very explicitly a method of differentiation" (215). Wollstonecraft suggests that for women to see and respond to one another's suffering, the power structures in which they are situated must be unsettled, and yet she acknowledges the risks that this unsettling entails.

Rather than a single ethnographer/teacher like Smith's Mrs. Woodfield or her own Mrs. Mason, Wollstonecraft includes three storytellers in *The Wrongs of Woman*, with class positions both above and below Wollstonecraft's own. Wollstonecraft invites us "to read beyond and between the lines of" these three narrators' stories (Rajan 229). Maria's and Jemima's narratives make visible both the social mechanisms by which women are oppressed and the two actions necessary to fight that oppression—women's witnessing of one another's suffering and their recognition of mutual dependence. Darnford's narrative offers an instructive counterpoint to Maria's and Jemima's that serves primarily to educate readers in a third major action necessary for fighting oppression—the ability to see the social context rather than the sentimental subject. Darnford's cavalier description of his reliance on prostitutes settles uncomfortably next to Jemima's unflinching portraits of women who desperately turn to prostitution in order to survive. In Darnford's passing references to "a creature [he is] ashamed to mention," "other women ... of a class of which [Maria] can have no knowledge," and London's "women of the town" whom he regards as "angels," the reader sees prostitutes whose stories are submerged and hidden in male desire, rather than given a voice as is Jemima's experience (*MTWW* 94, 97). Thus, Wollstonecraft simultaneously educates her readers about Darnford's character and demonstrates the need for what current anthropologists would describe as a "participant-observer ethnographer"—that is, a narrator like Jemima rather than Darnford, a narrator whose experience partially overlaps with the lives of those she describes.

The placement of Darnford's narrative within the novel further educates readers in the dangers of seeing sentimentally. Wollstonecraft reveals Maria's disastrous misapprehension of Venables's character after the reader has felt the disjunction between Darnford's story of his libertine life and Jemima's story of suffering, inviting the reader to mistrust Maria's perception in this second love affair (Johnson "Mary" 203, O'Quinn 769). Showing not just the disease of sentimentalism but also the cure, Wollstonecraft dramatizes for readers Maria's movement from seeing the sentimental subject (herself) to seeing the social context. Listening to Jemima's story in the company of Darnford, Maria emerges from her sentimental love cocoon to consider social issues:

Active as love was in the heart of Maria, the story she had just heard made her thoughts take a wider range. The opening buds of hope closed, as if they had put forth too early, and the happiest day of her life was overcast by the most melancholy reflections. Thinking of Jemima's peculiar fate and her own, she was led to consider the oppressed state of women, and to lament that she had given birth to a daughter. (*MTWW* 120)

Thus, Wollstonecraft places in explicit opposition Maria's participation in the sentimental love plot and her understanding of the social context of women's oppression. With these moments of communication among the narrators, Wollstonecraft illustrates the way in which fictional ethnography widens the reader's view by placing an individual portrait within a panoramic picture of society. Just as the reader begins to settle into a love story, Wollstonecraft interrupts the desire for sentimental consummation, not with an explicit critique of this form, but with a series of juxtapositions from which we must draw our own conclusions.

As in *Original Stories* and other didactic children's literature, Wollstonecraft stages dramatic moments of learning—including mistakes and misreadings—within the text in order to invite her readers to learn alongside the characters. When Mrs. Woodfield of *Rural Walks* corrects Caroline's mistaken impression that beggars have no right to aid, Smith invites the reader to learn compassion along with her young character. Similarly, when characters misunderstand one another in *The Wrongs of Woman*, Wollstonecraft invites the reader to learn from their mistakes along with the characters. Relating these misreadings to the interpretative possibilities inherent in abortion/miscarriage in the eighteenth century, Cooper argues: "The need to read failure and the slippages of meaning it makes possible are, as we will see, a pattern that Wollstonecraft exploits in *The Wrongs of Woman*" (759). Cooper points out that Darnford and Maria both respond to Jemima's narrative solely in terms of class oppression (769). Jemima, however, corrects them, helping them to see gender as an essential part of the equation. Detailing a washerwoman's physically punishing labor, Jemima describes the difference in jobs available to men and to women: "A man with half my industry, and, I may say, abilities, could have procured a decent livelihood" (*MTWW* 115–16). Maria's initial impulse to see Jemima's suffering as a problem only of class helps her (like Darnford) to feel protected from the problems Jemima faces. In contrast, acknowledging the role that gender plays in these troubles forces Maria to acknowledge her own vulnerability and thus the needs that she shares with Jemima.

In her characters' misreadings of one another and corrections to those misreadings, Wollstonecraft demonstrates both how much her social critique depends on her readers' ability to analyze social problems and how much more effective that analysis is when embarked upon as a collective experience. Myers notes that in the *Vindication of the Rights of Woman*, Wollstonecraft presents the ideal mother saying to her children: "when your mind arrives at maturity, you must only obey me, or rather respect my opinions, so far as they coincide with the light that is breaking in on your own mind" (Myers "Impeccable" 49). As in her children's literature, in *The Wrongs of Woman*, Wollstonecraft instructs us to read social issues by the light within and in good company.[13] When that company of collaborative viewers includes people of

_____

13 Cooper eloquently argues: "The text's revolutionary possibility lies not simply in what has been written, its substance and conclusions, but in how it openly engages societal

different classes, some restructuring of power relationships is required. Sam Haigh cites the work of Gayatri Spivak to comment on the ethnographer's negotiation of the power differential between the one who sees and the one who is seen:

> [The] displacement of authority is the best that can be hoped for by the intellectual trying to find evidence of, and write about, those subjugated and colonized ... peoples missing from official discourse. As is by now well known, Spivak's recommended practice is one of "constant vigilance"—a scrupulous self-awareness and self-reflexivity on the part of the intellectual with regard both to his or her own position and that of the "subaltern subject" or "native informant" about whom s/he is writing. This, alone, will ensure that untold stories are told—but only by working "at the silences between bits of language to see what will work as meaning." (77)

Seeing suffering—especially when there is class difference—requires "self-awareness and self-reflexivity" in order to make visible the invisible, give voice to the silences. Accordingly, Wollstonecraft presents adult learning in *The Wrongs of Woman* as a push-and-pull, a collective undertaking, an active negotiation between one's own experience and the experience of others.[14]

If, as Hoeveler points out, "sentimental and gothic heroines need a man, because without one they are missing ... victimization and abusive trauma," then children's literature—a world of women and children—offers a safe space from which to begin to build the more humane society Wollstonecraft imagines ("Reading" 401). The stories that Maria and Jemima tell across class transform the "place" of the asylum with its binaries between sane and insane, free and imprisoned, into a "space" of cross-class identification between women. The positive aspects of this confinement in the asylum recall the pleasure Wollstonecraft describes in *Letters from Norway* when she experiences the "confinement" of her cozy room in Tonsberg as a secure embrace that corresponds with the sheltering scene outside her window. Similarly combining security and identification, Jemima and Maria build a two-woman community based on their sympathetic witnessing and recognition of common dependence. However, their escape reveals the fragility of this community outside of the context of the "space" created in the asylum. As they flee the asylum, Maria is grabbed by a male maniac who asks, "'Woman ... what have I to do with thee?'" (190). Maria breaks his grasp, crying, "'[Y]ou have nothing to do with me'" and "throwing her arms around Jemima, crie[s], 'Save me!'" (*MTWW* 190). Jane Kromm argues that in this gothic moment, Wollstonecraft "demonstrates that it is the abusive potential of male, maniacal outbursts that remains unmonitored and unchecked in society, and that this danger persists despite the supposed moderating effect of

---

failure and reading practices through its structural workings ... . Instead of passing judgment, Wollstonecraft asks us repeatedly to attend to the processes by which judgments are made and to see how unstable and implicated they can be" (778). I would add that Wollstonecraft's attempt to teach the process of reading parallels the teacher's role in didactic children's literature.

14 My understanding of learning in *The Wrongs of Woman* as a collaborative negotiation, a process of misreading and re-reading, supports Lynch's assertion that "in romantic aesthetics we don't terminate interpretation," that characters revise their (often self) understandings in the second or third look at a place or another person (132).

sensibility on aggressive behavior in men" (371). I would add to Kromm's reading that the lack of recognition and disassociation between Maria and the male maniac is also meant to contrast with the mutual recognition and understanding Jemima and Maria create in the asylum. By inverting the world—the asylum begins to feel safe while the world feels threatening—Wollstonecraft demonstrates that the creation of a space in which a woman can name the darkest aspects of her oppression and have that oppression acknowledged is, simply put, *the* condition under which women's sanity is possible.

In *The Wrongs of Woman*, Wollstonecraft takes the ethic of sociability inherent in children's literature and transforms it into a call for women's collective activism. Wollstonecraft hoped that if sensibility would not encourage social justice, mutual sympathy and ethnographic vision might. Accordingly, she pushed the boundaries of narrative form in her effort to retrain the public's ability to see suffering. Just as I argue that Smith's children's literature be taken seriously for its intervention into social issues of her time, I suggest that Wollstonecraft's novel of social criticism be interpreted as an extension of children's literature. Her major revision to the Jacobin novel—the episodic organization of stories as in didactic children's literature— allows Wollstonecraft to refract her individual troubles through a number of fictional characters, thus transforming individual complaint into social critique. In addition, Wollstonecraft places these refracted portraits of her suffering among portraits of characters who experience degrees of oppression well beyond the author's own. In *Letters from Norway*, Wollstonecraft describes the way in which her suffering is temporarily alleviated by envisioning the physical manifestations of her pain and desire in the landscape—the sublime cascade, the sheltering scene. Similarly, Maria and Jemima are able to understand their own oppression more clearly when they see it manifested in other women's lives. Likewise, the reader is able to apprehend the social context of suffering when she views the common oppression of women in a variety of situations and from a range of socio-economic backgrounds. Seeing suffering ethnographically rather than sentimentally means placing individual suffering into a relational framework, while allowing each individual experience to reconstitute the collective picture. It is a deliberate, dynamic, and contingent process of seeing.

In this regard, the dialogic structure of the narratives is as important as is their episodic presentation. Through dialogue, characters discover in one another similar experiences, learn to reinterpret their misreadings, and slip out of their "proper" roles. It is in dialogue that "place" modulates into "space." Thus, the dialogue among characters also reveals the limitations of seeing through the lens of sensibility, a mode of vision that depends upon the distinction between the sympathetic viewer and the object of pity. In *Rural Walks*, Elizabeth's failed, imaginary appeal to Mrs. Wadford's sensibility displays the problems with this mode of seeing. Not inclined to be charitable, and denying that she has any vulnerability in common with Sarah Hobloun, Mrs. Wadford is blind to the ways in which she is implicated in the poor woman's suffering. Simply put, because she cannot see it, she cannot respond to her poor neighbor's suffering. Similarly, in *The Wrongs of Woman*, the dialogue and exchange of stories among the three narrators encourages the reader to see a social context for individual suffering. Jemima's and Maria's tales of their own and other women's oppression correct Darnford's self-absorbed narrative of the man of sensibility. Unlike the clueless Darnford, the reader might learn from the disjunctures among these narratives.

Wollstonecraft, then, criticizes the sentimental novel for translating suffering into self-absorption rather than into social action. James Averill describes the interest eighteenth-century characters such as Yorick, Tristram, Belford, Harley, and Rasselas show in suffering: "What distinguishes the sentimentalist is his profound interest in the man looking at the sorrow, in a word, himself" rather than the suffering person he observes (24). Authors like Laurence Sterne and Henry Mackenzie are "primarily interested in human misery for the response it evokes in observer and reader" (Averill 31). Averill argues that William Wordsworth draws on and modulates the sentimental mode by depicting an observer who responds to the suffering of others not with tears, but with calmness and a "revolution within the self" (13). Wollstonecraft's narrative focuses much more on the sufferer than do other sentimental texts, but *The Wrongs of Woman* also explores the revolution within the observing subject. This revolution of the self depends not upon objectification, but upon identification between the sufferer and the observer. Rather than moving the observer to calm, the sight of suffering in Wollstonecraft's novel moves the viewer into social action, laying the groundwork for an external revolution as well as an internal one.

Because Wollstonecraft presents Maria's and Jemima's episodic fictional ethnographies as a dialogue, she suggests that the healing of the individual and the healing of the social body are linked. If Wollstonecraft feels comfort in *Letters from Norway* when she imagines both herself and the landscape as maternal, vulnerable, and mutually sympathetic, this interaction is transferred to relationships among women in *The Wrongs of Woman*. Healing is possible only when women see one another's suffering and recognize their mutual dependence. Further, this witnessing and recognition is possible only when the social structure of patriarchal oppression—represented in the novel as the asylum—is made visible.

Afterword

This study's concern with vision and suffering ultimately engages two dialectics—empiricism vs. idealism, and materiality vs. transcendence. First, as I hope is obvious by now, I argue that Charlotte Smith, Mary Wollstonecraft, and Mary Shelley explore the nuanced middle ground between the empiricist's reliance on visual evidence and the idealist's commitment to internal vision, both compelling positions of inquiry and expression in the late eighteenth century. The cultural interest in visual, or empirical, proof not only informs the study of natural sciences, but also plays out politically as a profound trust in social transparency and readability, and a deep distrust of dissimulation and acting. In this model, we see "things as they are," an objective reality assumed to be implicitly and inevitably confirmed by what others see. At its most extreme, this position contradicts the idealist's notion that reality is inextricable from our internal vision. Scientific discoveries about the individual physiology of the eye in the late eighteenth century, however, deconstruct this opposition between empiricist and idealist perspectives. From a medical point-of-view, subjective vision cannot be understood as the abstract, internal vision of the idealist, but rather as embodied in the particularities of the individual seeing subject's eyes.

Thus, to come to the second binary, the materiality of embodied seeing resists the familiar Romantic model of transcendent vision because it always occurs in a changing body, a body that is both individually constituted and constantly responsive to the world around. This understanding of the physiology of the eye in the late eighteenth century, then, deflates the fantasy of transcendence, tethering vision to the material world. The idea that vision is subjective and material might suggest that what each person sees will be different from what others see, that reality will be unknowable in any collective sense. However, Donna Haraway's "situated knowledge(s)," a theory to which I refer several times in the preceding chapters, offers a vocabulary for conceptualizing the value of the "partial view," the idea that what we each see, though limited, offers us valid information about the external world. Furthermore, Kaja Silverman's construction of a "world spectator" posits that both the viewer and the objects seen come into being collaboratively. Thus, the materiality of the object seen is just as important as is the materiality of the seeing subject's vision. With embodied vision, a new way of thinking about the interaction between self and world emerges: the seeing subject might find healing in the external world. This healing occurs not by transcending either phenomenal forms or the body in pain, but rather by bringing the world into the body through the eyes, by interacting with natural structures like the sheltering scene, by allowing emotional memories to spill out into one's vision, and by inviting the objects in the world to organize one's mind while simultaneously looking at them through aesthetic or scientific systems of thought.

Exploring the cultural work accomplished by non-transcendent modes of vision, the first part of this book, "Illness," considers the conditions under which illness or difference becomes culturally visible. Smith claims melancholic genius for women by emphasizing its roots in both rational thought and deep feeling, and by repeatedly portraying melancholia as an embodied condition. In the *Elegiac Sonnets*, she creates a series of portraits of melancholic sufferers who present their bodies for view so that others may perceive their pain. Importantly, these sufferers also actively look at the world themselves. In these portraits, Smith expresses her desire for a sympathetic gaze, describes the therapeutic value of vision, and engages the persuasive power of multiple portrayals of individual suffering—three topics on which she would elaborate in the literature that followed the *Elegiac Sonnets*. In addition, she figures the loss of loved ones as the loss of the sight of them. Mary Shelley, in contrast, explores the conditions of sympathetic interaction that allow the sufferer not necessarily to be seen, but also or instead to tell the story of his/ her suffering. Mary Shelley has less faith than does Smith in the human ability to look past gender or ethnicity in order to sympathize—that is, less faith in the power of empirical evidence to change society. Instead, Mary Shelley explores the value of strategic invisibility for the potentially marked, or culturally invisible, suffering subject. In *Frankenstein*, she suggests that blindness to the physical evidence of difference is necessary for sympathetic communication. When one is marked by gender or ethnicity, invisibility—a condition which takes one out of the economy of sensibility, but also potentially out of the economy of racism and sexism—makes it possible to tell the story of one's suffering and enables others to hear that story.

The first two chapters in the section entitled "Healing" explain that both Smith and Wollstonecraft believed that viewing nature's order would help reorder their minds and thus alleviate their emotional suffering. Smith and Wollstonecraft emphasize the female sufferer's deep responsiveness to aesthetics—or ability to look actively rather than to be the passive object of someone else's vision. Thus, they claim immersion in sensibility as a position of strength for women and fight the man of sensibility's tendency to objectify and appropriate women's suffering. Wollstonecraft modifies the picturesque aesthetic to express her longing for a therapeutic, maternal embrace, and consequently imagines health as an exchange between solitude and sociability. Smith finds healing in her practice of botany, and models a language of suffering on this natural science. She collects and contextualizes individual experiences of suffering in order to name them in a relational framework. Thus, both Wollstonecraft and Smith seek company, companionship, and context in their desire for healing. In the third chapter of this section, we find that Mary Shelley offers a somewhat different perspective on healing. In *Rambles in Germany and Italy*, Mary Shelley— like her mother—refers to the therapeutic potential of the picturesque landscape, but resists the systematic and classificatory approach to healing espoused by her spa doctors, an approach that was intertwined with Germany's political agenda. She prefers instead to explore her traumatic past in the landscape and in conjunction with historical experiences of courageous suffering that are written on the land. Although all three writers rely to some extent on aesthetic or scientific frameworks to interact with the therapeutic landscape, in 1848, Mary Shelley finds it necessary to distinguish between aesthetic and political modes of categorization. More than the other two authors, Mary Shelley is committed to invisibility—a strategy that allows her both to escape judgment and external control and also to live within her own traumatic experience. At the same time, she wishes for the Italian struggle to be seen in the landscape.

The final section of this study, "Social Justice," introduces the term "fictional ethnography" to distinguish the visually based methodology of Wollstonecraft's and Smith's reformist literature from that of the Jacobin novel. Wollstonecraft's *Original Stories* and Smith's *Rural Walks* combine instruction with social criticism by developing three aspects of children's literature—the dialogic and visual structure of experiential learning, the plurality of scenes created in the episodic organization of stories, and the portrayal of powerful mother-teacher figures, who help train their children to see. These children's works enact the language of suffering that Smith develops from botany by offering to the reader's view a series of cases of the impoverished ill that intervene in discussions about the 1790s poverty crisis. These educational books train child and adult readers to see social problems, thus suggesting that productive, social vision must be learned. It is not enough, as in the Jacobin novel, to unveil corrupt social structures; it is also crucial to refine the visual acuity of those who look. Wollstonecraft takes the technique of fictional ethnography that she uses in *Original Stories* a step further in *The Wrongs of Woman* to convey the interdependence of individual healing and social change. The twenty-seven portraits of women suffering under patriarchy painted by this novel depict the complex relationships among gender, class, and poverty in the late eighteenth century. The collections of verbal portraits in these works encourage readers not to blame individual sufferers, but to see instead the social context and causes of their pain.

The three authors I discuss in this book respond to and shape a cultural moment in which the idea of embodied vision opened up possibilities for creative expression, healing, and social change. The connections among their ideas raise the question of how much they interacted with one another intellectually. The literary and familial relationship between Wollstonecraft and Mary Shelley has been discussed a great deal in scholarly literature, but the ways in which Smith's life intersected with Wollstonecraft's and with Mary Shelley's are less well known. Nonetheless, there is growing evidence that Smith and Wollstonecraft read and admired each other's work. Between 1788 and 1794, Wollstonecraft favorably reviewed five of Smith's novels in *The Analytical Review*.[1] Wollstonecraft also praised Smith's *Elegiac Sonnets*, using it as a model with which to compare other poetry collections she reviewed (*WMW* 7:72, 87). Likewise, Smith read both Wollstonecraft's and William Godwin's published works. In a letter written to Godwin shortly after Wollstonecraft's death in December of 1797, Smith quotes from her *Letters from Norway* (Clemit 34). Smith dedicated her novel *The Young Philosopher* (1798) to Wollstonecraft, commenting that "I may just mention that the incident of the confinement in a mad house of one of my characters was designed before I saw the fragment of 'The Wrongs of Woman,' by a Writer whose talents I greatly honoured, and whose untimely death I deeply regret; from her I should not blush to borrow, and if I had done so I would have acknowledged it" (Smith *YP* v). In a letter written on 1 September 1797, Smith informs Godwin that she is reading *Political Justice* (Clemit 33). Pamela Clemit's

---

1   See Wollstonecraft's review of *Emmeline* (*WMW* 7:22–27), review of *Ethelinde* (*WMW* 7:188–90), review of *Celestina* (*WMW* 7:388–89), review of *Desmond* (*WMW* 7:450–52), and review of *Marchmont* (*WMW* 7:485–86).

discovery of five letters from Smith to Godwin and Mary Jane Godwin reveals what Clemit terms "a pattern of mutual family support between the Smiths and the Godwins" (31). Smith sought to comfort Godwin after Wollstonecraft's death, noting that she "should have a melancholy pleasure in seeing the two poor little girls," that is, Fanny Imlay and the newborn Mary Godwin (Clemit 34). Additionally, the letters confirm that Godwin introduced Smith to Samuel Taylor Coleridge, and reveal that Mary Jane Godwin helped identify a governess for Smith's grandchildren. Although the link between seeing and suffering is, I argue, a general feature of Romantic-era literature, natural history, and social activism, these personal and intellectual exchanges also strongly support the particular lines of influence among the three authors explored in this study.

Read together, Wollstonecraft, Smith, and Mary Shelley offer a compelling and complex account of vision and suffering in multiple genres of Romantic-era literature. These three authors develop the potential for expression inherent in the culture's interest in embodied seeing and also focus on making visible the social structures that contribute to suffering. As a point of contrast, William Wordsworth embraces the relationship between visuality and individual subjectivity (most famously in his spots of time), yet invokes the connection between seeing and suffering only to dismiss the picturesque (that "strong infection of the age") (*The Prelude* XI.156). Most strikingly, these three authors offer models of collaborative perception in which multiple perspectives correct and temper one another. Smith depicts sympathetic seeing in the *Elegiac Sonnets* as multidirectional, occurring simultaneously among several bodies. In her works referencing botany, in *The Letters of a Solitary Wanderer*, and in her children's books, Smith suggests that we see the suffering of an individual most accurately in the context of multiple, collected portraits of individual suffering. Similarly, Wollstonecraft imagines wellness in *Letters from Norway* as a sociable rather than an individual state, characterizing both the viewer and the landscape as maternal, vulnerable, and mutually sympathetic. In addition, she posits collective vision as an essential step toward healing the social body. By creating two teacher figures rather than one in *The Wrongs of Woman*, Wollstonecraft calls for a collaborative investigation of oppression. Furthermore, she insists that this shared exploration and mutual support among women can only occur when patriarchal economic and social structures are explicitly exposed. Her desire to make oppressive social structures transparent coincides with her commitment to developing reciprocal identification and interdependence among women. She wishes for women to see one another and to see clearly the context of one another's experiences. Mary Shelley's *Frankenstein* also explicitly values communal narrative efforts: it relies on three narrators to tell the tale, credits evening conversations with others for its inspiration, and acknowledges Percy Bysshe Shelley's co-editing work. In *Rambles in Germany and Italy*, Mary Shelley describes yet another kind of co-operative vision. Internalizing the notion of collaborative perception, she re-approaches sites of traumatic memory in the company of those she has lost, signaling her incorporation of them by seeing as they would see.

If the desire for transcendence is a desire for psychic wholeness, then the kind of non-transcendent vision that Wollstonecraft, Smith, and Mary Shelley explore is a process that necessarily accepts the shadows, the partial, and the impure in order to see and be healed by the surrounding world. These authors do not ask—as does John Keats at the end of his transcendent reverie—"Was it a vision, or a waking dream? ... Do I wake or sleep?"—but instead ask other seeing subjects, "Do you see me? What does the world look like to you?" (ll.79–80). Collaborative rather than transcendent, embodied vision opens up the desire to be held in a loving gaze, to look through the eyes of lost loved ones, and to have one's vision refined by that of other seeing subjects. These authors suggest that the most ethical kind of authority rests finally in our own shared vision—in what we together are able to see both literally and in our mind's eye. It is important to note, however, that Mary Shelley's depiction of collective, embodied vision is much less hopeful than is that of the women of the generation before her. Both *Frankenstein* and *Rambles in Germany and Italy* explore the connection between seeing and suffering, yet Mary Shelley is more explicitly concerned about the danger of individual vision than are Smith and Wollstonecraft.

The dialectics that this book traces are visible in the works of subsequent women writers. In particular, post-Napoleonic women writers invoke collective vision—perhaps inspired by Smith's language of suffering based on collecting and naming—yet these works resonate more with Mary Shelley's cautious sociability than with Smith's and Wollstonecraft's reformist vision. Felicia Hemans's *Records of Woman* (1828), for example, might be analyzed as a poetic ethnography that presents multiple portraits of suffering and often suicidal women. However, the frequent displacement of women's experiences in the poems onto other cultures and time periods does not offer the contextualization of women's suffering within a specific cultural moment as do the texts by Wollstonecraft and Smith. Letitia Landon's *Subjects for Pictures* (1841), with its specific references to visuality and its recurrent theme of loss, would be a particularly rich text for extending this study's analysis of seeing and suffering.[2] The women characters in these poems written for annuals are paired with plates, visual representations of the speakers and their contexts. However, Hemans's and Landon's collections—published several decades later than Wollstonecraft's and Smith's literature, but between the two texts by Mary Shelley that I analyze—seem less a map for social change than a record of despair. In the post-Napoleonic period, it no longer felt inevitable that making suffering visible would be enough to inspire the social improvement necessary to relieve that suffering. Building on several of the rhetorical strategies and formal innovations highlighted in this study, this later literature has a different emotional tenor that perhaps does its own cultural work. Although these later works suggest that the late-eighteenth-century optimism for social reform could not be sustained based on the terms outlined in this study, it is worth remembering that there was a historical moment in which seeing suffering implied social change.

---

2 Landon's 41-page *Subjects for Pictures* was published in Laman Blanchard, *Life and Literary Remains of L.E.L.*, 2 vols., London: Colburn, 1841.

Bibliography

Abrams, M. H. *The Mirror and the Lamp*. Oxford: Oxford University Press, 1953.

Adams, Joseph. *Inquiry into the Laws of Epidemics; with Remarks on the Plans Lately Proposed for Exterminating the Small-Pox*. London: J. Johnson, 1809.

Aiken, John. *An Essay on the Application of Natural History to Poetry*. London: J. Johnson, 1777.

Aiken, John, and Anna Letitia Aiken. "An Inquiry into Those Kinds of Distress which Excite Agreeable Sensations." *Miscellaneous Pieces in Prose, by J. and A. L. Aikin*. Belfast: James Magee, 1774. 93–105.

Aiken, John, and Anna Letitia Barbauld. *Evenings at Home; Or, the Juvenile Budget Opened: Consisting of a Variety of Miscellaneous Pieces for The Instruction and Amusement of Young Persons*. 2nd edition. Vols. 4 and 5. London: J. Johnson, 1796, 1798. 6 vols.

Albert, Daniel M., and Diane D. Edwards, eds. *The History of Ophthalmology*. Cambridge, MA: Blackwell Science, 1996.

Andrew, Donna T. *Philanthropy and Police: London Charity in the Eighteenth Century*. Princeton: Princeton University Press, 1989.

Andrews, Malcolm. *The Search for the Picturesque: Landscape Aesthetics and Tourism in Britain, 1760–1800*. Stanford: Stanford University Press, 1989.

Annals of Natural History; Or, Magazine of Zoology, Botany, and Geology. Eds. Sir W. Jardine, P. J. Selby, Dr. Johnston, Sir W. J. Hooker, and Richard Taylor. Vol. 1. London: R. and J. E. Taylor, 1838.

Anonymous. *Identities Ascertained; Or, an Illustration of Mr. Ware's Opinion Respecting the Sameness of Infection in Venereal Gonorrhoea, and the Ophthalmia of Egypt: With an Examination of Affinity between Antient Leprosy and Lues*. London: J. Callow, 1808.

Arrington, George E. *A History of Ophthalmology*. New York: MD Publications, 1959.

Averill, James H. *Wordsworth and the Poetry of Human Suffering*. Ithaca: Cornell University Press, 1980.

Ball, John Clement. "Imperial Monstrosities: 'Frankenstein,' the West Indies, and V. S. Naipaul." *ARIEL* 32.3 (July 2001): 31–58.

Barker-Benfield, G. J. *The Culture of Sensibility: Sex and Society in Eighteenth-Century Britain*. Chicago: University of Chicago Press, 1992.

Barthes, Roland. "Image, raison, déraison." *Univers de l'Encyclopedie*. Eds. Roland Barthes, Robert Mauzi, and Jean-Pierre Seguin. Paris: Les Libraires Associés, 1964.

Batra, Nandita. "Animal Rights in the Romantic Period: Legal Jurisdiction in England and the Intellectual Milieu." *Atenea* 15.1–2 (1996): 99–113.

Batten, Guinn. *The Orphaned Imagination: Melancholy and Commodity Culture in English Romanticism*. Durham: Duke University Press, 1998.

Behar, Ruth, and Deborah A. Gordon, eds. *Women Writing Culture.* Berkeley: University of California Press, 1995.

Bentham, Jeremy. *An Introduction to the Principles and Morals of Legislation.* Eds. J. H. Burns and H. L. A. Hart. London: University of London, Athlone Press, 1970.

Berkeley, George. *Philosophical Works: Including the Works on Vision.* Ed. M. R. Ayers. London: Everyman's Library, 1975.

Bermingham, Ann. "System, Order, and Abstraction: The Politics of English Landscape Drawing around 1795." *Landscape and Power.* Ed. W. J. T. Mitchell. Chicago: University of Chicago Press, 1994. 77–101.

Bewell, Alan. *Romanticism and Colonial Disease.* Baltimore: Johns Hopkins University Press, 1999.

Black, Jeremy. *The British Abroad: The Grand Tour in the Eighteenth Century.* New York: St. Martin's Press, 1992.

Blake, William. Letter to Reverend Dr. Trusler, August 23, 1799. *The Complete Prose and Poetry of William Blake.* Ed. David V. Erdman. Rev. ed. Garden City, NJ: Doubleday, 1982. 702.

Bloom, Allan. Intro. *Emile or On Education.* By Jean-Jacques Rousseau. New York: Basic Books, 1979. 3–29.

Boerhaave, Herman. *Aphorisms: Concerning the Knowledge and Cure of Diseases* (1735). *The Nature of Melancholy from Aristotle to Kristeva.* Ed. Jennifer Radden. New York: Oxford University Press, 2000. 173–80.

Bohls, Elizabeth A. "Standards of Taste, Discourses of 'Race,' and the Aesthetic Education of a Monster: Critique of Empire in *Frankenstein.*" *Eighteenth-Century Life* 18 (November 1994): 23–36.

———. *Women Travel Writers and the Language of Aesthetics, 1716–1818.* Cambridge: Cambridge University Press, 1995.

Bostetter, E. E. *The Romantic Ventriloquists: Wordsworth, Coleridge, Keats, Shelley, Byron.* Seattle: University of Washington Press, 1963.

Braun, Julius, M.D. *On the Curative Effects of Baths and Waters, Being a Handbook to the Spas of Europe.* Ed. Hermann Weber, M.D. London: Smith, Elder, and Co., 1875.

Brennan, Matthew. *Wordsworth, Turner, and Romantic Landscape: A Study of the Traditions of the Picturesque and Sublime.* Columbia, SC: Camden House, 1987.

Brontë, Charlotte. *Villette.* London: Penguin Classics, 2004.

Brown, John. *The Elements of Medicine of John Brown, M.D. Translated from the Latin, with Comments and Illustrations, by the Author 1786. A New Edition, Revised and Corrected with a Biographical Preface by Thomas Beddoes, M.D.* London: J. Johnson, 1795.

Brownlee, Peter. "'The Economy of the Eyes': Ophthalmology and the Formation of the Modern Observer in Antebellum America." Unpublished paper presented to the McNeil Center for Early American Studies Seminar Series, College of Physicians of Philadelphia. 31 October 2003.

Buchan, William. "Cautions Concerning Cold Bathing and Drinking the Mineral Waters." *Domestic Medicine.* 9th ed. London: A. Strahan and T. Cadell, 1786.

————. *Domestic Medicine: Or, a Treatise on the Prevention and Cure of Diseases by Regimen and Simple Medicines*. 16th ed. London: A. Strahan and T. Cadell and W. Davies, 1798.

Burgess, Thomas. *Moral Annals of the Poor, and Middle Ranks of Society, in Various Situations of Good and Bad Conduct*. Durham: L. Pennington, 1793.

Burke, Edmund. *A Philosophical Enquiry into the Origin of Our Ideas of the Sublime and Beautiful*. Ed. James T. Boulton. Notre Dame: Notre Dame University Press, 1968.

Burton, Robert. *The Anatomy of Melancholy* (1621). Eds. Thomas C. Faulkner, Nicolas K. Kiessling, and Rhonda L. Blair. 6 vols. Oxford: Clarendon Press, 1989.

Bush, Donald. "Monstrosity and Representation in the Postcolonial Diaspora: *The Satanic Verses*, *Ulysses*, and *Frankenstein*." *Borders, Exiles, Diasporas*. Eds. Elazar Barkan and Marie-Denise Shelton. Stanford: Stanford University Press, 1998. 234–56.

Buzard, James. *Disorienting Fiction: The Autoethnographic Work of Nineteenth-Century British Novels*. Princeton: Princeton University Press, 2005.

Caldwell, Janis McLarren. "Sympathy and Science in *Frankenstein*." *The Ethics in Literature*. Eds. Andrew Hadfield, Dominic Rainsford, and Tim Woods. New York: St. Martin's Press, 1999. 262–74.

Caruth, Cathy. *Unclaimed Experience: Trauma, Narrative, and History*. Baltimore: Johns Hopkins University Press, 1996.

Chambers, John. *A Pocket Herbal: Containing the Medicinal Virtues and Uses of the Most Esteemed Native Plants; with Some Remarks on Bathing, Electricity, &c.* Bury: P. Gedge, 1800.

Cheyne, George. *The English Malady: Or, a Treatise of Nervous Diseases of All Kinds, as Spleen, Vapours, Lowness of Spirits, Hypochondriacal, and Hysterical Distempers, &c.* London: G. Strahan, 1733.

Clarke, Norma. "'The Cursed Barbauld Crew': Women Writers and Writing for Children in the Late Eighteenth Century." *Opening the Nursery Door: Reading, Writing and Childhood 1600–1900*. Eds. Mary Hilton, Morag Styles, and Victor Watson. London: Routledge, 1997. 91–103.

Clarkson, Thomas. *The History and the Rise, Progress, and Accomplishment of the Abolition of the African Slave-Trade, by the British Parliament*. 3 vols. New York: John S. Taylor, 1836.

Clemit, Pamela. "Charlotte Smith to William and Mary Jane Godwin: Five Holograph Letters." *Keats-Shelley Journal* 55 (2006): 29–40.

Coleridge, Samuel Taylor. Introduction to *Sonnets* by William Lisle Bowles (1796). *The Complete Poetical Works of Samuel Taylor Coleridge*. Ed. Hartley Coleridge. 2 vols. Oxford: Clarendon Press, 1912. 1139–40.

Conger, Syndy McMillen. "The Sorrows of Young Charlotte: Werther's English Sisters 1785–1805." *Goethe Yearbook* 3 (1986): 21–56.

Cooper, Christine M. "Reading the Politics of Abortion: Mary Wollstonecraft Revisited." *Eighteenth-Century Fiction* 16.4 (2004): 735–82.

Crompton, Louis. *Byron and Greek Love: Homophobia in Nineteenth-Century England*. Berkeley: University of California Press, 1985.

Crook, Nora. "'Meek and Bold': Mary Shelley's Support for the Risorgimento." *Mary Versus Mary.* Eds. Lilla Maria Crisafulli and Giovanna Silvani. Naples: Ligouri, 2001. 73–88.

———. "Pecksie and the Elf: Did the Shelleys Couple Romantically?" *Romanticism On the Net* 18 (May 2000) [4 November 2005] <http://users.ox.ac.uk/~scat0385/18crook.html>

Cruickshank, Joanna. "'Appear as Crucified for Me:' Sight, Suffering, and Spiritual Transformation in the Hymns of Charles Wesley." *Journal of Religious History* 30.3 (Oct. 2006): 311–30.

Curran, Stuart. "Charlotte Smith and British Romanticism." *South Central Review* 11.2 (Summer 1994): 64–78.

———. General introduction to *The Works of Charlotte Smith.* Vol. 1. London: Pickering and Chatto, 2005. vii–xxvii.

Daffron, Eric. "Male Bonding: Sympathy and Shelley's *Frankenstein.*" *Nineteenth-Century Contexts* 21 (1999): 415–35.

Davidson, Luke. "'Identities Ascertained': British Ophthalmology in the First Half of the Nineteenth Century." *The Society for the Social History of Medicine* 9.3 (1996): 313–33.

Dayes, Edward. *The Works of the Late Edward Dayes.* London: T. Maiden, 1805.

de Bolla, Peter. *The Discourse of the Sublime: Readings in History, Aesthetics and the Subject.* Oxford: Basil Blackwell, 1989.

de Certeau, Michel. *The Practice of Everyday Life.* Trans. Steven F. Rendall. Berkeley: University of California Press, 1984.

de Man, Paul. *The Rhetoric of Romanticism.* New York: Columbia University Press, 1984.

Descriptive Poetry: Being a Selection from the Best Modern Authors: Principally Having Reference to Subjects in Natural History. London: W. Savage, 1807.

Dolan, Elizabeth A. (as Beth Dolan Kautz). "Movement, Melancholia, and Madness: American and British Health Travelers in Post-Napoleonic Europe." *Revolutions and Watersheds: Transatlantic Dialogues 1775–1815.* Eds. W. M. Verhoeven and Beth Dolan Kautz. Amsterdam: Rodopi Press, 1999. 39–57.

———. "Spas and Salutary Landscapes: The Geography of Health in Mary Shelley's *Rambles in Germany and Italy.*" *Romantic Geographies: Discourses of Travel 1775–1844.* Ed. Amanda Gilroy. Manchester: Manchester University Press, 2000. 165–81.

Edmondston, Arthur. *A Treatise on the Varieties and Consequences of Ophthalmia. With a Preliminary Inquiry into its Contagious Nature.* London: Longman, Hurst, Rees, and Orme, 1806.

"Rev. of *Elegiac Sonnets, and Other Poems*, Vol. 2, by Charlotte Smith." *The Critical Review* 21 (1797): 149–51.

"Rev. of *Elegiac Sonnets, and Other Poems*, Vol. 2, by Charlotte Smith." *The Monthly Review* 24 (1797): 458–59.

Ellis, Carolyn, and Arthur P. Bochner. "Autoethnography, Personal Narrative, Reflexivity: Researcher as Subject." *Handbook of Qualitative Research.* 2nd ed. Eds. Normal K. Denzin and Yvonna S. Lincoln. Thousand Oaks, CA: Sage Publications, 2000. 733–68.

Ender, Evelyne. *Sexing the Mind: Nineteenth-Century Fictions of Hysteria*. Ithaca: Cornell University Press, 1995.

Erle, Sibylle. "Face to Face with Johann Caspar Lavater." *Literature Compass* 2:1 (2005). <http://www.blackwell-compass.com>

Everett, Nigel. *The Tory View of Landscape*. New Haven: Yale University Press, 1994.

Favret, Mary A. "*Letters Written During a Short Residence in Sweden, Norway and Denmark*: Traveling with Mary Wollstonecraft." *The Cambridge Companion to Mary Wollstonecraft*. Ed. Claudia Johnson. Cambridge: Cambridge University Press, 2002. 209–27.

———. *Romantic Correspondence: Women, Politics and the Fiction of Letters*. Cambridge: Cambridge University Press, 1993.

Fawcett, Benjamin. *Observations on the Nature, Causes, and Cure of Melancholy: Especially of That Which is Commonly Called Religious Melancholy*. London: J. Buckland and T. Longman, 1780.

Fay, Elizabeth A. *Becoming Wordsworthian: A Performative Aesthetics*. Amherst: University of Massachusetts Press, 1995.

Feibel, R. M. "John Vetch and the Egyptian Ophthalmia." *Surv. Ophthalmol.* 28.2 (1983): 128–34.

Fergus, Jan. "'My Sore-Throats, You Know, Are Always Worse Than Anybody's': Mary Musgrove and Jane Austen's Art of Whining." *Jane Austen's Business: Her World and Her Profession*. Ed. Juliet McMaster and Bruce Stovel. New York: Macmillan Press, 1996. 69–80.

Ferguson, Moira. *Animal Advocacy and Englishwomen, 1780–1900: Patriots, Nation, and Empire*. Ann Arbor: University of Michigan Press, 1998.

Fletcher, Loraine. *Charlotte Smith: A Critical Biography*. Basingstoke: Palgrave, 2001.

Foucault, Michel. *The Foucault Reader*. Ed. Paul Rabinow. New York: Pantheon Books, 1984.

———. *The Order of Things: An Archaeology of the Human Sciences*. New York: Vintage Books, 1994.

Frank, Arthur W. *The Wounded Storyteller: Body, Illness, and Ethics*. Chicago: University of Chicago Press, 1995.

Fyfe, Aileen. "Reading Children's Books in Late Eighteenth-Century Dissenting Families." *The Historical Journal* 43.2 (2000): 453–73.

Galperin, William H. *The Return of the Visible in British Romanticism*. Baltimore: Johns Hopkins University Press, 1993.

Gill, Stephen. *William Wordsworth: A Life*. Oxford: Clarendon Press, 1989.

Gilligan, Carol. *In a Different Voice*. Cambridge: Harvard University Press, 1982.

Gilman, Sander. *Seeing the Insane*. Lincoln, NE: University of Nebraska, 1982.

Gilpin, William. *Observations, on Several Parts of England, Particularly the Mountains and Lakes of Cumberland and Westmoreland, Relative Chiefly to Picturesque Beauty, Made in the Year 1772*. London, 1792.

———. *Observations on the River Wye* (1782). Oxford: Woodstock Books, 1991.

———. *Three Essays: On Picturesque Beauty: On Picturesque Travel: And on Sketching Landscape: With a Poem, on Landscape Painting*. 3rd ed. London: T. Cadell and W. Davis, 1808.

Gisborne, Thomas. *An Enquiry into the Duties of the Female Sex.* Philadelphia: James Humphreys, 1798.

Godwin, William. *Enquiry Concerning Political Justice.* Ed. K. Codell Carter. Oxford: Clarendon Press, 1971.

Goldsmith, Oliver. "The Traveller, or A Prospect of Society." *The Poems of Thomas Gray, William Collins, Oliver Goldsmith.* Ed. Roger Lonsdale. London: Longmans, Green and Co., 1969. 632–56.

Goldsmith, Steven. *Unbuilding Jerusalem: Apocalypse and Romantic Representation.* Ithaca: Cornell University Press, 1993.

Good, Byron J. *Medicine, Rationality, and Experience: An Anthropological Perspective.* Cambridge: Cambridge University Press, 1994.

Gordon, Lyndall. *Vindication: A Life of Mary Wollstonecraft.* New York: Harper Collins, 2005.

Gorin, George. *History of Ophthalmology.* Wilmington: Publish or Perish, 1982.

Granville, Augustus Bozzi. *The Spas of Germany.* 2nd ed. London: Henry Colburn, 1838.

Gray, Thomas. "Ode on a Distant Prospect of Eton College." *The Poems of Gray and Collins.* Ed. Austin Lane Poole. London: Oxford University Press, 1966. 29–35.

Grenby, M. O. "'Real Charity Makes Distinctions': Schooling the Charitable Impulse in Early British Children's Literature." *British Journal for Eighteenth-Century Studies* 25 (2002): 185–202.

Haigh, Sam. "Ethnographical Fictions/Fictional Ethnographies: Ina Césaire's *Zonzon Tête Carrée.*" *Nottingham French Studies* 40.1 (2001): 75–85.

Hall, Jason Y. "Gall's Phrenology: A Romantic Psychology." *Studies in Romanticism* 16 (1977): 305–17.

Hammond, J. L., and Barbara Hammond. *The Village Labourer 1760–1832: A Study in the Government of England before the Reform Bill.* London: Longmans, Green, and Co., 1920.

Haraway, Donna J. "Situated Knowledges: The Science Question in Feminism and the Privilege of Partial Perspective." *Simians, Cyborgs, and Women: The Reinvention of Nature.* New York: Routledge, 1991. 183–201.

Harrison, Faye V. "Writing Against the Grain: Cultural Politics of Difference in the Work of Alice Walker." *Women Writing Culture.* Eds. Ruth Behar and Deborah A. Gordon. Berkeley: University of California Press, 1995. 233–45.

Hartley, David. *Hartley's Theory of the Human Mind, on the Principle of the Association of Ideas; with Essays Relating to the Subject of It.* Ed. Joseph Priestley. 2nd ed. London: J. Johnson, 1790.

Hartman, Geoffrey H. "A Poet's Progress: Wordsworth and the *Via Naturaliter Negativa.*" *The Prelude 1799, 1805, 1850.* Eds. Jonathan Wordsworth, M. H. Abrams, and Stephen Gill. New York: Norton, 1979. 598–613.

Hastings, R. P. *Poverty and the Poor Law in the North Riding of Yorkshire, c. 1780–1837.* Leeds: Borthwick Papers, 1982.

Hawley, Judith. "Charlotte Smith's *Elegiac Sonnets*: Losses and Gains." *Women's Poetry of the Enlightenment, The Making of a Canon, 1730–1820.* Eds. Isobel Armstrong and Virginia Blain. New York: St. Martin's Press, 1999. 184–98.

Hayden, John. "Wordsworth, Hartley, and the Revisionists." *Studies in Philology* 81.1 (1984): 94–118.

Heilbrun, Carolyn G. *Writing a Woman's Life*. New York: Ballantine Books, 1988.

Heinroth, Johann Christian. *Textbook of Disturbances of Mental Life: Or Disturbances of the Soul and Their Treatment*. Trans. J. Schmorak. 2 vols. Baltimore: Johns Hopkins University Press, 1975.

Heydt-Stevenson, Jill. "Liberty, Connection, and Tyranny: The Novels of Jane Austen and the Aesthetic Movement of the Picturesque." *Lessons of Romanticism: A Critical Companion*. Eds. Thomas Pfau and Robert F. Gleckner. Durham: Duke University Press, 1998. 261–79.

The History of Little Good Two-Shoes; Otherwise Called, Mrs. Margery Two-Shoes. Attrib. to either Oliver Goldsmith or Giles Johns. London: T. Carnan and F. Newberry, 1772.

Hoeveler, Diane Long. "Fantasy, Trauma, and Gothic Daughters: *Frankenstein* as Therapy." *Prism(s): Essays in Romanticism* 8 (2000): 7–28.

——. "Reading the Wound: Wollstonecraft's *Wrongs of Woman, or Maria* and Trauma Theory." *Studies in the Novel* 31.4 (1999): 387–408.

——. "The Secularization of Suffering: Toward a Theory of Gothic Subjectivity." *The Wordsworth Circle* 35.3 (2004): 113–17.

Ingham, Patricia Clare. "Romancing Troy: Trauma, Desire, and the Problem of History." MLA Presentation. 27 December 2005.

Johnson, Claudia L. *Equivocal Beings: Politics, Gender, and Sentimentality in the 1790s: A Study of Wollstonecraft, Burney, and Austen*. Chicago: University of Chicago Press, 1995.

——. "Mary Wollstonecraft's Novels." *The Cambridge Companion to Mary Wollstonecraft*. Cambridge: Cambridge University Press, 2002. 189–208.

Johnson, James. *Change of Air, or the Philosophy of Travelling; Being Autumnal Excursions Through France, Switzerland, Italy, Germany, and Belgium; With Observations and Reflections on the Moral, Physical, and Medicinal Influences of Travelling-Exercise, Change of Scene, Foreign Skies, and Voluntary Expatriation. To Which Is Prefixed, Wear and Tear of Modern Babylon*. London: S. Highley, 1831.

Jones, Angela D. "'When a Woman So Far Outsteps Her Proper Sphere': Counter-Romantic Tourism." *Women's Life Writing: Finding Voice/Building Community*. Ed. Linda S. Colman. Bowling Green, OH: Bowling Green State University Press, 1997. 209–37.

Jones, Chris. *Radical Sensibility: Literature and Ideas in the 1790s*. London: Routledge, 1993.

Jones, Vivien. "Placing Jemima: Women Writers of the 1790s and the Eighteenth-Century Prostitution Narrative." *Women's Writing: The Elizabethan to Victorian Period* 4.2 (1997): 201–20.

Jordan, Elaine. "Criminal Conversation: Mary Wollstonecraft's *The Wrongs of Woman*." *Women's Writing* 4.2 (1997): 221–34.

Keats, John. "Ode to a Nightingale." *The Poems of John Keats*. Ed. Jack Stillinger. Cambridge, MA: Harvard University Press, 1978. 369–72.

Kelley, Theresa M. "Romantic Exemplarity: Botany and 'Material' Culture." *Romantic Science: The Literary Forms of Natural History*. Ed. Noah Heringman. Albany: State University of New York Press, 2003. 223–54.

———. *Wordsworth's Revisionary Aesthetics*. Cambridge: Cambridge University Press, 1988.

Kelly, Gary. *The English Jacobin Novel, 1780–1805*. Oxford: Clarendon Press, 1976.

———. "Politicizing the Personal: Mary Wollstonecraft, Mary Shelley, and the Coterie Novel." *Mary Shelley in Her Times*. Eds. Betty T. Bennett and Stuart Curran. Baltimore: Johns Hopkins University Press, 2000. 147–59.

———. *Revolutionary Feminism: The Mind and Career of Mary Wollstonecraft*. New York: St. Martin's Press, 1996.

Kharbutli, Mahmoud. "Locke and Wordsworth." *Forum for Modern Language Studies* 25.3 (1989): 225–37.

King, Steven. *Poverty and Welfare in England, 1700–1850: A Regional Perspective*. Manchester: Manchester University Press, 2000.

Kipp, Julie. *Romanticism, Maternity and the Body Politic*. Cambridge: Cambridge University Press, 2003.

Komisaruk, Adam. "The Privatization of Pleasure: 'CRIM. CON.' in Wollstonecraft's *Maria*." *Law and Literature* 16.1 (2004): 33–63.

Kristeva, Julia. "Stabet Mater." *The Kristeva Reader*. Ed. Toril Moi. New York: Columbia University Press, 1986. 160–86.

Kromm, Jane. "*Olivia furiosa*: Maniacal Women from Richardson to Wollstonecraft." *Eighteenth-Century Fiction* 16.3 (2004): 343–72.

Kuczynski, Ingrid. "'Only by the Eye'—Visual Perception in Women's Travel Writing in the 1790s." *Mary Wollstonecraft's Journey to Scandinavia: Essays*. Eds. Anka Ryall and Catherine Sandbach-Dahlström. Stockholm: Almqvist and Wiksell International, 2003. 25–52.

Kuhnke, Laverne. "Early Nineteenth-Century Ophthalmological Clinics in Egypt." *Clio Medica* 7.3 (1972): 209–21.

Labbe, Jacqueline M. *Charlotte Smith: Romanticism, Poetry and the Culture of Gender*. Manchester: Manchester University Press, 2003.

———. *Romantic Visualities: Landscape, Gender and Romanticism*. New York: St. Martin's Press, 1998.

———. "Selling One's Sorrows: Charlotte Smith, Mary Robinson, and the Marketing of Poetry." *The Wordsworth Circle* 25.2 (1994): 68–71.

———. "'Transplanted into More Congenial Soil': Footnoting the Self in the Poetry of Charlotte Smith." *Mar(k)ing the Text: The Presentation of Meaning on the Literary Page*. Eds. Joe Bray, Miriam Handley, and Anne C. Henry. Aldershot: Ashgate Press, 2000. 71–86.

Lamb, Jonathan. "Hartley and Wordsworth: Philosophical Language and Figures of the Sublime." *Modern Language Notes* 97 (1982): 1064–85.

Landry, Donna. "Green Languages? Women Poets as Naturalists in 1653 and 1807." *Forging Connections: Women's Poetry from the Renaissance to Romanticism*. Eds. Anne K. Mellor, Felicity Nussbaum, and Jonathan F. S. Post. San Marino, CA: Huntington Library, 2002. 39–61.

Langbauer, Laurie. "An Early Romance: Motherhood and Women's Writing in Mary Wollstonecraft's Novels." *Romanticism and Feminism*. Ed. Anne Mellor. Bloomington: Indiana University Press, 1988. 208–19.

Larrissy, Edward. *The Blind and Blindness in Literature of the Romantic Period.* Edinburgh: Edinburgh University Press, 2007.

Lavater, Johann Casper. *Essays on Physiognomy*. 3 vols. Trans. Thomas Holcroft. London: G. G. J. and J. Robinson, 1789.

Lawrence, Karen R. *Penelope Voyages: Women and Travel in the British Literary Tradition*. Ithaca: Cornell University Press, 1994.

Leask, Nigel. "Shelley's 'Magnetic Ladies': Romantic Mesmerism and the Politics of the Body." *Beyond Romanticism: New Approaches to Texts and Contexts, 1780–1832*. Ed. Stephen Copley. Syracuse: Syracuse University Press, 1991. 53–78.

Lee, Debbie. *Slavery and the Romantic Imagination*. Philadelphia: University of Pennsylvania Press, 2002.

Leinhardt, Godfrey. *Divinity and Experience: The Religion of the Dinka*. New York: Oxford University Press, 1961.

Rev. of *Letters of a Solitary Wanderer* by Charlotte Smith. *The Critical Review* 32 (May 1801): 35–42.

Lev, E. and E. Dolev. "Use of Natural Substances in the Treatment of Renal Stones and Other Urinary Disorders in the Medieval Levant." *American Journal of Nephrology* 22 (2002): 172–79.

Lew, Joseph W. "The Deceptive Other: Mary Shelley's Critique of Orientalism in *Frankenstein*." *Studies in Romanticism* 30 (Summer 1991): 255–83.

Liu, Alan. "The Politics of the Picturesque." *Wordsworth: The Sense of History*. Stanford: Stanford University Press, 1989. 61–137.

Lloyd, Genevieve. *The Man of Reason: "Male" and "Female" in Western Philosophy*. Minneapolis: University of Minnesota Press, 1984.

Logan, Peter. *Nerves and Narratives: A Cultural History of Hysteria in Nineteenth-Century British Prose*. Berkeley: University of California Press, 1997.

Lokke, Kari E. "'The Mild Dominion of the Moon': Charlotte Smith and the Politics of Transcendence." *Rebellious Hearts: British Women Writers and the French Revolution*. Eds. Adriana Craciun and Kari E. Lokke. Albany: State University of New York Press, 2001. 85–106.

London Times. 23 Sept. 1806: 3. 26 Sept. 1806: 2. 14 March 1808: 3. 2 April 1816: 3.

Lynch, Deidre Shauna. *The Economy of Character: Novels, Market Culture, and the Business of Inner Meaning*. Chicago: University of Chicago Press, 1998.

Malchow, H. L. "Frankenstein's Monster and Images of Race in Nineteenth-Century Britain." *Past and Present* 139 (May 1993): 90–130.

Malekin, Peter. "Wordsworth and the Mind of Man." *An Infinite Complexity: Essays in Romanticism*. Edinburgh: Edinburgh University Press, 1983. 1–25.

Mandeville, Bernard. *A Treatise of the Hypochondriack and Hysteric Passions, Vulgarly Call'd the Hypo in Men and Vapours in Women*. London: Dryden Leach and W. Taylor, 1711.

Marriott, John, and Masaie Matsumura, eds. *The Metropolitan Poor: Semifictional Accounts, 1795–1910*. Vol. 1. London: Pickering and Chatto, 1999. 6 vols.

Martin, Emily. *Flexible Bodies: The Role of Immunity in American Culture from the Days of Polio to the Age of AIDS.* Boston: Beacon Press, 1994.

Matthews, S. Leigh. "(Un)Confinements: The Madness of Motherhood in Mary Wollstonecraft's *The Wrongs of Woman.*" *Mary Wollstonecraft and Mary Shelley: Writing Lives.* Eds. Helen M. Buss, D. L. Macdonald, and Anne McWhir. Waterloo: Wilfrid Laurier University Press, 2001. 85–97.

Mavor, William. *The Lady and Gentleman's Botanical Pocket Book; Adapted to Withering's Arrangements of British Plants. Intended to Facilitate and Promote the Study of Indigenous Botany.* London: Joseph Banks, 1800.

McCarthy, William. "Mother of All Discourses: Anna Barbauld's *Lessons for Children.*" *The Princeton University Library Chronicle* 60 (1999): 196–219.

McGann, Jerome. *The Poetics of Sensibility: A Revolution in Literary Style.* Oxford: Clarendon Press, 1996.

McGonegal, Julie. "Of Harlots and Housewives: A Feminist Materialist Critique of the Writings of Wollstonecraft." *Women's Writing* 11.3 (2004): 347–62.

McGrew, Roderick E., and Margaret P. McGrew. *Encyclopedia of Medical History.* New York: McGraw-Hill, 1985.

Mellor, Anne K. "A Novel of Their Own: Women's Fiction, 1790–1830." *Columbia History of the British Novel.* Ed. John Richetti. New York: Columbia University Press, 1994. 327–51.

———. "*Frankenstein*, Racial Science and the Yellow Peril." *Nineteenth-Century Contexts* 23 (2001): 1–28.

———. "Possessing Nature: The Female in *Frankenstein.*" *Romanticism and Feminism.* Ed. Anne K. Mellor. Bloomington: Indiana University Press, 1988. 220–32.

Miall, David S. "'I See It Feelingly': Coleridge's Debt to Hartley." *Coleridge's Visionary Languages.* Eds. Tim Fulford and Morton D. Paley. Cambridge: D. S. Brewer, 1993. 151–63.

Michaelson, Patricia Howell. "*The Wrongs of Woman* as a Feminist *Amelia.*" *The Journal of Narrative Technique* 21.3 (1991): 250–61.

Minois, George. *History of Suicide: Voluntary Death in Western Culture.* Trans. Lydia G. Cochrane. Baltimore: Johns Hopkins University Press, 1999.

Mitchell, W. J. T. "Visible Language: Blake's Wond'rous Art of Writing." *Romanticism and Contemporary Criticism.* Eds. Morris Eaves and Michael Fischer. Ithaca: Cornell University Press, 1986. 46–95.

More, Hannah. *Strictures of the Modern System of Female Education; with a View of the Principles and Conduct Prevalent Among Women of Rank and Fortune.* (1799). *The Complete Works of Hannah More.* Vol. 6. New York: Harper and Brothers, 1835. 1–265. 7 vols.

Morris, David. "The Plot of Suffering." *Illness and Culture in the Postmodern Age.* Berkeley: University of California Press, 1998. 190–217.

Morton, A. G. *History of Botanical Science: An Account of the Development of Botany from Ancient Times to the Present Day.* London: Academic Press, 1981.

Moskal, Jeanne. "Gender and Italian Nationalism in Mary Shelley's *Rambles in Germany and Italy.*" *Romanticism* 5.2 (1999): 188–201.

————. "Introductory Note." *Rambles in Germany and Italy*. Jeanne Moskal, ed. *Travel Writing*. Vol. 8 of *The Novels and Selected Works of Mary Shelley*. Gen. ed. Nora Crook, with Pamela Clemit. London: Pickering and Chatto, 1996. 49–57.

————. "Mary Shelley's *Rambles in Germany and Italy* and the Discourses of Race and National Manners." *La questione romantica; rivista interdisciplinare di studi romantici* 3–4 (1997): 205–12.

————. "The Picturesque and the Affectionate in Wollstonecraft's *Letters from Norway*." *Modern Language Quarterly* 52.3 (1991): 263–94.

————. "Speaking the Unspeakable: Art Criticism as Life Writing in Mary Shelley's *Rambles in Germany and Italy*." *Mary Wollstonecraft and Mary Shelley: Writing Lives*. Eds. Helen M. Buss, D. L. Macdonald, and Anne McWhir. Waterloo: Wilfrid Laurier University Press, 2001. 189–216.

————. "Travel Writing." *The Cambridge Companion to Mary Shelley*. Ed. Esther Schor. Cambridge: Cambridge University Press, 2003. 242–58.

Murray, Charlotte. *The British Garden. A Descriptive Catalogue of Hardy Plants, Indigenous or Cultivated in the Climate of Great-Britain. With Their Generic and Specific Characters, Latin and English Names, Native Country, and Time of Flowering. With Introductory Remarks*. 2 vols. Bath: S. Hazard, 1799.

Murray, E. B. "Shelley's Contribution to Mary's *Frankenstein*." *Keats-Shelley Memorial Bulletin* 19 (1978): 50–68.

Myers, Mitzi. "Impeccable Governesses, Rational Dames, and Moral Mothers: Mary Wollstonecraft and the Female Tradition in Georgian Children's Books." *Children's Literature* 14 (1986): 31–59.

————. "Little Girls Lost: Rewriting Romantic Childhood, Righting Gender and Genre." *Teaching Children's Literature: Issues, Pedagogy, Resources*. Ed. Glenn Edward Sadler. New York: Modern Language Association, 1992. 131–42.

————. "Pedagogy as Self-Expression in Mary Wollstonecraft: Exorcising the Past, Finding a Voice." *The Private Self: Theory and Practice of Women's Autobiographical Writings*. Ed. Shari Benstock. Chapel Hill: University of North Carolina Press, 1988. 192–210.

————. "Unfinished Business: Wollstonecraft's *Maria*." *The Wordsworth Circle* 11 (1980): 107–14.

Neff, D. S. "Hostages to Empire: The Anglo-Indian Problem in *Frankenstein, The Curse of Kehama*, and *The Missionary*." *European Romantic Review* 8.4 (1997): 386–408.

New General History of the World. 6 vols. London: W. Owen, 1762.

Newman, Gerald. *Britain in the Hanoverian Age, 1714–1837*. New York: Garland Publishing, 1997.

Nitchie, Elizabeth. "Mary Shelley, Traveler." *Keats-Shelley Journal* 10 (1961): 29–42.

O'Quinn, Daniel. "Trembling: Wollstonecraft, Godwin and the Resistance to Literature." *ELH* 64.3 (1997): 761–88.

Orr, Clarissa Campbell. "Mary Shelley's *Rambles in Germany and Italy*, the Celebrity Author, and the Undiscovered Country of the Human Heart." *Romanticism On the Net* 11 (August 1998) [4 November 2005] <http://users.ox.ac.uk/~scat0385/rambles.html>

Pascoe, Judith. "Female Botanists and the Poetry of Charlotte Smith." *Revisioning Romanticism, 1776–1837*. Eds. Carol Shiner Wilson and Joel Haefner. Philadelphia: University of Pennsylvania Press, 1994. 193–209.

Perkins, David. "Compassion for Animals and Radical Politics: Coleridge's "To a Young Ass." *ELH* 65.4 (1998): 929–44.

———. *Romanticism and Animal Rights*. Cambridge: Cambridge University Press, 2003.

Perry, Seamus. "Coleridge, Wordsworth, and Other Things." *The Wordsworth Circle* 29.1 (1998): 31–41.

Pinch, Adela. *Strange Fits of Passion: Epistemologies of Emotion, Hume to Austen*. Stanford: Stanford University Press, 1996.

Polwhele, Richard. *The Unsex'd Females: A Poem*. 1798. Intro. Gina Luria. New York: Garland Publishing, 1974.

Poovey, Mary. "Mary Wollstonecraft: The Gender of Genres in Late Eighteenth-Century England." *Novel: A Forum on Fiction* 15.2 (1982): 111–26.

———. *The Proper Lady and the Woman Writer: Ideology as Style in the Works of Mary Wollstonecraft, Mary Shelley, and Jane Austen*. Chicago: University of Chicago Press, 1984.

Pope, Alexander. "Eloisa to Abelard." *The Twickenham Edition of the Poems of Alexander Pope*. Gen. ed. John Butt. Vol 2. New Haven: Yale University Press, 1940. 291–349. 6 vols.

Porter, Roy. *Health for Sale: Quackery in England 1660–1850*. Manchester: Manchester University Press, 1989.

Poynter, J. R. *Society and Pauperism: English Ideas on Poor Relief, 1795–1834*. London: Routledge, 1969.

Pratt, Kathryn. "Charlotte Smith's Melancholia on the Page and Stage." *Studies in English Literature, 1500–1900* 41.3 (Summer 2001): 563–81.

Pratt, Mary Louise. *Imperial Eyes: Travel Writing and Transculturation*. London: Routledge, 1992.

Radcliffe, Ann. *The Mysteries of Udolpho*. Oxford: Oxford University Press, 1983.

Radden, Jennifer, ed. *The Nature of Melancholy from Aristotle to Kristeva*. New York: Oxford University Press, 2000.

Rajan, Tilottama. "Wollstonecraft and Godwin: Reading the Secrets of the Political Novel." *Studies in Romanticism* 27 (1988): 221–51.

"Rev. of *Rambles in Germany and Italy in 1840, 1842, and 1843*, by Mary Wollstonecraft Shelley." *The Athenaeum* (10 Aug. 1844): 725–27.

———. *The Critic* (2 Sept. 1844): 35–39.

———. *The Literary Examiner* (27 July 1844): 467–68.

———. *The Morning Chronicle* (23 August 1844): 3.

———. *Tait's Edinburgh Magazine* (11 Nov. 1844): 729–40.

Relihan, Constance C. *Cosmographical Glasses: Geographic Discourse, Gender, and Elizabethan Fiction*. Kent: Kent State University Press, 2004.

Richardson, Alan. *British Romanticism and the Science of the Mind*. Cambridge: Cambridge University Press, 2001.

———. "Romanticism and the Body." *Literature Compass* 1.1 (2004). <http://www.blackwell-compass.com>

Richey, William. "The Rhetoric of Sympathy in Smith and Wordsworth." *European Romantic Review* 13 (2002): 427–43.

Ridley, Glynis. "Injustice in the Works of Godwin and Wollstonecraft." *Women, Revolution, and the Novels of the 1790s.* Ed. Linda Lang-Peralta. East Lansing, MI: Michigan State University Press, 1999. 69–88.

Roach, John. *Social Reform in England, 1780–1880.* New York: St. Martin's Press, 1978.

Robbins, Sarah. "*Lessons for Children* and Teaching Mothers: Mrs. Barbauld's Primer for the Textual Construction of Middle-Class Domestic Pedagogy." *The Lion and the Unicorn* 17 (1993): 135–51.

Rose, Gillian. *Feminism and Geography: The Limits of Geographical Knowledge.* Minneapolis: University of Minnesota Press, 1993.

Rose, Michael E. *The English Poor Law 1780–1930.* New York: Barnes and Noble, 1971.

Rosen, George. *The Specialization of Medicine with Particular Reference to Ophthalmology* (1944). New York: Arno Press, 1972.

Ross, Marlon B. *The Contours of Masculine Desire: Romanticism and the Rise of Women's Poetry.* New York: Oxford University Press, 1989.

Rousseau, Jean-Jacques. *Emile or On Education.* Intro. and trans. Allan Bloom. New York: Basic Books, 1979.

———. *Letters on the Elements of Botany. Addressed to a Lady.* Trans. with notes and twenty-four additional letters by Thomas Martyn. 4th ed. London: B. and J. White, 1794.

———. *Reveries of the Solitary Wanderer.* Trans. and intro. by Peter France. Middlesex: Penguin, 1979.

Rev. of *Rural Walks* by Charlotte Smith. *The Analytical Review* 21 (1795): 548–49.

———. *The Critical Review* 18 (1796): 445–49.

———. *The Monthly Review* 17 (1795): 349–50.

———. *New Annual Register* 16 (1795): 283.

Ruwe, Donelle R. "Benevolent Brothers and Supervising Mothers: Ideology in the Children's Verses of Mary and Charles Lamb and Charlotte Smith." *Children's Literature* 25 (1997): 87–115.

———. "Charlotte Smith's Sublime: Feminine Poetics, Botany, and *Beachy Head*." *Prism(s): Essays in Romanticism* 7 (1999): 117–32.

Scarry, Elaine. *The Body in Pain: The Making and Unmaking of the World.* Oxford: Oxford University Press, 1985.

Schiebinger, Londa. *The Mind Has No Sex? Women in the Origins of Modern Science.* Cambridge, MA: Harvard University Press, 1989.

Schiesari, Juliana. *The Gendering of Melancholia: Feminism, Psychoanalysis, and the Symbolics of Loss in Renaissance Literature.* Ithaca: Cornell University Press, 1992.

Schor, Esther H. "Mary Shelley in Transit." *The Other Mary Shelley: Beyond Frankenstein.* Eds. Audrey A. Fisch, Anne K. Mellor, and Esther H. Schor. Oxford: Oxford University Press, 1993. 235–57.

Shakespeare, William. *The Life and Death of King John. The Riverside Shakespeare.* Ed. G. Blakemore Evans. Boston: Houghton Mifflin, 1974. 765–99.

Shelley, Mary. *The Journals of Mary Shelley: 1814–1844*. Eds. Paula R. Feldman and Diana Scott-Kilvert. Baltimore: Johns Hopkins University Press, 1987.

———. *The Letters of Mary Wollstonecraft Shelley*. Ed. Betty T. Bennett. 3 vols. Baltimore: Johns Hopkins University Press, 1980–1988.

———. *The Novels and Selected Works of Mary Shelley*. Gen. Ed. Nora Crook. 8 vols. London: Pickering and Chatto, 1996.

Sherman, Paul D. *Colour Vision in the Nineteenth Century: The Young-Helmhotz-Maxwell Theory*. Bristol: Adam Hilger, 1981.

Showalter, Elaine. *Hystories: Hysterical Epidemics and Modern Culture*. New York: Columbia University Press, 1997.

Shteir, Ann B. *Cultivating Women, Cultivating Science: Flora's Daughters and Botany in England 1760–1860*. Baltimore: Johns Hopkins University Press, 1996.

Sickles, Eleanor M. *The Gloomy Egoist: Moods and Themes of Melancholy from Gray to Keats*. New York: Columbia University Press, 1932.

Silverman, Kaja. *World Spectators*. Stanford: Stanford University Press, 2000.

Smith, Charlotte. *The Collected Letters of Charlotte Smith*. Ed. Judith Phillips Stanton. Indianapolis: Indiana University Press, 2003.

———. *The Poems of Charlotte Smith*. Ed. Stuart Curran. New York: Oxford University Press, 1993.

———. *The Works of Charlotte Smith*. Gen. ed. Stuart Curran. 14 vols. London: Pickering and Chatto, 2006–07.

Smyth, James Carmichael. *The Effect of the Nitrous Vapour in Preventing and Destroying Contagion; ... With an Introduction Respecting the Nature of Contagion, Which Gives Rise to the Jail or Hospital Fever*. Philadelphia: Thomas Dobson, 1799.

Spivak, Gayatri Chakravorty. "Three Women's Texts and a Critique of Imperialism." *Critical Inquiry* 12 (Autumn 1985): 243–61.

Stanton, Judith Phillips. "Charlotte Smith and 'Mr. Monstroso': An Eighteenth-Century Marriage in Life and Fiction." *Women's Writing* 7.1 (2000): 7–22.

———. "Charlotte Smith's 'Literary Business.'" *The Age of Johnson* 1 (1987): 375–401.

St. Clair, William. *The Reading Nation in the Romantic Period*. Cambridge: Cambridge University Press, 2004.

Sterne, Laurence. *A Sentimental Journey Through France and Italy.* (1768). Ed. Graham Petrie. London: Penguin Books, 1987.

Sullivan, Zohreh T. "Race, Gender, and Imperial Ideology in the Nineteenth Century." *Nineteenth-Century Contexts* 13.1 (Spring 1989): 19–31.

Sunstein, Emily. *Mary Shelley: Romance and Reality*. Baltimore: Johns Hopkins University Press, 1989.

Swaab, Peter. "Romantic Self-Representation: The Example of Mary Wollstonecraft's *Letters in Sweden.*" *Mortal Pages, Literary Lives: Studies in Nineteenth-Century Autobiography*. Eds. Vincent Newey and Philip Shaw. Aldershot, UK: Scolar Press, 1996. 13–30.

Tauchert, Ashley. *Mary Wollstonecraft and the Accent of the Feminine*. New York: Palgrave, 2002.

Taylor, Barbara. *Mary Wollstonecraft and the Feminist Imagination*. Cambridge: Cambridge University Press, 2003.

Tedlock, Barbara. "Ethnography and Ethnographic Representation." *Handbook of Qualitative Research*. 2nd edition. Eds. Norma K. Denzin and Yvonna S. Lincoln. Thousand Oaks, CA: Sage Publications, 2000. 455–86.

Thomas, Helen. *Romanticism and Slave Narratives*. Cambridge: Cambridge University Press, 2000.

Thomas, Keith. *Man and the Natural World: Changing Attitudes in England, 1500–1800*. Oxford: Oxford University Press, 1983.

Thomson, James. *The Seasons and The Castle of Indolence*. Ed. James Sambrook. Oxford: Clarendon Press, 1972.

Todd, Janet. *Mary Wollstonecraft: A Revolutionary Life*. New York: Columbia University Press, 2000.

———. *Sensibility: An Introduction*. London: Methuen & Co., 1986.

Tomalin, Claire. *The Life and Death of Mary Wollstonecraft*. New York: Harcourt Brace Jovanovich, 1974.

Tong, Rosemary Putnam. *Feminist Thought: A More Comprehensive Introduction*. 2nd ed. Boulder: Westview Press, 1998.

Trimmer, Sarah. *Fabulous Histories. Designed for the Instruction of Children, Respecting Their Treatment of Animals*. London: T. Longman, 1786.

Trotter, Thomas. *A View of the Nervous Temperament; Being a Practical Inquiry into the Increasing Prevalence, Prevention, and Treatment of Those Diseases Commonly Called Nervous; Bilious, Stomach, and Liver Complaints; Indigestion; Low Spirits; Gout, &c*. 3rd ed. London: Longman, Hurst, Rees, Orme, and Brown, 1812.

Turner, Rufus Paul. *Charlotte Smith (1749–1806): New Light on Her Life and Literary Career*. University of Southern California Diss., 1966.

Ty, Eleanor. "'The History of My Own Heart': Inscribing Self, Inscribing Desire in Wollstonecraft's *Letters from Norway*." *Mary Wollstonecraft and Mary Shelley: Writing Lives*. Eds. Helen M. Buss, D. L. Macdonald, and Anne McWhir. Waterloo: Wilfrid Laurier University Press, 2001. 69–84.

———. *Unsex'd Revolutionaries: Five Women Novelists of the 1790s*. Toronto: University of Toronto Press, 1993.

Tytler, Graeme. "Lavater and Physiognomy in English Fiction 1790–1832." *Eighteenth-Century Fiction* 7.3 (1995): 293–310.

Vetch, John. *An Account of the Ophthalmia Which Has Appeared in England since the Return of the British Army from Egypt*. London: Longman, Hurst, Rees and Orme, 1807.

Wagemans, Marianne, and O. Paul Van Bijsterveld. "The French Egyptian Campaign and Its Effects on Ophthalmology." *Documenta Ophthalmologica* 68 (1998): 135–44.

Wardle, Ralph M. *Mary Wollstonecraft: A Critical Biography*. Lincoln: University of Nebraska Press, 1951.

Wardrop, James. *Essays on the Morbid Anatomy of the Human Eye*. London: John Murray, 1808.

Ware, James. *Chirurgical Observations Relative to the Epiphora, or Watery Eye, the Scrophulous and Intermittent Ophthalmy, the Extraction of the Cateract, and the Introduction of the Male Catheter*. London: C. Dilly, 1792.

———. "To The Editor of the Times." *London Times*. 11 August 1806: 2.

White, Daniel E. "Autobiography and Elegy: The Early Romantic Poetics of Thomas Gray and Charlotte Smith." *Early Romantics: Perspectives in British Poetry from Pope to Wordsworth*. Ed. Thomas Woodman. New York: St. Martin's Press, 1998. 57–69.

Whytt, Robert. *Observations on the Nature, Causes, and Cure of Those Disorders, Which Have Been Commonly Called Nervous, Hypochondriac, or Hysteric. To Which Are Prefixed, Some Remarks on the Sympathy of the Nerves*. London: T. Maiden, 1797.

———. *The Works of Robert Whytt, M.D. Published by His Son*. Edinburgh: Balfour, Auld, and Smellie, 1768.

Wilberforce, William. *A Letter on the Abolition of the Slave Trade; Addressed to the Freeholders and Other Inhabitants of Yorkshire*. London: T. Cadell and W. Davies, 1807.

Williams, Helen Maria. *Letters Written in France, In the Summer 1790, to a Friend in England; Containing Various Anecdotes Relative to the French Revolution*. Eds. Neil Fraistat and Susan C. Lanser. Peterborough, Ontario: Broadview Press, 2001.

Withering, William. *An Arrangement of British Plants, According to the Latest Improvements of the Linnaean System; with an Easy Introduction to the Study of Botany. Illustrated with copper plates*. 3rd, 6th, 7th ed. 4 vols. London: C. J. G. and F. Rivington, et al., 1796, 1818, 1830.

———. *A Botanical Arrangement of All the Vegetables Naturally Growing in Great Britain with Descriptions of Genera and Species, According to the System of the Celebrated Linnaeus. Being an Attempt to Render Them Familiar to Those Who Are Unacquainted with the Learned Languages*. 1st ed. 2 vols. London: T. Cadell and P. Elmsley, 1776.

———. *A Botanical Arrangement of British Plants: Including the Uses of Each Species, in Medicine, Diet, Rural Economy and the Arts: With an Easy Introduction to the Study of Botany. Illustrated by copper plates*. 2nd ed. 3 vols. London: J. Balfour, 1787/92.

Wolf, Margery. *A Thrice-Told Tale: Feminism, Postmodernism, and Ethnographic Responsibility*. Stanford, CA: Stanford University Press, 1992.

Wollstonecraft, Mary. *The Collected Letters of Mary Wollstonecraft*. Ed. Janet Todd. New York: Columbia University Press, 2000.

———. *Mary and The Wrongs of Woman*. Ed. Gary Kelly. Oxford: Oxford University Press, 1976.

———. "On Poetry, and Our Relish for the Beauties of Nature." *Brown University Women Writer's Project*, 1993.

———. *Posthumous Works of the Author of A Vindication of the Rights of Woman*. 4 vols. Ed. William Godwin. London: J. Johnson, 1798.

———. *The Works of Mary Wollstonecraft*. Ed. Janet Todd and Marilyn Butler. 7 vols. New York: New York University Press, 1989.

Wordsworth, William. *The Fourteen Book Prelude.* Ed. W. J. B. Owen. *The Cornell Wordsworth.* Gen. ed. Stephen Parrish. Ithaca: Cornell University Press, 1985.

———. *Lyrical Ballads, and Other Poems, 1797–1800.* Ed. James Butler and Karen Green. *The Cornell Wordsworth.* Gen. ed. Stephen Parrish. Ithaca: Cornell University Press, 1992.

———. *The Prelude, 1799, 1805, 1850.* Eds. Jonathan Wordsworth, M. H. Abrams, and Stephen Gill. New York: Norton, 1979.

———. *The Prose Works of William Wordsworth.* Eds. W. J. B. Owen and Jane Worthington Smyser. 3 vols. London: Oxford University Press, 1974.

Young, Thomas. *On The Mechanism of the Eye.* London: Bulmer, 1801.

Yousef, Nancy. "Wollstonecraft, Rousseau and the Revision of Romantic Subjectivity." *Studies in Romanticism* 38.4 (1999): 537–58.

Zimmerman, Sarah. "Charlotte Smith's Letters and the Practice of Self-Presentation." *Princeton University Library Chronicle* 53.1 (Autumn 1991): 50–77.

Zingeser, James A. "Sight for Sore Eyes." *Natural History Magazine.* Dec. 2004–Jan. 2005. <http://www.naturalhistorymag.com/1204/1204_feature2.html> On-line extra feature. 6 February 2006.

Index